International Series on Sport Sciences
Volume 21

Biochemistry of Exercise VII

Edited by:

Albert W. Taylor, PhD, Philip D. Gollnick, PhD, Howard J. Green, PhD,
C. David Ianuzzo, PhD, Earl G. Noble, PhD, Guy Métivier, PhD,
and John R. Sutton, MD

Human Kinetics Books
Champaign, Illinois

Library of Congress Cataloging-in-Publication Data

International Biochemistry of Exercise Conference (7th : 1988 :
    London, Ont.)
    Biochemistry of exercise VII / edited by Albert W. Taylor.
        p.   cm. -- (International series on sport sciences. ISSN
    0160-0559 ; v. 21)
        "Proceedings of the 7th International Biochemistry of Exercise
    Conference held on June 1-4, 1988 in London, Ontario, Canada"--T.p.
    verso.
        Includes bibliographical references.
        ISBN 0-87322-260-1
        1. Exercise--Physiological aspects--Congresses.   2. Muscles-
    -Physiology--Congresses.   I. Taylor, Albert W.   II. Title.
    III. Series.
        [DNLM: 1. Biochemistry--congresses.   2. Exercise--congresses.
    3. Muscles--metabolism--congresses.   WE 103 I543b 1988]
    QP301.I536   1988
    612'.044--dc20
    DNLM/DLC
    for Library of Congress   89-24627
                                                           CIP

ISBN: 0-87322-260-1
ISSN: 0160-0559

Copyright © 1990 by Human Kinetics Publishers, Inc.

Proceedings of the 7th International Biochemistry of Exercise Conference held on June 1-4,
1988 in London, Ontario, Canada.

Developmental Editor: Kathy Kane
Production Director: Ernie Noa
Copyeditor: Peter Nelson
Assistant Editors: Julia Anderson and Robert King
Proofreader: Pamela Johnson
Typesetters: Sandra Meier, Brad Colson, and Cindy Pritchard
Text Design: Keith Blomberg
Text Layout: Jill Wikgren and Denise Lowry
Printer: Braun-Brumfield

Printed in the United States of America

10 9 8 7 6 5 4 3 2 1

Human Kinetics Books
A Division of Human Kinetics Publishers, Inc.
Box 5076, Champaign, IL 61825-5076
1-800-747-4HKP

Contents

Program and Organizing Committees

Dr. Philip D. Gollnick
Department of Veterinary and
  Comparative Anatomy, Pharmacology
  and Physiology
Washington State University
Pullman, WA
USA

Dr. Howard Green
Department of Kinesiology
University of Waterloo
Waterloo, Ontario
Canada

Dr. C. David Ianuzzo
Departments of Biology and Physical
  Education
York University
Downsview, Ontario
Canada

Dr. Guy Métivier
School of Human Kinetics
University of Ottawa
Ottawa, Ontario
Canada

Dr. Earl Noble
Faculty of Physical Education
The University of Western Ontario
London, Ontario
Canada

Dr. John Sutton
Department of Medicine
McMaster University
Hamilton, Ontario
Canada

Dr. A.W. Bert Taylor (Chairman)
Department of Physiology and Faculty
  of Physical Education
The University of Western Ontario
London, Ontario
Canada

Research Group: Biochemistry of Exercise

Dr. Jacques Poortmans (President)
Chimie Physiologique
Inst. Super. Educ. Phys. Kines.
Université Libre de Bruxelles
28 Avenue P. Héger
B-1050 Bruxelles
Belgium

Dr. Jidi Chen
Research Division of Sports
  Biochemistry
Institute of Sports Medicine
Beijing Medical College
Beijing - 100083
China

Dr. Pietro di Prampero
Universita Degli Studi Di Udine
Istituto Di Biologia
Facolta Di Medicina E. Chirurgia
Udine, Italy
33100

Dr. Henrik Galbo
Institute of Medical Physiology B
The Panum Institute, bygn. 18
University of Copenhagen
Blegdamsvej 3C
DK-2200 Copenhagen
Denmark

Dr. Philip D. Gollnick
Department of Veterinary and
  Comparative Anatomy, Pharmacology
  and Physiology
College of Veterinary Medicine
Washington State University
Pullman, Washington
USA 99164-6520

Dr. Jan Henriksson
Department of Physiology III
Karolinska Institutet
1 Lidingovagen
S-114 33 Stockholm
Sweden

Dr. John O. Holloszy
Section of Applied Physiology
Department of Internal Medicine
Washington University School of
  Medicine
4566 Scott Avenue - Box 8113
St. Louis, Missouri
USA 63110

Dr. Hans Howald
Institut de Recherche
Ecole Federale de Gymnastique et Sport
CH-2532 Macolin
Switzerland

Dr. Nicolas N. Jakovlev
Pudozskaja ul.; 3/2, Kv 20
197110 Leningrad, USSR

Dr. Joseph Keul
Abt. Sportsmedizin
Universitatsklinik
55 Hugstetterstrasse
D-7800 Freiburg im Bresgau
FRG

Dr. Howard G. Knuttgen
Sargent College of Allied Health
  Professions
Boston University
36 Cummington Avenue
Boston, Massachusetts
USA 02215

Dr. Guy Métivier
Ecole des Sciences de l'Activite Physique
Universite d'Ottawa
35 McDougal
Ottawa, Ontario
K1N 6N5 Canada

Dr. Eric Newsholme
Department of Biochemistry
University of Oxford
South Parks Road
GB - Oxford
0X1 3QU
England

Dr. Albert W. Taylor
Faculty of Physical Education
The University of Western Ontario
Thames Hall
London, Ontario
N6A 3K7 Canada

Dr. Alexander Tsopanakis
Department of Biochemistry
Hellenic Sports Research Institute
37 Kifissas Ave Maroussi
GR - 151 53 Athens
Greece

Preface

This volume represents the proceedings of the seventh in a series of international meetings pertaining to the biochemistry of exercise and has been organized through the Research Group of the International Council of Sport and Physical Education, which is sponsored by UNESCO. Previous symposia have been held in Brussels, Belgium (1968), Magglingen, Switzerland (1973), Quebec City, Canada (1976), Brussels, Belgium (1979), Boston, U.S.A. (1982), and Copenhagen, Denmark (1985). The Research Group was formed with the objectives of furthering the knowledge of exercise in order to better understand the basic biological and biochemical mechanisms involved and to provide information of practical value to clinicians, scientists, and educators.

The 1988 Conference, hosted by the Faculty of Physical Education, was held in London, Canada, June 1-4. The format included a set of seven symposia with four or five invited papers dealing with aspects of muscular fatigue, the role of functional demand in regulating gene expression, determinants of compensatory muscular growth, muscle bioenergetics, extramuscular substrate utilization, and ion regulation with exercise and training.

It is anticipated and hoped that conference proceedings of symposia format will prove to be most useful to young scientists as a learning tool and for established investigators as a means to synthesize and record the current state of knowledge in a particular interest area. Most important is the need to demonstrate the metabolic mechanisms regulating the practical application of exercise.

Albert W. Taylor

Acknowledgments

Major financial support for the Conference was provided by:
Canadian Oxygen Limited
Fitness Canada
Government of Ontario—Hospitality Committee
National Sciences and Engineering Research Council of Canada (NSERC)
Ontario Ministry of Health
Ontario Ministry of Tourism and Recreation
Sport Canada
The Lawson Foundation
The University of Western Ontario
University Hospital

The Organizing Committee also wishes to acknowledge the contributions of the following:
Air Canada
Chateau Gai
Frito Lay
Holiday Inn City Centre
Human Kinetics Publishers
Labatts Ontario Breweries
Pathfinder Beverages
Perez Corporation
St. Joseph's Health Centre
Victoria Hospital Corporation
Wintergreen Graphics and Designs

The Conference could not have been successful without the artistic, technical, clerical, and secretarial assistance of the following:
University of Western Ontario Graphics Department
  Mr. Alex Hamilton
  Ms. Vickie Hughes
  Mr. Steve Smith
  Mr. Tony Nicoletti

Faculty of Physical Education, University of Western Ontario
  Miss Wanda Burns
  Mrs. Jean Neal

Ambassador Travel
  Ms. Monique Powell

Secretary General
  Mrs. Carole J. Taylor

Conference Welcome

Today we are celebrating the 20th birthday of our symposia. Indeed, 20 years ago the First International Symposium on Biochemistry of Exercise was held in Belgium, and this meeting led to the creation of the Research Group on Biochemistry of Exercise, which was rapidly admitted by the International Council of Sport Science and Physical Education at UNESCO. For those who attended this meeting (Phil Gollnick, Guy Métivier, Bengt Saltin, Charles Tipton), these days were particularly hot, not because of the nice weather we had in early June, but because of the May 1968 student antiestablishment rebellion on Belgian campuses. We managed to hold the Symposium throughout the local riots. Since then, five more symposia were held in different cities: Magglingen, Québec, Brussels, Boston, and Copenhagen. The aims of these symposia were, and still are, to bring together scientists working in the same area, sharing the same enthusiasm, in order to stimulate discussions and to clarify ideas in this particular growing field of human activities. The number of participants and papers submitted to these meetings have increased almost fourfold since the first event. The participation as lecturers of two Nobel Prize winners and the quality of contributions have reinforced the Proceedings of these symposia, which are commonly cited in the sports medicine literature. Besides the high-level meetings, the Research Group has organized three courses devoted to those who are beginners in the field of biochemistry of exercise or who belong to other science areas, such as psychology, sports medicine, or coaching. France, Italy, and Greece were the host countries of these refresher courses.

The theme of the 7th Symposium, which has become a Conference, is devoted to biochemical strategies in response to altered functional demand. This knowledge will fill the gap between normal conditions observed in equilibrated organisms and the adaptation to stressful situations found in performance athletes. It also may attempt to throw a bridge between ingenious animal adaptation to uncommon survival and the protection of human tissues from hypoxia and hyperthermia. Let us remember we have many things to learn from the animal kingdom besides social behavior. Before closing, I would like to congratulate Professor Taylor and his local organizing committee for the marvelous job achieved to prepare this conference. As well, my thanks are extended to the secretarial staff and especially to Carol Taylor. I am convinced we will be listening to provoking and stimulating presentations during the following days.

Jacques R. Poortmans

The Biochemical Limits of Muscle Work

Peter W. Hochachka
University of British Columbia, Vancouver, Canada

In an Olympic year, exercise biochemists may be more interested than ever in the question of biochemical limits to muscle work or in how these limits might be extended. When a group of my students and I first began exploring this question (12), we were surprised by the lack of theoretical frameworks for guiding our work. We reasoned that to probe this question in proper context, we needed to consider the expression and organization of metabolism over broader ranges than are commonly available to exercise biochemists. That is why we chose size and exercise as the two key variables giving us the range we were seeking. On average, maximum aerobic metabolic rate, or $\dot{V}O_2$max, exceeds resting metabolic rate (RMR) by about an order of magnitude, and this seems independent of animal size (27). On the other hand, the mass-specific metabolic rates of very small animals (say, hummingbirds and shrews) exceed the predicted value for the largest mammals (10^5-kg blue whales) by about 1000-fold (1, 23). Thus, by combining the two variables, we find a range of aerobic metabolic rates in mammals that can differ by about a 10^4 factor (the lowest values being the mass-specific RMR of blue whales, the highest values known being those for $\dot{V}O_2$max of hummingbirds; see 26).

The metabolic biochemistry underlying these extremes of metabolism, while not fully explored, is nevertheless extensive enough to allow some important insights. For example, a study of 13 species of teleosts found that the catalytic activities of oxidative enzymes per g muscle decreased systematically with body mass. In contrast, there was a direct relationship between body mass and the catalytic potential of enzymes working in anaerobic muscle metabolism (24). At the same time, Emmett (4) independently studied a series of 10 species of mammals, varying in size by a factor of between 10^5 and 10^6. He showed that the catalytic activities of muscle anaerobic enzymes (in μmol g^{-1} min^{-1} or Units $[U]g^{-1}$) scale directly with body mass, whereas the catalytic activities of muscle oxidative enzymes scale inversely (5). More recently, we concluded (12) that enzymes in aerobic metabolism of cardiac muscle in U g^{-1} also scale with similar negative slopes. Thus, in overall organization, the anaerobic potential of muscle increases with animal size, whereas the aerobic potential per g muscle decreases. Volume densities of the sarcoplasmic reticulum (SR)— including the junctional SR, the terminal cisternae, and the transverse tubules—are about 1.5 to 2 times greater in fast muscles than in slow muscles and also tend to increase in small animals (see 3, 15, and discussion below).

Two Potential Strategies for Scaling
of Energy Metabolism

At the outset it is clear that in theory two different mechanisms could be utilized to account for the allometric scaling of metabolic rates and of metabolic enzyme activities: Either enzyme efficiency could be adjusted (k_{cat} adaptation of muscle enzymes), or the number of copies of specific muscle enzymes could be adjusted as a function of body size. Of these two alternatives, the latter seems to be favored by nature. Thus, although k_{cat} adaptations to temperature and pressure are known, this characteristic seems to be otherwise fairly conservative for homologous enzymes wherever they are found (see 14). This conclusion is well illustrated in recent studies of mitochondrial ATP synthase; assayed in vitro as an ATPase, its activity per mg of heart mitochondrial protein is found to be the same in mammals ranging in size by about 10^5 (21). Similarly, muscle citrate synthetase k_{cat} values are the same in the shrew as in the ox, indicating that the large difference in enzyme activity per g muscle is due to the amount of enzyme rather than to its catalytic efficiency (Emmett, unpublished data).

Elegant in vivo studies of this problem conclude that a given volume of muscle mitochondria consumes a similar amount of O_2 (4-5 ml O_2 min^{-1} ml mitochondria^{-1}) irrespective of source, again over a very broad body-size range (see 27). This means that muscles in small homeotherms have very high metabolic capacities compared to large animals because they amplify the number of copies of mitochondria, not because their mitochondria are catalytically more efficient. Making more copies of basic metabolic machinery, rather than adjusting k_{cat} values, is also the scaling strategy for glycolytic enzymes, which display similar turnover numbers irrespective of source (14), apparently as well as in amplification of sarcoplasmic reticulum (SR) in going from large to small mammals (7). This, too, is the widely accepted mechanism of training improvement of muscle biochemical performance not involving fiber-type adjustments; it accounts for most of the difference between elite animal athletes and their more sluggish relatives (see 11).

Upper Limits in Oxidative Enzyme Scaling Patterns

In considering the upper limits to copy-number adaptations, we will assume only three basic units of muscle performance: the contractile machinery per se, the SR, and the enzyme machinery for generating ATP. Our question then reduces itself to a seemingly simple one of how these are maximally upward regulated. Nature may have come close to an upper packing limit in the design of the fastest muscles currently known, the tymbal muscles of cicadas. These muscles can operate at contraction frequencies of 550 Hz and may well be at a functional limit determined by the approximately 1:1:1 volume density ratios of mitochondria:SR:myofilaments (16). We suggest that any further increase in oxidative enzyme capacity (i.e., in mitochondrial volume densities) would be counterproductive because it would simultaneously require reductions in either SR or myofilaments. The 1:1:1 ratio observed represents a classic example of compromise and coadaptation where contraction frequency is the property under selective pressure. In mammals, a similar optimization point seems to be selected in bats in the cricothyroid muscle, which operates at up to 200 Hz in sound production during echolocation of prey (20).

The ultrastructures of skeletal muscle and heart of the smallest mammal (the shrew) and of the smallest bird (the hummingbird) also indicate amplification of mitochondria and SR toward an optimization point. Although the three volume densities (mitochondria, SR, and myofilaments) have not been quantified systematically, most workers in this field estimate mitochondrial volume density at about 45%, about equal to that of the myofilaments and consistent with recent measurements of very high levels of oxidative enzymes (26). This allows for a volume density for SR approaching 10% (7), a value substantially lower than for the fast tymbal muscles of cicadas or other very fast vertebrate muscles.

The difference in ultrastructural design of the two muscle types can be rationalized in terms of their different functions. In heart and skeletal muscles of the smallest homeotherms, maximum oxidative metabolism (and presumably maximum power output) is achieved during hummingbirds' hovering flight at contraction frequencies of about 20 Hz for the heart and about 60-80 Hz for flight muscle (see 26 for literature in this area). The sound-generating muscles of bats and cicadas, on the other hand, are adapted for much higher contraction frequency; however, power output apparently is *not* high, presumably because these muscles need not shorten by more than a fraction of that required in hummingbird or shrew muscles (16, 23). Because of the role of the SR in modulating Ca^{2+} fluxes during contraction-relaxation cycles, maximizing muscle for frequency in this system would be expected to require SR amplification: The limit appears to be close to the 1:1:1 ratios observed in bats and cicadas.

By similar reasoning, I conclude that the mitochondrial volume densities in hummingbird and shrew muscles also are close to their upper limits; further up-regulation would require decreases in myofilament or SR volume densities. The former would reduce the maximum forces that could be exerted, whereas the latter would reduce contraction frequencies that are possible. Thus, there seems to be very little room left for adaptation (at least expressed as upward regulation of mitochondrial abundance). If this conclusion is correct, it supplies another reason why hummingbirds and shrews are at the lower size limit for homeotherms; additional reductions in size would require qualitative adjustments either in skeletal muscle or in cardiac muscle design. Many workers believe that even attaining their current small size requires added physiological adjustments; in particular, the time required for the systole-diastole cycle must be minimized (this requires about 50 msec and sets the maximum contraction frequency at 20 Hz, substantially *less* than can be achieved by the flight muscle), the mass ratio of heart:body is elevated, and the blood O_2 carrying capacity is tightly (if precariously) balanced with respect to viscosity (23).

Design Principles for Upward Regulation of Oxidative Capacities

From my analysis, so far it appears that the design of muscle for ever higher rates of aerobic work and ATP turnover requires the "tuning up" of three main metabolic building blocks: (a) myofilaments; (b) oxidative metabolism (mitochondria + input pathways); and (c) SR, including junctional SR and (in mammals) transverse tubules. Protein isoforms may be involved in these coadaptations (11), but improving catalytic efficiency (i.e., having enzymes with higher turnover numbers) is not the most basic strategy of adaptation. Instead, in any muscle type, all fundamental building units between species seem to be inherently similar; coadaptation simply involves coordinated change in their abundance. If glucose is used as the fuel and about 1/3 of the available energy is partitioned for the SR (19), one metabolic flux unit (forming 36 ATP) at steady state would be functionally coupled with 24 actomyosin ATPase flux units and with 12 SR CA^{2+} ATPase units. To move from standard mammalian muscles to the hummingbird extreme (3, 6) requires a doubling of SR (from less than 5% to close to 10% volume density) but as much as a 5- to 6-fold increase in mitochondrial volume densities (from about 8% to over 40%). The upper limits for aerobic muscle work therefore requires the coadaptation of mitochondria and myofilaments toward 1:1 volume densities, which probably reflect actual ATP flux ratios that deviate from 1:1 only by the percentage of ATP required for SR function.

Upper Limits in Glycolytic Scaling Patterns

Just as in the case of oxidative fibers, the question arises of how far large mammals can go in upward scaling of activities of enzymes in anaerobic metabolism, such as muscle lactate dehydrogenase (LDH). What factors account for the upper limits for muscle glycolytic capacity? As in our analysis of oxidative fibers, the answers depend upon whether selection is for high-frequency, lower power-output performance, or for low-frequency, high–power-output performance. With respect to the former, one of the fastest anaerobically powered vertebrate muscles is the sound-producing muscle of toadfish (6, 18). With drastic reductions in mitochondrial volume densities, this muscle may well be near its own inherent limit of about 1:1:1 volume density ratios of myofilaments:SR:"metabolic machinery." However, metabolic machinery here is formed predominantly by enzymes in anaerobic metabolism (29) plus glycogen granules as endogenous substrate. It would appear that any further upward scaling of glycolytic capacity would be counterproductive because of a consequent reduction either in SR or contractile protein functions. Either adjustment would have a negative impact on speed, the parameter presumably being selected.

In contrast, most anaerobic skeletal muscles are designed more for power output than for the speed with which contraction-relaxation cycles can be completed, so the factors determining glycolytic limits are different. The main difference is in the amount of SR, which, compared to the sound-producing muscles, is drastically reduced. Typical values for SR volume densities are in the 4-5% range for fast mammalian muscles, only marginally higher than in slow muscles (3). In contrast to reductions in SR and mitochondrial volume densities, the concentrations of glycolytic enzymes are increased in fast-twitch skeletal muscles. The relative directions and magnitudes of these coadaptations can be gleaned by comparative analyses. Thus, in moving from a slow- to a fast-twitch type of mammalian muscle, SR volume densities increase by less than 2-fold, whereas glycolytic enzyme concentrations may increase by 4-5 times (see 10). Assuming that glycogen is used as the fuel and that SR function costs 30% of the maximum muscle glycolytic ATP synthesized, then the upper limit for ATP turnover and power output would be attained at 4:8:4 ratios of glycolytic flux to actomyosin ATPase flux to Ca^{2+} ATPase flux. That is, at steady state, for each 4 glucosyls (from glycogen) converted to lactate, 12 ATPs would be made, 8 of which would be available for actomyosin ATPase while 4 would be available for Ca^{2+} ATPase. Assuming for the moment identical k_{cat} values, the molar ratios required (expressed as μmol substrate converted g^{-1} min^{-1}) would be 1 glycolysis unit (producing 3 ATPs) to 2 actomyosin ATPase units to 1 Ca^{2+} ATPase unit. There would be little or no room left for any further upward adjustment of these three functional units of muscle.

To see whether this limit can be attained, let us consider relative concentrations. In rabbit psoas, a predominantly fast-type muscle, myosin concentrations are about 100 μM, and actin is at about 300 μM (30); these constitute about 85% of the volume density of the muscle cell (3). The k_{cat} for actomyosin is about 10 μmol ATP hydrolyzed per μmol actomyosin ATPase per s; thus, an in vivo maximum value might be about 50 units of ATPase (50 μmol ATP g^{-1} min^{-1}). If glycolytic enzymes had similar turnover numbers, their concentrations would only have to be about 1/2 that of myosin, or about 50 μM, to be able to pace maximum muscle work (assuming, as above, that 2 of each 3 ATPs are available for actomyosin ATPase). Because the k_{cat} values for most glycolytic enzymes are substantially higher than that for actomyosin ATPase, the actual concentrations of glycolytic enzymes in theory could be even lower, in some cases well below 1 μM.

Paradoxically, however, the concentrations of glycolytic enzymes in fast mammalian muscles are typically 10 to 100 times higher than these minimally expected values (25). If the muscle is made faster or the animal bigger, even more glycolytic enzymes are packed in. To confound the problem, these same muscles seem to pack in less glycogen than they could in theory hold. Generally, vertebrate skeletal muscles contain on the order of 100 μmol glycogen (glucosyl) g^{-1}. In contrast, it is possible to pack in glycogen to well over 1 M levels, as is commonly observed in hypoxia-tolerant animals (14). Thus, we are faced with an interesting paradox: Fast muscles seemingly pack in more glycolytic enzymes than are needed, while packing in glycogen far below possible levels. We feel that this paradox can be resolved in terms of two key features of glycolysis—the accelerator and brake functions—that seem to be under selective pressure in muscle tissue. The accelerator feature is expressed as high activities of glycolytic enzymes, far higher than found in any other tissues of the vertebrate body. From what we know of the kinetic and regulatory properties of muscle glycolytic enzymes (14), these high activities allow (a) rapid flare-up of the pathway and (b) high flux rates, even though most intermediates of the pathway occur at low concentrations, well below apparent K_m values.

On the other hand, because glycogenolysis in activated muscle may well operate as an essentially closed system potentially capable of generating harmful end products, it is necessary to maintain the system under close control. Numerous regulatory mechanisms (allosteric enzymes) and defense mechanisms (such as high buffering capacities) have evolved and together may well constitute the overriding brake feature of the pathway. A final safety feature (or emergency brake?) may well be the limited amount of stored glycogen; when this is used up, no matter what else prevails, the pathway must grind to a halt. Whatever brake mechanisms are used, glycolysis must be switched down or even off before end product accumulation leads to (a) undesirable acidification, (b) osmotic perturbation, or (c) uncontrollable side reactions. In tissues (such as the liver) that contain enormously high amounts of storage glycogen, the end product of glycogen mobilization is glucose, not lactate; there is no net generation of protons, and enzyme activities are low. Because the accelerator of muscle glycolysis is absent, the emergency brake also can be slackened.

This analysis suggests that several properties—stored glycogen, catalytic capacities of glycolytic enzymes, actomyosin ATPase capacities (or volume densities of myofilaments), and muscle buffering power—all coadapt; upward or downward adjustments in any one of these parameters means proportionate adjustment in them all (10). That is why it appears that the upper limit for anaerobic work capacity in muscle must represent a kind of balancing process that maximizes the amounts of actomyosin ATPase and glycolytic enzymes in appropriate proportions while minimizing the risk by maintaining the right (modest) amount of glycogen and the right (large) amount of intracellular H^+ buffering capacity. At a theoretical upper limit, any further upward adjustment of glycolytic capacity may well require compromise in one of the other coadapting properties, which would be counterproductive. We do not know whether such a theoretical limit is approached or actually reached in the muscles of the largest whales. However, this limit clearly is not reached in fin whales of about 3×10^4 kg in size: The LDH levels in their muscles can be surpassed by performance adaptation of white muscles in very fast-swimming fishes (9, 10).

Lowest Observed Limits
to Glycolytic Enzyme Scaling Patterns

In contrast to the large animals, are there limits to how *low* muscle glycolytic enzyme levels can be reduced in small homeotherms? Hummingbird and shrew skeletal muscles retain some LDH activity, for example, so it is useful to inquire why these kinds of enzymes are not deleted. Because such deletion of LDH in fact occurs in some insect flight muscles (22), we may conclude that muscle cells can work perfectly well without any LDH. However, in insect flight muscle, LDH deletion is considered particularly crucial because these muscles depend upon alpha-glycerophosphate dehydrogenase (α-GPDH) for cycling reducing equivalents from NADH into the mitochondria. Under aerobic conditions it is imperative to avoid α-GPDH–LDH competition for NADH because, with glucose as carbon source, a 50:50 split of NADH between these two reaction pathways would mean zero net ATP formation in glucose conversion to lactate (see 9, 14).

In contrast, vertebrate skeletal muscles, including hummingbird and shrew muscles, seem to depend mainly upon the malate-aspartate cycle for shuttling hydrogen between cytosol and mitochondria (see 26 for relative enzyme activities). Connett et al. (2) argue that in these muscle types, the LDH reaction serves as a kind of safety mechanism buffering the cytosolic NADH/NAD$^+$ ratios during activated aerobic muscle metabolism. Such an aerobic function for LDH (which may be exaggerated in the phenomenal rest-to-work transitions typical of hummingbird flight muscle) may well explain why this enzyme is retained even in muscles as aerobic as those of the shrew and the hummingbird. The above redox buffering function proposed for LDH during otherwise totally oxidative work is analogous to the function proposed for creatine phosphokinase (CPK) in buffering the cell's ATP reserves during rest-to-work transitions (see 17). Again, the need for this function may be exaggerated in muscles of very small homeotherms, which may explain why hummingbird flight muscle sustains some 2,000 U of CPK g^{-1} (26), a level clearly at variance with the scaling patterns for ezymes that are normally thought to be mainly involved in anaerobic metabolism.

Lower Limits in Aerobic Enzyme Scaling Patterns

Finally, just as scaling studies raise the question of lower limits to size, they also raise the question of upper limits to the size of homeotherms. Is there a minimum level of mass-specific oxidative metabolism beyond which homeotherms cannot grow? These questions are much more difficult to address than the minimum size one: The answers may depend on the state of the organism or on environmental conditions, and some systems can go fully ametabolic (see 13).

Although direct measurements are unavailable, extrapolations indicate that the mass-specific $\dot{V}O_2$ of a 10^8-g whale is already down to 0.02 ml O_2 $g^{-1}h^{-1}$. That is equivalent to an ATP turnover rate of 0.013 μmol ATP g^{-1} min^{-1}. By comparison, the resting metabolic rate of a human turns over ATP about 10 times faster (0.14 μmol ATP g^{-1} min^{-1}). Running marathoners turn over muscle ATP at about 30 μmol ATP g^{-1} min^{-1}, whereas the muscles of a hovering hummingbird turn over ATP at over 600 μmol g^{-1} min^{-1} (26), or nearly 50,000 times faster than expected in the whale. How much bigger could a mammal be? How much more could it slow down? Although we cannot know for sure, there are again reasons for thinking that the largest whales are close to a lower metabolic limit. In fact, at this rate of oxidative energy metabolism, the normally expected metabolic differences between ectotherms and endotherms begin to get blurry. Two examples illustrate the point. In the first place, whereas the mass-specific metabolic rate at 3° C of a torpid turtle (one of the most hypometabolic vertebrates known) is about 0.001 ml O_2 $g^{-1}h^{-1}$ (8), that of a 100-g iguanid is 20 times higher and not too different from the above projected estimate for whales of 10^5 kg mass or from permanently hypometabolic midwater fishes (28).

Secondly, reptiles—excluding varanids, which display unusually high metabolic rates for reptiles, and snakes, which display unusually low metabolic rates—are thought to display resting metabolic rates about 1/4 to 1/3 of those of mammals of the same size. The allometric exponent, on the other hand, is generally higher than in mammals (see 12 for literature in this area). It is thus possible that log-log plots of mass-specific metabolic rate versus body mass for mammals and reptiles would intersect at about the mass of the largest dinosaurs or of whales (between 10^5 and 10^6 kg). If whales slowed down much further, they might find themselves in another phylogenetic class.

Conclusion

1. Mass-specific metabolic rates in the smallest homeotherms are over 1,000 times higher than estimated rates in 10^8-g whales, the largest animals ever to have lived on the planet.
2. Upper and lower limits to aerobic metabolism and work seem to be reached or closely approached by the smallest and largest homeotherms, respectively.
3. Mass-specific activities of muscle glycolytic enzymes such as LDH scale directly with body mass; their upper and lower limits probably are not reached by the biggest and smallest homeotherms, respectively.

References

1. Calder, W.A. Size, function, and life history. Cambridge, MA: Harvard Univ. Press; 1984.
2. Connett, R.J.; Gayeski, T.E.J.; Honig, C.R. Energy sources in fully aerobic rest-work transit: a new role for glycolysis. Am. J. Physiol. 248:H922-H929; 1985.
3. Eisenberg, B. Quantitative ultrastructure of muscle. Handbook of physiology—skeletal muscle. Am. Phys. Soc. 1983:85-98.
4. Emmett, B. The metabolic biochemistry of the wandering shrew (*Sorex vagrans*). Vancouver: Univ. of British Columbia; 1980. M. S. thesis.
5. Emmett, B.; Hochachka, P.W. Scaling of oxidative and glycolytic enzyme in mammals. Respir. Physiol. 45:261-272; 1981.
6. Franzini-Armstrong, C. Structure and function of membrane systems of skeletal muscle cells. Handbook of physiology—skeletal muscle. Am. Phys. Soc. 1983:23-71.
7. Franzini-Armstrong, C.; Nunzi, M.G. Junctional feet and particles in the triads of a fast-twitch muscle fibre. J. Muscle Res. Cell Motil. 4:233-252; 1983.
8. Herbert, C.V.; Jackson, D.C. Temperature effects on the responses to prolonged submergence in the turtle Chrysemys picta bellii. II. Metabolic rate, blood acid-base and ionic changes, and cardiovascular function in aerated and anoxic water. Physiol. Zool. 58:670-681; 1985.
9. Hochachka, P.W. Living without oxygen. Cambridge, MA: Harvard Univ. Press; 1980.
10. Hochachka, P.W. Fuels and pathways as designed systems for support of muscle work. J. Exp. Biol. 115:149-164; 1985.
11. Hochachka, P.W.; Dobson, G.P.; Mommsen, T.P. Role of isozymes in metabolic regulation during exercise: insights from comparative studies. In: Rattazzi, M.C.; Scandalius, J.G.; Whitt, G.S., eds. Isozymes: current topics in biol. & med. res. New York: Alan R. Liss, Inc.; 1983:91-113 (Vol. 8).

12. Hochachka, P.W.; Emmett, B.; Suarez, R.K. Limits and constraints in the scaling of oxidative and glycolytic enzymes in homeotherms. Can. J. Zool 66:1128-1138; 1988.

13. Hochachka, P.W.; Guppy, M. Metabolic arrest and the control of biological time. Cambridge, MA: Harvard Univ. Press; 1987.

14. Hochachka, P.W.; Somero, G.N. Biochemical adaptation. Princeton, NJ: Princeton Univ. Press; 1984.

15. Hoppeler, H. Exercise-induced ultrastructural changes in skeletal muscle. Int. J. Sports Med. 7:187-204; 1986.

16. Josephson, R.K.; Young, D. A synchronous insect muscle with an operating frequency greater than 500 Hz. J. Exp. Biol. 118:185-208; 1985.

17. Kushmerick, M. Patterns in mammalian muscle energetics. J. Exp. Biol. 115:165-177; 1985.

18. Nunzi, M.G.; Franzini-Armstrong, C. Trabecular network of adult skeletal muscle. J. Ultrastruct. Res. 73:21-26; 1980.

19. Rall, J.A. Energetic aspects of skeletal muscle contraction: implication of fiber types. Exerc. Sport Sci. Rev. 13:33-74; 1985.

20. Revel, J.P. The sarcoplasmic reticulum of the bat cricothyroid muscle. J. Cell Biol. 12:571-588; 1962.

21. Rouslin, W. The mitochondrial ATPase in slow and fast heart rate hearts. Am. J. Physiol. 252:H622-H627; 1987.

22. Sacktor, B. Biochemical adaptations for flight in the insect. Biochem. Soc. Symp. 41:111-131; 1976.

23. Schmidt-Nielsen, K. Scaling: Why is size so important? Cambridge, England: Cambridge Univ. Press; 1984.

24. Somero, G.N.; Childress, J.J. A violation of the metabolism-size scaling paradigm: activities of glycolytic enzymes in muscle increase in larger-size fish. Physiol. Zool. 53:322-337; 1980.

25. Srivastava, D.K.; Bernhard, S.A. Metabolite transfer via enzyme-enzyme complexes. Science 234:1081-1086; 1986.

26. Suarez, R.K.; Brown, G.S.; Hochachka, P.W. Metabolic sources of energy for hummingbird flight. Annu. Rev. Physiol. 251:R537-R542; 1986.

27. Taylor, C.R. Structural and functional limits to oxidative metabolism: insights from scaling. Annu. Rev. Physiol. 49:135-146; 1987.

28. Torres, J.J.; Belman, B.W.; Childress, J.J. Oxygen consumption rates of mid-water fishes off California. Deep-Sea Res. 26A:185-197; 1979.

29. Walsh, P.J.; Bedolla, C.; Mommsen, T.P. Reexamination of metabolic potential in the toadfish sonic muscle. J. Exp. Zool. 241:133-136; 1987.

30. Yates, L.D.; Greaser, M.L. Quantitative determination of myosin and actin in rabbit skeletal muscle. J. Mol. Biol. 168:123-141; 1983.

PART I

Biochemistry of Muscle Fatigue

Manifestations and Sites of Neuromuscular Fatigue

Howard J. Green

University of Waterloo, Waterloo, Ontario, Canada

For the researcher, unraveling the mechanistic basis of fatigue in skeletal muscle is a task of substantial proportions. Not only must the specific site be identified among a myriad of special tissues and structures involved in excitation and contraction, but the specific rate-limiting process within each site must also be determined. By and large, investigations in this area have had to rely on in vitro preparations and simulated conditions. To what degree a specific site and mechanism can be implicated in fatigue so evident during repetitive voluntary contraction in vivo, is an issue of a decidedly different dimension. Indeed, the term *fatigue* is itself complex, encompassing a variety of different behaviors that are unique to each situation. The likelihood that deterioration in such a wide spectrum of motor behavior can be traced to a single common event or process and mediated by some singular disturbance appears naive.

This introductory paper is an attempt to bridge the gap between in vitro investigations designed to delineate the functional limitations of a specific process, on the one hand, and the role of different excitation and contraction processes in the etiology of fatigue, at least as expressed voluntarily. Four aspects of this problem will be considered. First, the nature of fatigue will be briefly examined with a view to determining the implication of different expressions of fatigue to different sites and mechanisms. Second, the developments and problems associated with the identification of specific fatigue sites during performance will be explored. Third, an overview of research completed to date will be presented in an attempt to determine how definitive the evidence is in support of specific fatigue sites. Finally, potential compensating strategies will be examined in order to determine whether they are beneficial and under what circumstances.

The Nature of Fatigue

For simplicity, the term *muscle fatigue* will be restricted only to those behaviors that are observable and can be measured physically. In the intact conscious organism, the behavior measured can in the main be a product of the collective function of the thousands of motor units comprising a single muscle or a group of synergistic muscles, and as modified by biomechanical considerations. Present methods by and large preclude measurement of the mechanical behavior of individual motor units and muscle fibers during voluntary effort.

13

Muscular fatigue is most frequently operationally defined as an inability to generate a required or expected force (26). With this definition, a specific force criterion is established, and fatigue is defined as that point at which a particular force level can no longer be maintained. The criterion force level established, whether maximal or submaximal, and the contraction schedule used to induce the fatigue are inconsequential to the definition. Moreover, some have differentiated weakness from fatigue (23).

Weakness has been defined as a failure to generate maximal force, whereas fatigue is a failure to sustain a given level of power output during repetitive contraction (22, 27). Davies and White (23) have concluded that contractile activity can induce weakness but not alter the rate of force loss (fatigability) following a repetitive task. This distinction, intended to differentiate between the immediate and more persistent effects of the repetitive exercise, remains confusing. During a voluntary task, weakness and fatigability can be synonymous. As an example, during a task requiring repeated generation of maximal force, the resulting loss of the ability to generate maximal force is by definition fatigability. Similarly, during a repetitive task requiring a submaximal force level, the inability to generate the criterion force is by definition both weakness and fatigability. Davies and White (23), it appears, incorporate a new and important observation, namely, that an exercise-induced muscle weakness need not be accompanied by a greater relative force loss. Obviously, the rate of force loss would be decidedly different if the task required the generation of the same absolute force by the fresh compared to the weakened muscles.

The quest for the mechanistic nature of fatigue also requires that the physical entity used to define fatigue, force, be further examined. Force loss can occur during both isometric or isotonic conditions. Further, either concentric or eccentric contractions may be involved. It is generally acknowledged that the amount of isometric force developed is directly related to the number of attached cross-bridges. A reduction in the number of cross-bridges could conceivably be due to exercise-induced damage and disorientation of the cross-bridges (77) or to metabolic factors such as the concentration of phosphate or hydrogen ion the muscle (19). With fatigue resulting from eccentric work, the metabolic alterations are not as pronounced, and it is probable the force loss accompanying eccentric exercise may relate more to damage of the contractile proteins or to some process involved in excitation. Eccentric exercise is known to cause extensive muscle damage and necrosis (68). If the criteria for fatigue is based on isotonic considerations, velocity is involved. In this case, the loss of force may have a decidedly different mechanistic origin. At least in high velocities, and specifically Vmax, performance is related to the rate of cross-bridge cycling, which can be altered by both ADP and hydrogen ion concentration (19). The effects of the different products of ATP hydrolysis on contractile function have been discussed in detail by Cooke and Pate (19). The points to be emphasized are that a variety of different mechanical properties may be disturbed and that the specific mechanism depends on which property is altered.

Other expressions of performance deterioration, perhaps not so obvious to the physiologist, may also be an integral component of fatigue behavior. Loss of accuracy, position sense, and tremor, for example, may also have different mechanistic origins.

One is overwhelmed by the complexity of possibilities particularly during gross body activity where virtually every muscle is involved, each fulfilling a specific function as dedicated by the requirements of the task. The isolation of the "weak link," or a specific failing process, may be fortuitous at best.

Measurement and Identification of Fatigue Sites

At the most fundamental level, voluntary fatigue can be quantified by measuring force loss resulting in a muscle or group of synergistic muscles acting over one or more joints, the conditions being rigidly standardized. However, such a measurement fails to differentiate between force loss occurring as a result of inadequate activation of the muscle by the neural network (central) and loss as a result of deterioration in excitation–contraction processes within the muscle itself (peripheral). For investigations oriented toward determining the cause of the force loss, the necessary first step is to be able to differentiate between central and peripheral failure. Two different approaches have been employed. One approach, which is amenable only to selected muscles, involves determining the muscle compound action potential (M wave). Where accessibility of the motor nerve is possible, as with the triceps surae and the adductor pollicis, M waves can be elicited by supramaximal stimulation of the nerve during voluntary contraction. Measurement of selected M wave characteristics from the muscle surface, such as amplitude and area (using electromyographic techniques), can then be used to evaluate the integrity of the neuromuscular junction and the sarcolemma. Where M wave alterations occur during voluntary force loss, these sites must be considered along with the neural drive as possible candidates in accounting for the fatigue that results (16). Where no alteration in M wave properties occur, the force loss can be attributed to sites peripheral to the sarcolemma. An alternative method for separation of peripheral from central determinants of force is the interpolated twitch (10). This involves superimposing a single supramaximal stimulus on a maximal voluntary contraction (MVC). If no measurable increase in force results, maximal activation is believed to have occurred. Again, this technique includes both the neuromuscular junction and the sarcolemma as potential candidates to explain the force loss. This is true whether the nerve is stimulated directly or transcutaneous muscle stimulation is used. Hultman et al. (40), using curare, have shown that transcutaneous stimulation of the muscle activates the motor nerve endings in the muscle and not the muscle directly.

Although both of these approaches have proved useful in selected experimental situations, they are not without limitations. In the case of the M wave, the motor nerve is accessible for stimulation in only a few muscles. Further, for example, in the case of the femoral nerve, all muscles of the quadriceps femoris are activated (vastus lateralis, vastus medialis, vastus intermedius, and rectus femoris), precluding the possibility of isolating peripheral disturbances to a single muscle. M wave measurements are also highly variable, necessitating constant repositioning of the stimulating electrode to ensure maximization of the M wave response. Standardization of preexperimental or baseline measurements are also a significant problem because M wave potentiation can occur (31). Temperature also appears to elicit changes in M wave amplitude, probably due to alterations in impedance and current to the motor nerve (MacNabb, unpublished). Interpretation of the alterations in the M wave response is also difficult even under valid measurement conditions. The selection of a criterion property or properties of the M wave is uncertain, as is the magnitude of the relative change in appropriate properties needed to unequivocally implicate the M wave as contributing to the force impairment (61).

In the case of the interpolated twitch, contamination of the force produced can occur from factors other than those resulting from fatigue. The twitch response is extremely sensitive to the contractile history and may be influenced by potentiation, particularly in muscles containing a high percentage of fast-twitch fibers (81). Consequently, with repetitive maximal contractions, potentiation may offset the actual reduction in the superimposed twitch occurring as a result of fatigue. Where neural activation is maximal, this is not a problem. However, where neural drive is not maximal, quantification of the significance of the central component is difficult (10).

Involuntary techniques alone, such as electrical stimulation via the nerve directly or transcutaneously over the muscle, have also been employed to determine the inability of the neuromuscular system to generate a required or expected force. Edwards et al. (28) have employed high- and low-frequency stimulation to determine the specificity of force loss resulting from increased muscle usage. Based on several different exercise protocols, they have concluded that force loss at low frequency (10 to 20 Hz) may be independent of force loss at high frequency (50 to 100 Hz). These two types of fatigue, operationally defined as low- and high-frequency fatigue, respectively (28), relate only to the method of determination and not to the type of activity or impulse pattern used to induce the fatigue.

The identification of these two types of fatigue is not without controversy. This is particularly so in muscles (such as the quadriceps) where submaximal stimulation conditions must be used to determine the nature of peripheral fatigue. To characterize this type of fatigue, Edwards et al. (28) have used the ratio of the force produced at low frequencies to the force produced at high frequencies. The ratio was used to stabilize the measure because variability in force output can result because of changes in impedance resulting from variable electrode position, surface preparation, temperature, and so on. It is also assumed that high-frequency fatigue returns to preexercise levels within seconds following the end of the repetitive contraction. However, the validity of this procedure has been challenged by Davies et al. (22). These investigators have presented evidence, using the triceps surae, that force increases elicited via submaximal electrical stimulation following increases in temperature are frequency dependent. Consequently, a ratio cannot be used to define low-frequency fatigue because the denominator is affected to a different degree than the numerator. In a follow-up investigation, Edwards and Newham (29) have challenged the conclusions of Davies et al. (22). They have presented evidence demonstrating that the ratio of the forces obtained at low and high frequencies (20 Hz and 50 Hz) were relatively constant over a wide range of submaximal stimulation voltages.

However, these results obtained from the inactive quadriceps muscle (29) do not address the probable impedance changes in muscle during prolonged exercise. These impedance changes could potentially occur as a result of changes in the skin and/or muscle due to variations in temperature, blood flow, or a host of other factors. Our laboratory has examined the question of quadriceps fatigue in prolonged, one-legged exercise (1). Following an initial reduction in force elicited at both low and high frequencies of stimulation, force progressively increased, attaining levels that exceeded the preexercise state, particularly with high-frequency stimulation. The effect of using the ratio of low to high frequency force outputs to characterize low-frequency fatigue was to produce a pronounced low-frequency fatigue. In this case, the appearance of "low-frequency" fatigue was mediated in large part by the elevation in force occurring at high stimulation frequencies. Because force during a maximal voluntary contraction declined substantially, it is unlikely that force output at high stimulation frequency would increase if the stimulating current was unchanged.

Although we have found highly reproducible absolute torque outputs for a range of submaximal stimulation frequencies in the unexercised quadriceps both within and between days (42), such may not occur following a period of contractile activity. The appearance of reductions in force output at low frequencies in the absence of changes in force output at high frequencies, as found by Edwards et al. (28), could be due to the filter characteristics of the muscle. The electrical properties of the tissue (muscle, skin, fat) can be modeled as a low-pass filter. If these characteristics changed differentially for the muscle versus skin and fatty tissue, one effect could be to reduce the activation to the muscles and, therefore, the number of motor units recruited. Fewer motor units would be recruited, even though the current is the same, because of alterations in the parallel components of the tissue circuitry, resulting in disproportionally more current being directed superficially to the skin and fatty tissue. Corrections for impedance, such as to maintain a constant current, would not help in this instance because it would not compensate for the shunting effect.

The potential impact of these considerations—particularly at low-frequency stimulation in submaximally stimulated muscle—would be to exaggerate the expression of fatigue because the change in impedance, if as indicated, would add to any real fatigue occurring as a result of contractile activity. These problems seriously challenge the results of studies using submaximal measurement conditions to evaluate the specificity of fatigue.

The time taken to standardize the subject position, prepare the instrumentation, and measure the torque output of the contracting muscle poses another serious limitation. Recent studies (63, 64) have described three phases of recovery following maximal-fatiguing isometric contraction. The first phase appears to be complete within 20 s following postexercise, although the full return of force to preexercise levels (at least with the fatiguing protocol employed) may take several minutes. In studies that attempt to measure fatigue immediately after repetitive isometric contractions, such as where the subject remains positioned ready for measurement, force changes can be immediately recorded. However, in order to investigate the fatigue occurring in other types of ergometry such as cycling or treadmill running, the subject is normally repositioned for the measurement (28). The time taken precludes the detection of the initial phase of fatigue, which, depending on the exercise challenge, may be the cause of the impaired performance. What is measured is a more persistent type of fatigue, which may be related to the concept of weakness as defined by Davies et al. (22). Consequently, in experiments where the subject must be repositioned for measurement, energy imbalance or the by-products resulting from ATP and creatine phosphate hydrolysis probably do not represent a serious consideration in attempting to describe the mechanisms of fatigue.

Collectively, the considerations cited are of paramount importance in attempting to elucidate the mechanisms for a failing performance in the exercising in vivo state. For all excitation–contracting sites to be considered as potential candidates to explain deteriorating performance, it is necessary to obtain rapid measurements of functional characteristics immediately following the cessation of exercise.

Sites of Fatigue

Conceptually, the failure to produce a given or expected force can be localized to one or more of several sites. In general, fatigue has been subdivided into central and peripheral components, based on whether the impairment is within the central nervous system or within the muscle itself. Perturbations in central motor drive resulting in suboptimal activation of the muscle can result from an altered excitability of the motoneuron itself or from an inability of the motor nerve to conduct a repetitive action potential to the presynaptic side of the neuromuscular junction (Figure 1). Alterations in motoneuron excitability resulting in either elimination or reduction of motoneuron discharge rates can occur as a result of several factors. These include the intrinsic properties of the motoneurons themselves, higher centers, feedback mechanisms from the muscle, and recurrent inhibition. Branch point failure, or a failure of the action potential to regenerate in all branches of the motor nerve, has also been identified as a cause of failure of the action potential to invade the presynaptic area (18).

At the level of the skeletal muscle fiber, potential fatigue sites are numerous (Figure 2). These processes have been commonly subdivided into either excitation or contraction processes. Excitation processes include failure of the sarcolemma and/or the T tubule to conduct a regenerative action potential, failure of the coupling between the T tubule and the sarcoplasmic reticulum, and failure at the level of the sarcoplasmic reticulum itself. The effect of a failure at any one of these sites would be to reduce the amount of calcium in the cytosol for activation of the myofibrillar complex. Contraction failure can range from disturbances at the level of the regulatory proteins troponin and tropomyosin to failure at the level of the force-generating

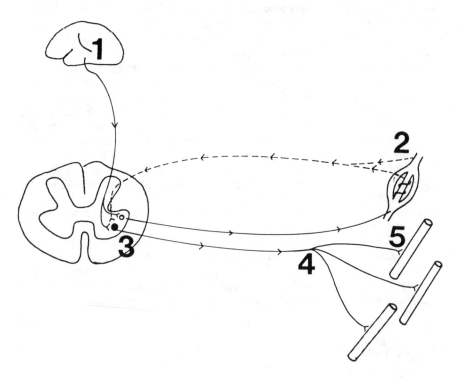

Figure 1. Central fatigue sites: (1) supraspinal failure, (2) segmental afferent inhibition, (3) depression of motoneuron excitability, (4) loss of excitation at branch points, and (5) presynaptic failure.

proteins actin and myosin. Collectively, the contraction processes, acting either singularly or in concert, could result in depressions in force either in response to a given submaximal activating stimulus or in response to a maximal activating stimulus. In the case of a submaximal activating stimulus, reductions in force could occur because of change in sensitivity of the regulatory proteins to bind calcium, resulting in an inability to maintain the force at a given cytosolic calcium concentration.

Impairment in mechanical function may also result from changes in the recovery following the cessation of the activating stimulus and the change in the return of force to prestimulation levels. As an example, alterations in the kinetics of calcium release from troponin, change in the rate at which actin disengages from myosin, and/or change in the capabilities of the sarcoplasmic reticulum for calcium reaccumulation could affect the rate at which force returns to the preactivated or rest

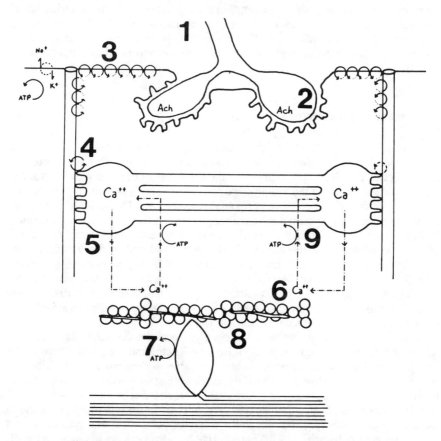

Figure 2. Peripheral fatigue sites: (1) presynaptic failure, (2) inability to develop an action potential at motor end plate, (3) failure of sarcolemma to sustain an action potential, (4) loss of coupling of excitation between T tubule and sarcoplasmic reticulum, (5) depressed Ca^{2+} release from sarcoplasmic reticulum, (6) reduced binding affinity of troponin for Ca^{2+}, (7) a failure in cross-bridge cycle, (8) delayed cross-bridge dissociation, and (9) depressed Ca^{2+} reaccumulation by sarcoplasmic reticulum.

level. The impact of alterations in recovery would depend on the contractile property under study. Prolongations in relaxation would serve to enhance isometric force output, particularly at submaximal activating levels and subtetanic force outputs. However, in the case where isotonic contractions are involved, the velocity generated would be expected to be compromised. These considerations suggest a paradox. What may be construed as a failing process by the biochemist may in effect be a potentiating process when viewed by the muscle physiologist.

An additional process that could conceivably be responsible for a reduction in performance is the neuromuscular junction. The neuromuscular junction couples central drive to peripheral activation. As previously described, detecting functional abnormalities in the neuromuscular junction is particularly difficult and can be accomplished only with pharmacologic agents such as curare (16). In practice, the neuromuscular junction has been characterized as either a central or a peripheral component, depending on the measurement protocol. As an example, electrical stimulation under maximal conditions in order to detect fatigue includes the neuromuscular junction as a peripheral process. Where the EMG is used to evaluate central drive, this neuromuscular junction has been included as a component of the central processes (16).

Fatigue and Central Drive

In general, the majority of investigations conducted to date on fatigue have focused on peripheral sites and have excluded central considerations. This is unfortunate, in fact, because such an approach denies the involvement of a complex central network capable of altering the motor drive and of optimizing neuromuscular performance in the face of progressive peripheral disturbances. The strategy that occurs in the central nervous system during the progression of fatigue is also of fundamental importance in evaluating the significance of disturbances in different excitation-contraction processes in the muscle. Disturbances induced in the muscle cell by artificial patterns of electrical stimulation used to induce fatigue may well be responsible for a deterioration in contractile behavior. When the normal pattern of innervation is expressed during voluntary activity, the magnitude of the disturbances may never be realized. This may be a result of a protective responsibility afforded by the central nervous system on the muscle (3, 10).

Recently, an increased emphasis has been given to the central basis of fatigue, mediated primarily through the work of Bigland-Ritchie and her group (7, 16). This group, using isometric contractions, has been able to demonstrate that failure in central drive can occur that appears to be specific both to the muscle and to the characteristics of the contractile activity. Using an abbreviated schedule of maximal isometric contractions, central fatigue has been detected in the quadriceps (13) and in the big toe extensors (33), but not in the adductor pollicis (8) and plantar flexors (51). Pronounced disturbances in central drive has also been documented in the diaphragm during loaded breathing (3). With prolonged submaximal static contractions, central impairment appears to occur in the plantar flexors, and particularly in the soleus (10), but not in the quadriceps (9, 10).

Alterations in central drive characterized by a reduction in firing frequencies have been repeatedly documented during sustained isometric contractions with both maximal and submaximal activity (9, 16). The reduction in firing rate, however, does not result in impaired activation but rather has been postulated to prevent supratetanic stimulation, given the alterations in contractile speed that occur in the muscle (16). The decreases in contractile speed, mediated primarily by increases in relaxation time, have been suggested to be intimately linked with the reduction in firing rate that occurs in the individual motor units (12). The reduction in firing rate could serve to protect the neuromuscular junction and the sarcolemma from failure (16), at the same time activating the muscle at a level consistent to exploit the mechanical capabilities given the disturbed intracellular environment. If this is the case—and considerably more experimentation is needed to confirm such a hypothesis—then the site of fatigue would be peripheral in nature. This could be due either to a lowered cytosolic calcium concentration or to an inability of the contractile network to translate the activating stimuli into an expected force. A depressed cytosolic calcium concentration could conceivably be due to failure in T tubule–sarcoplasmic reticulum coupling or within the sarcoplasmic reticulum itself. Further research using different contractile schedules is needed to determine whether the alterations in contractile function is irrevocably linked to reduced motor drive and whether the motor drive is in fact optimal under the circumstances.

Perhaps of more appeal to the biochemist is the isolation of the metabolic signal or signals arising from the muscle and the afferent pathways used to conduct these inhibitory signals to the alpha motoneurons. Recent emphasis has focused on group III and group IV afferents possibly being stimulated by some by-product of energy metabolism (34, 45, 46). In order to link the motoneuron excitabilty with the contractile changes in the muscle, the metabolic by-products that excite the afferent should be the same ones that are responsible for the altered mechanical behavior. In the case of prolongation of the relaxation time, a close relationship has previously been shown between resynthesis of creatine phosphate in the muscle and normalization of the relaxation time (76). This relationship, in conjunction with previous studies implicating changes in ADP and hydrogen ion concentration in the relaxation processes, has prompted these investigators to suggest that changes in the ionic species of ADP may be important, particularly the amount of the pronated form of ADP. It appears that the metabolic by-product is related to the anaerobic state of the muscle because recovery of firing rate patterns in a fatigued muscle is aerobic dependent (86).

How the afferent information is conveyed to the alpha motoneuron is uncertain. Recent experiments (50, 51, 58) have focused on recurrent inhibitory pathways via Renshaw cells, and evidence has been presented to demonstrate increases in excitability of Renshaw cells during both maximal (50) and submaximal (58) sustained isometric contraction. Changes in supraspinal command and other segmental influences may also be operative. Indeed, the reductions in the motoneuron firing rate could simply be controlled by the intrinsic properties of the motoneuron itself (47).

Fatigue and the Neuromuscular Junction and Sarcolemma

A key question is whether during sustained activity the neuromuscular junction and the sarcolemma can continue to translate the neural command into an appropriate intracellular stimulus for contraction without any impairment. To detect failure at these points, electromyographic techniques such as the surface action potential (M wave) have been employed. Alterations in muscle electrical activity observed in response to the superimposition of a stimulus applied to the nerve during the activity, have been used to indicate failure at one or both of these sites. The observation of a normal M wave is evidence that the functional integrity of both of these processes has been preserved and that, consequently, they are not limiting the mechanical behavior of the muscle.

It is generally accepted that failure of the neuromuscular junction and/or the sarcolemma can readily be induced through selected patterns of electrical stimulation of the muscle, particularly at high frequency (14, 41, 65, 74). Under these circumstances, force loss is accompanied by pronounced reductions in both the amplitude and the area of the action potential. Edwards et al. (28) as well as others (63) have used this type of evidence to suggest that a component of the force loss measured following sustained activity in response to high-frequency stimulation (50 Hz to 100 Hz) is due to failure at the level of the sarcolemma. This component of fatigue is characterized by a rapid recovery, appearing to be complete within seconds (26, 63).

The significance of alterations in the M wave in sarcolemma function and the role of these alterations in the progress of and recovery from fatigue have been challenged on several grounds. Metzger and Fitts (61, 62) have employed both high- and low-frequency stimulation to investigate sarcolemma action potentials and force loss in the in vitro rat phrenic nerve diaphragm. These investigators found extensive perturbations in sarcolemma action potentials induced with both stimulation protocols. However, the different stimulation protocols resulted in widely different force losses. These results, in conjunction with the observed dissociation between action potential recovery and recovery of force, have been used to suggest that events distal to the sarcolemma are responsible for fatigue from low- or high-frequency stimulation (61). Duchateau and Hainaut (25) have arrived at the same conclusion by using varied stimulation protocols delivered to the human ulnar nerve. Although the stimulation protocols employed resulted in similar reductions in force in the adductor pollicis, changes in the surface action potential were substantially different. Further support has also been provided by a recent study by Garland et al. (30), who found that fatigue in the dorsi flexor muscles of the human ankle was not due to impaired excitation regardless of whether a protocol using 15 Hz or 30 Hz was employed.

Although these results do not preclude the possibility that electrical failure can result in electrically stimulated muscle, they do suggest that an association between changes in the sarcolemma action potential and changes in force are insufficient to conclude a mechanistic link. Other strategies such as the use of pharmacologic agents, including caffeine, appear necessary to isolate the site of fatigue.

Until recently, the majority of evidence has failed to implicate the neuromuscular junction and/or the sarcolemma as the cause of fatigue either during voluntary sustained isometric maximal contractions or during submaximal contractions. This general position has been strongly influenced by the earlier results of Merton (60). More recently, Bigland-Ritchie and colleagues have found that in brief sustained maximal contractions resulting in force losses of between 30% and 50%, no convincing reductions in M wave amplitude or area were found in either the adductor pollicis (14, 15) or the first dorsal interosseus muscle (15). Similarly, no decline in M wave amplitude was found in the diaphragm during voluntary overload breathing where substantial fatigue was demonstrated (3). The absence of electrical failure during fatigue has also been suggested for the quadriceps during both maximal (13) and submaximal intermittent contractions (10). However, the inability to invoke maximal M waves in this muscle makes such conclusions tenuous. The primary evidence used in these circumstances to implicate only peripheral processes in fatigue was the progressive increase in target force IEMG to the initial control IEMG during an MVC (10). On the basis of the isometric fatiguing protocols employed and the muscles studied, Bigland-Ritchie et al. (8) have concluded that force production during fatigue is not limited by failure at the neuromuscular junction (or the sarcolemma).

However, a recent provocative study (4) has refuted this conclusion. These investigators used the adductor pollicis muscle, in which the ulnar nerve is readily accessible for inducing a maximal evoked M wave. They found that when fatigue was induced by sustained maximal voluntary contractions, the M wave during both contraction and recovery changed in parallel with muscle force. It was suggested that using a single interpolated nerve stimulus, evoking a single M wave, can be misleading because the background of firing activity in the already activated muscle may bias the characteristics of the M wave. The use of paired stimuli, similar to that previously employed by Stephens and Taylor (78), has been suggested to avoid the problems of background activity because the antidromic volley set up by the first impulse collides with the background activity and prevents interference with the subsequent impulse.

Bigland-Ritchie et al. (11) proposed that the natural fall in motoneuron firing rates during the progression of fatigue continues to result in maximal activation of the muscle, given the reduction in contractile speed, and at the same time prevents action potential failure. Although such a strategy may be critical in delaying the involvement of the neuromuscular junction and the sarcolemma in the force loss that ultimately occurs, it still does not preclude ultimate failure occurring at these processes. If the findings of Bellemare and Garzaniti (4) are correct and the pronounced changes in M wave amplitude are in fact sufficient to account for the force decay, electrical activation may remain as a primary failure point in most muscles.

There is extensive experimental evidence to indicate that alterations in the electrical properties of the sarcolemma do occur during sustained activity resulting from both electrically induced activity (44, 52, 59, 61, 71) and voluntary activity (75). These changes apparently involve both a reduction in the resting membrane potential and a change in the action potential waveform (52, 61). The electrical disturbances appear to be related, at least in part, to the loss of intracellular potassium from the contracting muscle (36, 44, 75). The potential mechanisms to explain the potassium loss and the complex interrelationships between the transsarcolemmal flexes of the various ionic species and the metabolic state of the muscle is the focus of the paper by Tibbits (80) entitled "Role of the Sarcolemma in Muscle Fatigue."

A critical issue from the perspective of muscle function and fatigue is whether or not these electrical disturbances are sufficient to impair activation, particularly during different tasks involving voluntary activity. Sjøgaard (75) has investigated electrolyte changes in the vastus lateralis muscle during both maximal and submaximal exercise and has calculated that reductions in intracellular potassium and the resting membrane potential occur during both types of exercise. Both types of exercise are also accompanied by an approximate 15% increase in total muscle water content. On the basis of these findings, Sjøgaard (75) has concluded that reductions in intracellular potassium concentration may be a major factor in the development of fatigue. However, such a conclusion is tenuous. Although a reduction in work performance in association with a reduction in the resting membrane potential creates the probability that the two may be mechanistically linked, the relationship does not establish cause. Indeed Vøllestad and Sejersted (83) have reasoned that the magnitude of the potassium loss is probably of minimal importance in effecting disturbances in sarcolemmal excitability.

However, there remains the issue of the degree of disturbance in the sarcolemma action potential waveform necessary to effect changes in intracellular activation. It has been suggested that decreases in the action potential amplitude could also be reflected in alterations in T tubular depolarization (44) and that the associated reduction in T tubular action potential amplitude could result in a reduction in the amount of calcium released from the sarcoplasmic reticulum (83). These issues must be resolved before M wave alterations can be employed as definitive markers of failure at the sarcolemma as a cause of fatigue. A distinguishing characteristic of the electrical changes that occur in the sarcolemma with repeated activity is that they are readily reversible, displaying a recovery that occurs within seconds or minutes after the cessation of the activity (44, 71). In addition, the recovery appears to parallel the intracellular restoration of potassium (44). An association between the early phase of force recovery, which occurs within the first 20 s after the last contraction, and recovery in membrane potential has been observed by Mainwood and Renaud (59) using the in vitro rat diaphragm preparation. In human skeletal muscle, Edwards et al. (28) have found that a rapid recovery of force at high stimulation frequencies (50 Hz to 100 Hz) also occurs during this time period. In addition, Miller et al. (63) have reported an early recovery of force and restoration of M wave characteristics following exhausting voluntary contractions, suggestive of restoration of muscle membrane excitability and impulse propagation. However, full recovery of the M wave took approximately 4 min. These investigators (64) have concluded that the significance of membrane electrical disturbances during fatigue depends on both the degree and duration of force impairment as well as on the intrinsic properties of the muscle.

Although these observations provide further evidence of impairment in sarcolemma function, at least during specific types of repetitive activity, it remains to be demonstrated that the alterations are of sufficient magnitude to ultimately result in impairment in activation of the contractile apparatus. To have physiological relevance, the impairment must be specific to the range of submaximal stimulation frequencies leading to full activation of the muscle. Because the experiments used to induce abnormalities in sarcolemma electrical properties have generally employed high-intensity activity, a metabolic acidosis and consequent slowing of the contractile speed of the muscle would be expected (59). Under these circumstances, lower motoneuron firing frequencies may elicit full activation of the muscle. Indeed, if Bigland-Ritchie et al. (11) are correct, sarcolemma failure does not result, because firing rates are reduced as the muscle contractile speed is decreased. On the other hand, if it can be demonstrated that the sarcolemma is involved in the force loss that occurs with repetitive activity, postulations regarding the significance of the reduction in firing rate must be questioned.

Fatigue and the Sarcoplasmic Reticulum

The sarcoplasmic reticulum (SR) is of primary significance in controlling the contraction-relaxation cycle in skeletal muscle. Following depolarization of the sarcolemma and the T tubules, calcium is released from an intracellular pool located in the terminal cisternae of the SR. The resulting rise in cytosolic free calcium concentration initiates the contractile process, ultimately leading to engagement of the cross-bridges. When stimulation ceases, calcium is sequestered back in the sarcoplasmic reticulum, and cross-bridge dissociation and relaxation occur. It is not surprising, therefore, that the sarcoplasmic reticulum is being increasingly implicated in fatigue (49).

Alterations in cytosolic calcium concentration can affect the mechanical behavior of the muscle in a number of ways. During repetitive stimulation at constant length, reductions in the steady state levels of cytosolic calcium could result in reduced binding of calcium to the regulatory protein subunit, troponin C, ultimately resulting in fewer cross-bridges and lower isometric force. The magnitude of the effect may well depend on the stimulation frequency. At threshold frequency, where intracellular calcium concentration is just sufficient to produce full activation, a reduction in calcium release by the SR in the absence of any compensatory changes would be expected to result in subtetanic force output. During nonfused tetanic contractions, both the kinetics of release as well as the amount of calcium released from the SR appear important to the rate and magnitude of force development (57). Similarly, alterations in reaccumulation of the calcium by the SR would be expected to alter the relaxation characteristics. During a nonfused tetanus, both contraction and relaxation kinetics are important parameters to the peak force that is realized.

A major problem in implicating the SR as a site of fatigue is one of measurement. To isolate the role of the SR, it must be demonstrated that the reduction in force with repetitive activity is due to reduced cytosolic calcium levels and that the reduced cytosolic calcium is mediated by the SR. Accurate measures of cytosolic calcium concentration in intact contracting skeletal muscle fibers have been most difficult to obtain and consequently have added little to our understanding. With the new generation of calcium-sensitive microelectrodes and fluorescent dyes (53, 72), this situation should soon change. Measurements of SR function have depended upon in vitro preparations made on the fractionated SR following sustained activity. Although these preparations provide evidence of exercise-induced alterations in calcium reaccumulation by the SR, they do not indicate how release of calcium from the SR is affected. Although the skinned fiber technique offers the possibility of studying SR function more stringently, its use appears to be limited in fatigue studies, given the time and problems associated with this type of preparation (19). Even with the techniques available, surprisingly few studies have been completed examining SR function during fatigue (2, 49).

A major paper that has had considerable impact in increasing awareness of the potential role of the SR in fatigue was published by Edwards et al. in 1977 (28). These authors found that a variety of sustained voluntary exercise tasks resulted in a long-lasting form of fatigue that was evident only at submaximal stimulation frequencies. At high stimulation frequencies, the force loss induced by the exercise recovered more quickly to normal levels. Because the force loss occurred only at submaximal stimulation frequencies (up to 20 Hz), this form of fatigue was labeled "low frequency fatigue." It was suggested by these authors that "low frequency fatigue," because it occurs at submaximal activation levels, results from impaired excitation-contraction coupling, namely, from a reduced calcium release from the sarcoplasmic reticulum per stimulation pulse. The collective effect would be a lower cytosolic calcium concentration and lower isometric force. Support for the role of the SR in "low frequency fatigue" also comes from the fact that the maximal force-generating capacity of the muscle need not be affected, and if it is, the impairment of force production at low-frequency stimulation is also greater than during maximal activating conditions (28).

The suggestion of a separate and discrete form of fatigue specific only to submaximal activating conditions has raised many questions. Consistent reproducibility of this form of fatigue has not always proved possible, a factor acknowledged by Edwards et al. (28). Because measurement of this type of fatigue depends on using submaximal conditions and specifically nonsaturating stimulus frequencies, alterations in tissue impedance induced during the activity could conceivably alter current patterns and result in variable stimulation conditions prior to and following the fatiguing exercise (23). This is of particular concern where submaximal voltages must be employed, as during fatigue protocols using large muscles such as the quadriceps (28). If the results of Davies et al. (22) are correct, the use of a ratio involving the force output at low to high frequencies does not correct this problem because the effects of temperature on impedance are specific for different frequencies.

Despite these problems, the general weight of evidence supports the existence of a low-frequency form of fatigue. This form of fatigue has been repeatedly demonstrated in small muscle groups where supramaximal voltages (20, 28, 66, 85) or voltages near supramaximal levels (23, 37) have been employed. This type of fatigue has also been demonstrated in large muscles, such as the quadriceps, using supramaximal twitches (9, 17). Further, there is evidence, from both in vitro preparations (43, 48, 56) and human in vivo studies (55), that methylxanthines known to stimulate calcium release from the SR can overcome or partially overcome this form of fatigue. Although the human studies are not all consistent in demonstrating the reversal of low-frequency fatigue with methylxanthines (54, 85), part of the discrepant results could be explained by the dosages of caffeine employed (85).

Reductions in cytosolic calcium levels could also explain the loss of force-generating capacity under normal activating conditions following repeated stimulation. Studies have been published to indicate that near-complete reversal of force loss can occur in in vitro preparations following the addition of caffeine to the incubating medium (48, 67, 84). It is unknown how long this impairment persists and how long this type of disturbance has impact on low-frequency fatigue. Available evidence suggests that the time courses of recovery of force measured with low- and high-frequency stimulation are independent (28). In this regard, the physiological significance of the recovery from the two different stimulation protocols may be fundamentally different. Stimulation of frequencies up to 25 to 30 Hz appear to lead to full activation of the human muscles regardless of fiber composition (5). Accordingly, low-frequency fatigue may disturb force output over most of the physiological range leading up to maximal voluntary contraction. Stimulation at higher frequencies (50 to 100 Hz), as used by Edwards et al. (28), appears to be quite unphysiological and, as suggested, to result in cytosolic calcium concentrations in excess of that needed for maximal activation. Although a depression in cytosolic calcium levels may occur with fatigue—in particular, low-frequency fatigue—the reduction may not be sufficient to affect the maximal activation of the fiber.

Conceivably, reductions in intracellular calcium levels during or following repetitive activity could result from impaired release of calcium from the SR, accelerated uptake by the SR, or both. If release is affected, the problem could occur with impaired signal transmission in the transverse tubules (assuming the functional integrity of the sarcolemma has been preserved), impaired transverse tubule–sarcoplasmic reticulum coupling (T tubule–SR coupling), or a defect at the level of the SR itself due either to depletion in calcium stores or to disruptions in the calcium release channel itself. The question of the role of the SR in controlling intracellular free calcium levels must be added to the contribution of the various cytosolic calcium-binding proteins as affected by their individual calcium-binding and calcium-release kinetics (73).

Dr. Donaldson (24), in her provocative paper on "Fatigue and Sarcoplasmic Reticulum," has examined the potential role of excitation-contraction coupling as a determinant of impaired force generation, particularly during submaximal activation. Previous work (6) has implicated the T tubule, due to its ability to accumulate calcium during stimulation, as a failure point. Regardless of what site is involved in the intracellular activation of the contractile proteins, it would appear that a number of criteria must be satisfied, consistent with the observational data, to demonstrate the involvement of a particular site. First, it must be demonstrated that the impairment results in a reduction in calcium release per stimulation pulse and that the reduction persists over a wide range of submaximal stimulation frequencies. Second, it must be shown that such a reduction does not occur at high stimulation frequencies, and that if it does, it does not affect the maximal activation of the fiber. Third, it must be demonstrated that the impairment is reversible but with a long recovery time course extending for up to 24 to 48 hours (28).

Fatigue and the Contractile Proteins

To establish that the contractile protein network is the ultimate site of failure, it must be demonstrated that at given levels of cytosolic calcium concentration, either submaximal or saturating force levels are reduced. At present the only definitive way to measure force output at controlled calcium levels in skeletal muscle cells is with the skinned fiber preparation; as previously indicated, however, such a preparation is not amenable to detection of force loss induced acutely in the intact fiber. In practice, methylxanthines have been used to implicate the contractile process. Incomplete reversal of force loss during maximal activation would indicate a problem distal to the sarcoplasmic reticulum. However, reversal of force levels at submaximal activation with methylxanthine does not necessarily absolve the contractile system as a participant in the fatigue observed. The effect of the methylxanthines may well result in intracellular calcium levels above that induced by the stimulation prior to the fatiguing exercise. If such is the case, the role of the contractile proteins would be masked.

As a result of these technical difficulties, few studies are available to demonstrate force failure as a result of contractile protein dysfunction, particularly in the exercising human. However, there is accumulating evidence to suggest problems at this level. Eccentric work, for example, has been shown to produce a profound and persistent fatigue that may extend for several days (69). This type of work is also accompanied by extensive myofibrillar disorganization, as determined ultrastructurally (68). Muscle fiber damage and necrosis have also been demonstrated with other work tasks, in particular with prolonged running (35, 77).

A number of sites could impair force generation by the myofibrillar complex. These sites include a number of possibilities ranging from reduced binding sensitivity and capacity of Troponin C for calcium, altered troponin-tropomyosin interaction to impaired binding, and force generation by actin and myosin. Virtually no information is available directly linking any one of these sites. Fatigue at this level certainly appears plausible, as discussed in the paper by Cooke and Pate (19) on "The Inhibition of Muscle Contraction by the Products of ATP Hydrolysis."

Mechanisms of Fatigue

Once a specific site of fatigue has been identified, the challenge is to elucidate the mechanisms responsible for the loss of functional integrity. A number of possibilities exist. These range from an alteration in the composition and structure of the membranes or myofibrillar complex (80), to alterations in ionic balance (75), to reductions in free energy availability (38), and to specific processes being directly inhibited as a result of elevation in the concentration of metabolic by-products (19). The particular impact of any one of these changes may well be specific to particular sites and processes.

The factor that has been most often implicated in the mechanism of fatigue has been the cell's impaired energy balance's being mediated as a result of ATP hydrolysis exceeding the rate of ATP regeneration. However, at least in voluntary activity, reductions in ATP concentration exceeding 30-40% of the resting concentration have rarely been reported even in the most challenging tasks. Recently, attention has focused on metabolic by-products as potential inhibitors of specific excitation-contraction processes. Potential candidates have included ADP, AMP, IMP, P_i, H^+, NH_3^{2+} or any one of a number of glycolytic intermediates (19). These metabolic by-products could potentially result in a feedback inhibition of metabolic pathways involved in ATP regeneration, such as anaerobic glycolysis (39), or by direct inhibition of the excitation or contraction process itself. Regarding the significance of inhibition of energy-producing metabolic pathways in creating an energy imbalance, the evidence is very tenuous. Some investigators have assumed such significance because reductions in force output are invariably caused by impaired energy availability. However, these conclusions may not be justified. If the cause of the force loss is more central, for example, resulting from inhibition of the motoneuron, the activation of the muscle cell would be reduced. Reductions in activation would result in reductions in actin-myosin turnover, with consequent reductions in energy expenditure. The depressed glycolysis may well be a response to a reduced energy demand rather than an inability of glycolysis to respond to an increased challenge. The ultimate criterion would be to demonstrate that the reductions in ATP that occur with this type of challenge are not detrimental to the force ouput of the muscle.

There is increasing evidence to indicate that, in vitro, the by-products produced by different energy metabolic reactions may bear significantly on the loss of force-generating capacity by the muscle. Cooke and Pate (19) have conducted an elegant series of experiments using the skinned fiber preparation to systematically investigate not only the effect of the by-products of ATP hydrolysis but the effect of MgATP itself on actomyosin function. The work provides the essential framework on which to model the significance of intracellular changes occurring in vivo on the mechanical alteration occurring during fatiguing exercise.

Fatigue and Compensatory Strategies

Another major obstacle in isolating the cause of fatigue to specific sites is the wide number of compensatory adjustments that may be invoked during sustained activity in order to minimize the impact of a failing process and to maximize work tolerance. Depending on the type of task and the specific criteria used to measure fatigue, the potential strategies include altering rate coding and recruitment within a muscle and rotating between different synergistic muscles (70). Potential strategies may also extend to different excitation and contraction processes within the muscle. For example, Bigland-Ritchie et al. (11) have emphasized the potential role of exercise-induced decreases in contractile speed as a method of allowing maximal activation of the fibers at reduced firing rates. The reduction in firing rates could serve to minimize premature failure at the neuromuscular junction and/or the sarcolemma. The reductions in contractile speed, mediated in large part by prolongations in relaxation time, probably result from reductions in the rate of calcium uptake by the sarcoplasmic reticulum. Clamann (18) has also introduced the concept of muscle hysteresis, or memory in which selective motor units appear to possess the property of maintaining force in the face of varying stimulus rates. These findings support the idea that intracellular modifications can result such that force output or mechanical behavior becomes uncoupled from the specific stimulus conditions.

The number of compensatory opportunities or degrees of freedom afforded to the neuromuscular system depends on the nature of the task. Tasks performed at maximal force levels offer little opportunity for manipulation of rate coding, recruitment, or synergistic muscle interactions. On the other hand, repetitive tasks performed at submaximal work outputs can potentially exploit a number of possibilities, both intracellular and extracellular.

Low-frequency fatigue, as an example, may be one such condition where compensatory strategies are involved. When the muscle is artificially stimulated, low-frequency fatigue occurs at firing frequencies below that needed for maximal activation. To sustain force output in the face of low-frequency fatigue, extracellular strategies could include increasing firing frequency or increasing motor unit recruitment both within and between muscles. Regardless of the strategy, the inability to sustain force output would eventually occur. Increasing recruitment would be only temporarily successful because further low-frequency fatigue would be expected in the newly recruited motor units. Increasing rate coding may result in fatigue at another site, such as the neuromuscular junction or the sarcolemma.

Another potential approach is to compensate for the reduced force output by intracellular mechanisms. One such possibility might be to use the phenomenon of post-tetanic potentiation, shown to be effective in enhancing force levels at submaximal activation (79). Alternatively, fatigue of this type might be avoided by altering the kinetics of calcium removal so as to maintain a prefatigue level of cytosolic calcium in the face of a reduced release from the sarcoplasmic reticulum per pulse. Although the mechanism appears to be unclear at this time, we have shown that a brief potentiating stimulus can overcome low-frequency fatigue observed during recovery (32). The concept of low-frequency fatigue is gaining increasing popularity.

However, we have little insight as to its cause or whether the muscle is capable of resisting it in the expression of normal voluntary activity.

The intracellular strategies may be most conspicuous in fast twitch muscles. Unfatigued fast twitch muscles require considerably more energy to sustain an isometric force. However, with sustained activity fast twitch muscles are able to greatly decrease the energy cost per unit force per cross-sectional area of the holding economy. This adaptation may be a fundamental way work tolerance can be enhanced in the fatigue-sensitive fast twitch fibers.

In summary, the quest for mechanisms to explain neuromuscular fatigue will undoubtedly consume our efforts for years to come. Impressive progress has been made. Further progress will continue to depend on intimate dialogue between the biochemist "employing in vitro techniques" and the physiologist attempting to relate findings to the multiple expressions of activity characteristic of the voluntarily exercising human.

References

1. Ball, M.E.; Green, H.J.; Houston, M.E. Metabolic correlates of muscle fatigue. Can. J. Appl. Sports Sci. 7(4):245; 1982.
2. Belcastro, A.N.; MacLean, I.; Gilchrist, J. Biochemical basis of muscular fatigue associated with repetitious contractions of skeletal muscle. Int. J. Biochem. 17(4):447-453; 1985.
3. Bellemare, F.; Bigland-Ritchie, B. Central components of diaphragmatic fatigue assessed by phrenic nerve stimulation. J. Appl. Physiol. 62(3):1307-1316; 1987.
4. Bellemare, F.; Garzaniti, N. Failure of neuromuscular propagation during human maximal voluntary contraction. J. Appl. Physiol. 64:1084-1093; 1988.
5. Bellemare, F; Woods, J.J.; Johansson, R.; Bigland-Ritchie, B. Motor unit discharge rates in maximal voluntary contractions of three human muscles. J. Neurophysiol. 50(6):1380-1392; 1983.
6. Bianchi, C.; Narayan, S. Muscle fatigue and the role of the transverse tubules. Science 215:295-296; 1982.
7. Bigland-Ritchie, B. EMG and fatigue of human voluntary and stimulated contractions. In: Porter, R.; Whelan, J., eds. Human muscle fatigue: physiologic mechanisms. London: Pitman Medical; 1981:130-148.
8. Bigland-Ritchie, B.; Bellemare, F.; Woods, J.J. Excitation frequencies and sites of fatigue. In: Jones, N.; McCartney; McComas, A., eds. Human muscle power. Champaign, IL: Human Kinetics Publishers, Inc.; 1986:197-213.
9. Bigland-Ritchie, B.; Cafarelli, E.; Vøllestad, N.K. Fatigue of submaximal static contractions. Acta Physiol. Scand. 128(Suppl. 556):137-148; 1986.
10. Bigland-Ritchie, B.; Furbush F.; Woods, J.J. Fatigue of intermittent submaximal voluntary contractions: central and peripheral factors. J. Appl. Physiol. 61(2):421-429; 1986.

11. Bigland-Ritchie, B.; Johansson, R.; Lippold, O.J.C.; Smith, S.; Woods, J.J. Changes in motoneuron firing rates during sustained maximal voluntary contractions. J. Physiol. (Lond.) 340:335-346; 1983.

12. Bigland-Ritchie, B.; Johansson, R.; Lippold, O.J.C.; Woods, J.J. Contractile speed and EMG changes during sustained maximal voluntary contractions. J. Neurophysiol. 50:313-324; 1983.

13. Bigland-Ritchie, B.; Jones, D.A.; Hosking, G.P.; Edwards, R.H.T. Central and peripheral fatigue in sustained maximal voluntary contractions of human quadriceps muscle. Clin. Sci. Mol. Med. 54:609-614; 1978.

14. Bigland-Ritchie, B.; Jones, D.A.; Woods, J.A. Excitation frequency and muscle fatigue: electrical responses during human voluntary and sustained contractions. Exp. Neurol. 64:414-427; 1979.

15. Bigland-Ritchie, B.; Kukula, C.G.; Lippold, O.C.J.; Woods, J.J. The absence of neuromuscular transmission failure in sustained maximal voluntary contractions. J. Physiol. (Lond.) 330:265-278; 1982.

16. Bigland-Ritchie, B.; Woods, J.J. Changes in muscle contractile properties and neural control during human muscular fatigue. Muscle Nerve 7:691-699; 1984.

17. Bigland-Ritchie, B.R.; Dawson, N.J.; Johansson, R.S.; Lippold, O.C.J. Reflex origin of the slowing of motoneuron firing rates in fatigue of human voluntary contractions. J. Physiol. (Lond.) 379:451-459; 1986.

18. Clamann, H.P. Fatigue mechanisms and contractile changes in motor units of the cat hindlimb. In: Jacobs, I., ed. Human adaptation to prolonged activity. Can. J. Sport Sci. 12(Suppl. 1):20s-25s; 1987.

19. Cooke, R.; Pate, E. The inhibition of muscle contraction by the products of ATP hydrolysis (this volume).

20. Cooper, R.G.; Edwards, R.H.T.; Gibson, H.; Stokes, M.J. Human muscle fatigue: frequency dependence on excitation and force generation. J. Physiol. (Lond.) 397:585-599; 1988.

21. Crow, M.T.; Kushmerick, M.J. The relationship between initial chemical charge and recovery chemical input in isolated hind limb muscles of the mouse. J. Gen. Physiol. 79: 147-166, 1982.

22. Davies, C.T.M.; Mecrow, I.K.; White, M.J. Contractile properties of the human triceps surae with some observations on the effects of temperature and exercise. Europ. J. Appl. Physiol. 49:255-269; 1982.

23. Davies, C.T.M.; White, M.J. Muscle weakness following dynamic exercise in humans. J. Appl. Physiol.: Respir. Environ. Exerc. Physiol. 53:236-241; 1982.

24. Donaldson, S. Fatigue and sarcoplasmic reticulum: Failure of excitation–contraction coupling in skeletal muscle (this volume).

25. Duchateau, J.; Hainaut, K. Electrical and mechanical failures during sustained and intermittent contractions in human. J. Appl. Physiol. 58(3):942-947; 1985.

26. Edwards, R.H.T. Human muscle function and fatigue. In: Porter, R.; Whelan, J., eds. Human muscle fatigue: physiological mechanisms. London: Pitman Medical; 1981:1-18.

27. Edwards, R.H.T. New techniques for studying human muscle function, metabolism and fatigue. Muscle Nerve 7:599-609; 1984.

28. Edwards, R.H.T.; Hill, D.K.; Jones, D.A.; Merton, P.A. Fatigue of long duration in human skeletal muscle after exercise. J. Physiol. (Lond.) 272:769-778; 1977.

29. Edwards, R.H.T.; Newham, D.J. Force frequency relationship determined by percutaneous stimulation of the quadriceps muscle. J. Physiol. (Lond.) 353:128P; 1984.

30. Garland, S.J.; Granger, S.H.; McComas, A.J. Relationship between numbers and frequencies of stimuli in human muscle fatigue. J. Appl. Physiol. 65(1):89-93; 1988.

31. Garner, S.; Hicks, A.; McComas, A.J. M-wave potentiation during muscle fatigue and recovery in man and rat. J. Physiol. (Lond.) 377:108P; 1986.

32. Green, H.; Jones, S.; Mills, D. Interactive effects of post tetanic potentiation on low frequency fatigue in human muscle. Fed. Proc. 46(3):640; 1987.

33. Grimby, L.; Hannerz, J.; Hedman, B. The fatigue and voluntary discharge properties of single motor units in man. J. Physiol. (Lond.) 316:545-554; 1981.

34. Hayward, L.; Brietbach, D.; Rymer, W.Z. Increased inhibitory effects on a close synergist during muscle fatigue in the decerebrate cat. Brain Res. 440:199-203; 1988.

35. Hikida, R.; Staron; Hagerman, F.; Sherman, W.; Costill, D. Muscle fiber necrosis associated with human marathon runners. J. Neurol. Sci. 59:185-203; 1983.

36. Hnik, P.; Uysolil; Ujec, E.; Vejsasa, R. Work-induced potassium loss from skeletal muscles and its physiological implications. Int. Ser. Sport Sci. 16:345-364; 1986.

37. Hughson, R.L.; Green, H.J.; Alway, S.E.; Patla, A.E.; Frank, J.S. Observations on human muscle fatigue by electrical stimulation following exercise with β-blockade. Clin. Physiol. 7:133-150; 1987.

38. Hultman, E.; Bergström, M.; Spriet, L.; Söderland, K. Energy metabolism and fatigue. Proceedings of the seventh international biochemistry of exercise conference; 1988 June 1-4; London, Ontario.

39. Hultman, E.; Sjöholm, H. Electromyogram, force and relaxation time during and after continuous electrical stimulation of human skeletal muscle in situ. J. Physiol. (Lond.) 339:33-40; 1983.

40. Hultman, E.; Sjöholm, H.; Jäderholm-Fk, I.; Kaynicki, J. Evaluation of methods for electrical stimulation of human skeletal muscle in situ. Pflügers Arch. 398:139-141; 1983.

41. Jones, D.A. Muscle fatigue due to changes beyond the neuromuscular junction. In: Porter, R.; Whelan, J., eds. Human muscle fatigue: physiological mechanisms. London: Pitman Medical; 1981:178-198.

42. Jones, D.A.; Howell, S.; Roussos, C.; Edwards, R.H.T. Low-frequency fatigue in isolated skeletal muscles and the effects of methylxanthines. Clin. Sci. 63:161-167; 1983.

43. Jones, S.; Green, H.; Houston, M. Reproducibility of muscle force output during transcutaneous stimulation. Med. Sci. Sports Exerc. 15(2):146; 1983.

44. Juel, C. Potassium and sodium shifts during in vitro isometric muscle contraction, and the time course of the ion-gradient recovery. Pflügers Arch. 406:458-463; 1986.

45. Kaufman, M.P.; Rybicki, K.J.; Waldrup, T.G.; Ordway, G.A. Effect of ischemia on responses of group III and IV afferents to contraction. J. Appl. Physiol. 57(3):644-650; 1984.

46. Kaufman, M.P.; Waldrup, T.G.; Rybicki, K.J.; Ordway, G.A.; Mitchell, J.E. Effects of static and rhythmic twitch contractions on the discharge of group III and IV muscle afferents. Cardiovasc. Res. 18:663-668; 1984.

47. Kernell, D.; Monster, A.W. Motoneuron properties and motor fatigue. Exp. Brain Res. 46:197-204; 1982.

48. Khan, A.R.; Bengtsson, B. Fatigue in frog skeletal muscle fibres and effects of methylxanthine derivates. Acta Physiol. Scand. 124:35-41; 1985.

49. Klug, G.F.; Tibbits, G.F. The effects of activity in calcium mediated events in striated muscle. In: Pandolf, K., ed. Exercise and sport science reviews. New York: Macmillan Publishing Co.; 1988:1-59.

50. Kukula, C.G.; Moore, M.A.; Russel, A.G. Changes in α-motoneuron excitability during sustained isometric contractions. Neurosci. Lett. 68:727-733; 1986.

51. Kukula, C.G.; Russel, A.G.; Moore, M.A. Electrical and mechanical changes in human soleus muscle during sustained isometric contractions. Brain Res. 362:47-54, 1986.

52. Lännergren, J.; Westerblad, H. Action potential fatigue in single skeletal muscle fibres of Xenopus. Acta Physiol. Scand. 129:311-318; 1987.

53. Lee, C.O. Measurement of cytosolic calcium: fluorescent calcium indicators. Miner. Electrolyte Metab. 14:15-21; 1988.

54. Lewis, M.I.; Bleman, M.J.; Sieck, G.S. Aminophylline and fatigue of sternomastoid muscle. Am. Rev. Respir. Dis. 133:672-675; 1986.

55. Lopes, J.M.; Aubier, M.; Jardin, J.; Varenda, J.; Macklem, P.T. Effect of caffeine on skeletal muscle function before and after fatigue. J. Appl. Physiol. 54:1303-1305; 1983.

56. MacIntosh, B.R.; Gardiner, P.F. Post-tetanic potentiation and skeletal muscle fatigue: interactions with caffeine. Can. J. Physiol. Pharmacol. 65:260-268; 1987.

57. MacIntosh, B.R.; Kupsch, C.C. Staircase, fatigue and caffeine in skeletal muscle in situ. Muscle Nerve 10:717-722; 1987.

58. MacNabb, N.J. Recurrent inhibition during sustained submaximal contraction in humans. Waterloo, Ontario: University of Waterloo; 1988. Thesis.

59. Mainwood, G.W.; Renaud, J.M. The effect of acid-base balance on fatigue of skeletal muscle. Can. J. Physiol. Pharmacol. 63:403-416; 1985.

60. Merton, P.A. Voluntary strength and fatigue. J. Physiol. (Lond.) 128:533-564; 1954.

61. Metzger, J.M.; Fitts, R.H. Fatigue from high and low frequency muscle stimulation: role of sarcolemma action potentials. Exp. Neurol. 93:320-333; 1986.

62. Metzger, J.M.; Fitts, R.H. Fatigue from high and low frequency muscle stimulation: contractile and biochemical alterations. J. Appl. Physiol. 62(5):2075-2082; 1987.

63. Miller, R.G.; Gianninin, D.; Milner-Brown, H.S.; Layzer, R.B.; Koretsky, A.P.; Hooper, D.; Weiner, M.W. Effects of fatiguing exercise on high-energy phosphates, forces and EMG: evidence for three phases of recovery. Muscle Nerve 10:810-821; 1987.

64. Milner-Brown, H.S.; Miller, R.G. Muscle membrane excitation and impulse propagation velocity are reduced during fatigue. Muscle Nerve 9:367-374; 1986.

65. Moritani, T.; Muro, M.; Kijima, A. Electromechanical changes during electrically induced and maximal voluntary contractions: electrophysiologic responses of different muscle fiber types during sustained contractions. Exp. Neurol. 88:471-483; 1984.

66. Moxham, J.; Wiles, C.M.; Newham, D.; Edwards, R.H.T. Sternomastoid muscle function and fatigue in man. Clin. Sci. 59:463-468; 1980.

67. Nassar-Gentina, V.; Passonneau, J.V.; Rapoport, J.I. Fatigue and metabolism of frog muscle fibers during stimulation and in response to caffeine. Am. J. Physiol. 241:C160-C166; 1981.

68. Newham, D.J.; McPhail, G.; Mills, K.R.; Edwards, R.H.T. Ultrastructural changes after concentric and eccentric contractions of human muscle. J. Neurol. Sci. 61:109-122; 1983.

69. Newham, D.J.; Mills, K.R.; Quigley, B.M.; Edwards, R.II.T. Pain and fatigue after concentric and eccentric muscle contractions. Clin. Sci. 64:56-62; 1983.

70. Patla, A.E. Some neuromuscular strategies characterizing the adaptation process during prolonged activity in human. Can. J. Sport Sci. (Suppl. 1): 7S-19S; 1987.

71. Renaud, J.M.; Mainwood, G.W. The effects of pH on the kinetics of fatigue and recovery in frog sartorius muscle. Can. J. Physiol. Pharmacol. 63:1435-1443; 1985.

72. Rink, T.J. Measurement of cytosolic calcium: fluorescent calcium indicators. Miner. Electrolyte Metab. 14:7-14; 1988.

73. Robertson, S.P.; Johnson, J.D.; Potter, J.D. The time-course of Ca^{2+} exchange with calmodulin, troponin, parvalbumin and myosin in response to transient increases in Ca^{2+}. Biophys. J. 34:559-569; 1981.

74. Sandercock, R.T.G.; Faulkner, J.A.; Albers, J.W.; Albrecht, P.H. Single motor unit and fiber action potentials during fatigue. J. Appl. Physiol. 58(4):1073-1079; 1985.

75. Sjøgaard, G. Water and electrolyte fluxes during exercise and their relation to muscle fatigue. Acta Physiol. Scand. 128(Suppl. 556):129-136; 1986.

76. Sjöholm, H.; Sahlin, K.; Edström, L.; Hultman, E. Quantitative estimation of anaerobic and oxidative energy metabolism in intact human skeletal muscle in response to electrical stimulation. Clin. Physiol. 3:227-239; 1983.

77. Sjöström, M., Fridén, J.; Ekblom, B. Endurance, what is it? Muscle morphology after an extremely long distance run. Acta Physiol. Scand. 130:513-520; 1987.

78. Stephens, J.A.; Taylor, A. Fatigue of maintained voluntary muscle contraction in man. J. Physiol. (Lond.) 320:1-18; 1972.

79. Sweeney, H.G.; Stull, J.T. Phosphorylation of myosin in permeabilized mammalian cardiac and skeletal muscle cells. Am. J. Physiol. 250:C657-C660; 1986.

80. Tibbits, G.F. Role of the sarcolemma in muscle fatigue (this volume).

81. Vandervoort, A.A.; Quinlan, A.J.; McComas, A.J. Twitch potentiation after voluntary contraction. Exp. Neurol. 81:141-152; 1983.

82. Vergera, J.; Benzanilla, F.; Salzberg, B.M. Nile blue fluorescence signals from cut muscle fibers under voltage or current clamp conditions. J. Gen. Physiol. 72:775-800; 1978.

83. Vøllestad, N.K.; Sejersted, O.M. Biochemical correlates of fatigue. Eur. J. Appl. Physiol. 57:336-347; 1988.

84. Westerblad, H.; Lännergren, J. Tension restoration with caffeine in fatigued Xenopus muscle fibres of various types. Acta Physiol. Scand. 130:357-358; 1987.

85. Wiles, C.M.; Moxham, J.; Newham, D.; Edwards, R.H.T. Aminophylline and fatigue of adductor pollicis in man. Clin. Sci. 64:547-550; 1983.

86. Woods, J.J.; Furbush, F.; Bigland-Ritchie, B. Evidence for a fatigue-induced reflex inhibition of motoneuron firing rates. J. Neurophysiol. 58:125-137; 1987.

Role of the Sarcolemma in Muscle Fatigue

Glen F. Tibbits
Simon Fraser University, Burnaby, British Columbia, Canada

The plasma membrane of skeletal muscle has been frequently implicated in the process of fatigue, which leads to a reduction in the ability of muscle to produce force (12, 24). Although the basis for this conclusion is often lacking evidence that is more than circumstantial, the sarcolemma appears to be a prime candidate in the etiology of fatigue. Almost without exception, the problem is due to failure of excitation itself, or to the failure of excitation to elicit contraction, and is dependent on the rate of stimulation (8, 12). Because the mandate of this paper is to discuss the role of the sarcolemma in fatigue, all aspects of sarcolemmal function with the potential to be involved in the etiology of fatigue, with the exception of the motor end plate, will be discussed. As such, the role of sarcolemma in muscle fatigue will be discussed from a perspective of its function in the regulation of metabolism, intracellular activities of H^+ and Ca^{2+}, and excitability.

It is difficult to discuss the role of the sarcolemma in muscle fatigue as an organelle distinct from other cellular processes or organelles. It is well known, for example, that sarcolemma structure and integrity can be affected by the metabolic state of the cell. Phospholipases can be activated, and active oxygen (free radicals) species can be generated, under cellular conditions that are consistent with those observed in certain types of fatigue. These molecular species can have a profound effect on the lipid bilayer and protein structure of the sarcolemma. Furthermore, the intimate interaction of the sarcolemma with other organelles, such as the junctional sarcoplasmic reticulum (JSR), makes it difficult for one to draw the line between these two membrane systems. The subsequent paper in this symposium by Dr. Sue Donaldson will discuss the role of the sarcoplasmic reticulum per se in muscle fatigue.

Sarcolemmal Function in Muscle

The sarcolemma can serve to regulate metabolism in several ways. The first is by virtue of the substrate transporters in sarcolemma, some of which have been reasonably well described (e.g., d-glucose), whereas the characterization of others (free fatty acid and amino acid) is in the formative stages. The second way occurs through regulation of these transporters by other sarcolemmal proteins, such as the insulin and adrenergic receptors, which may act through second messengers (e.g., cAMP, IP_3 and Ca^{2+}). There is little evidence, however, to suggest that the substrate transporters are deficient or compromised in any way during the fatiguing process.

The maintenance of pH_i in muscle around 7.0 is both critical for normal cell function and complex. During intense exercise, of course, pH_i falls by as much as one pH unit (10). This profound state of acidosis has been implicated by numerous investigators in the etiology of fatigue under these conditions. The factors contributing to acidosis during fatiguing conditions, however, are not entirely understood. The most commonly cited mechanism of acidosis, increased lactate production as a consequence of anaerobiosis, has been challenged on several grounds. It has also been suggested that changes in the strong ion differences, as proposed by Stewart (42), are largely responsible for the acidosis observed in high-intensity fatigue (29). This concept is the subject of an entire symposium at this conference; the reader is directed to those papers for a more detailed discussion. Although the sarcolemma also serves as an important regulator of pH_i, this organelle has been ignored, for the most part, in the literature on muscle fatigue. The importance is illustrated, in part, by the fact that even in the quiescent muscle H^+ is not at passive electrochemical equilibrium across the plasma membrane (37). If one takes, for example, H^+ activities of $10^{-7.4}$ and $10^{-7.0}$ M for the extra- and intracellular compartments, respectively, then an equilibrium potential of approximately -23 mV is calculated for H^+. In the normally polarized (~ -80 mV) quiescent muscle, therefore, a very strong inwardly directed electrochemical potential for H^+ exists. A simple calculation shows that the intracellular pH is about one pH unit more alkaline than expected; thus, H^+ must be actively transported out of the cell to maintain this pH so far removed from equilibrium. In the experiments of Aicken and Thomas (1) using mouse soleus muscle, the reversal of intracellular acidification caused by application and removal of NH_4Cl was slowed in the presence of amiloride, a reasonably potent inhibitor of the electroneutral Na^+/H^+ antiporter. In myoblasts from chick pectoralis muscle (45), the amiloride-sensitive Na^+ uptake into the muscle was stimulated by high pH_i and, conversely, Na^+ efflux was stimulated by low pH_o. In these experiments, the Na^+/H^+ antiporter had a K_m for Na^+ of 25 mM. Similar results have been obtained with cardiac sarcolemma vesicles (34), which provide a means of more accurately determining kinetic parameters of transport. The evidence suggests the transporter is regulated by both E_{Na} and E_H as well, perhaps, as by other regulatory factors that have yet to be characterized.

The nonspecific anion (or Cl^-/HCO_3^-) exchanger, which is inhibited by SITS, was found to play only a minor role in the reversal of intracellular acidification observed in the experiments of Aicken and Thomas (1). Similarly, Juel (26) showed that SITS had little effect on the recovery of muscle pH_i that had dropped in response to fatiguing stimulation. It appears, therefore, that this antiporter is relatively unimportant in the physiological regulation of pH_i in skeletal muscle and will not be discussed further.

A sarcolemmal protein that may be of paramount importance during intense exercise is the lactate transporter. Evidence from erythrocytes (11), intact muscle fibers (26), and isolated cardiac sarcolemmal vesicles (43) strongly suggest that both efflux and influx of lactate is carrier-mediated. Considering that the pK_a for lactic acid is approximately 3.9, at physiological pH more than 99% will be in the form of lactate$^-$, a charged species that does not readily permeate sarcolemma. The evidence for facilitated diffusion comes from the demonstration that lactate transport shows saturation in skeletal muscles of a variety of species, including humans, and isolated heart and isolated cardiac sarcolemmal vesicles. In addition to saturation (with an apparent K_m of about 20 mM), it has been demonstrated in vitro that lactate transport exhibits competition: Other monocarboxylic acids, such as pyruvate, compete with lactate. It also exhibits stereospecificity: l-lactate is transported more readily than d-lactate (43). Overall, the data from erythrocytes (23) and cardiac muscle (43) strongly suggest that this carrier functions as a lactate$^-$/H$^+$ symport. The transport kinetics, including direction, are dictated, therefore, by both the lactate and proton gradients across the sarcolemma. In muscle fatigued by intense exercise, the intracellular accumulation of both lactate$^-$ and H$^+$ promotes efflux as the symport is driven by the outwardly directed electrochemical potentials for both ions. This evidence suggests that the lactate transporter plays a role in muscle fatigue induced by intense work by both the regulation of pH$_i$ (by contributing to the efflux of H$^+$) and perhaps the rate of glycolysis by reducing [lactate$^-$]$_i$. This carrier in vitro is not inhibited by the appropriate concentrations of SITS or other inhibitors of the nonspecific anion transporter. However, there are inhibitors specific to the lactate transporter, including derivatives of cinnamic acid and isobutylcarbonyllactylanhydride (iBCLA). Although the latter compound is not available commercially, it can be readily synthesized (23). It has been shown that iBCLA is a potent inhibitor of lactate transport in erythrocytes (11, 23) and isolated sarcolemmal vesicles (Tibbits, unpublished observations) with a K_i in the low μM range.

Virtually nothing is known about the effect of intense exercise or exercise training on the sarcolemmal transport proteins that play a role in the regulation of pH$_i$. In addition to the metabolic factors that contribute to increased proton production during intense exercise, the profound drop in pH$_i$ must also be the consequence of failure of these sarcolemmal proteins to transport H$^+$ out of the cell at rates comparable to production. One could view the acidosis produced during high-intensity fatigue as a process by which H$^+$ ions are allowed to approach equilibrium across the plasma membrane.

Like in other excitable tissues, there are at least three proteins regulating trans-sarcolemmal Ca^{2+} fluxes in skeletal muscle: (a) voltage-dependent Ca^{2+} channels (41), (b) Ca^{2+} ATPase (5), and (c) Na$^+$/Ca^{2+} exchange (17). Under physiological conditions, the latter two transporters are likely to contribute only to Ca^{2+} efflux, whereas the Ca^{2+} channel contributes only to influx. Although there is little doubt of a trans-sarcolemmal Ca^{2+} influx during contraction, its role in excitation–contraction coupling has remained controversial. In part because the force output of muscle can be modified by varying the extracellular [Ca^{2+}], several investigators have suggested that the Ca^{2+} influx is critical in the SR release of calcium (9). A calcium influx associated with contraction was estimated by Curtis and Eisenberg (9) to be on the order of 1.5 pmol per fiber per min. Several lines of experimental evidence, however, speak against the notion of this Ca^{2+} influx initiating contraction. First, although the Ca^{2+} influx is linked to contraction, it occurs after K$^+$-induced contracture (13) and amounts to less than 1 Ca^{2+} ion per s per foot process of the junctional sarcoplasmic reticulum (JSR) complex and cannot, therefore, be causally related to contraction. Second, by depolarizing to membrane potentials exceeding the equilibrium potential for Ca^{2+} and thereby causing an efflux of Ca^{2+}, the magnitude of the intracellular Ca^{2+} transient was largely unaffected (7) and contraction still ensued. Even though the Ca^{2+} transient is decreased when extracellular [Ca^{2+}] is reduced, no more than 5% could be attributed to the decrease in I$_{Ca}$ (6). If this Ca^{2+} influx is not for the initiation of contraction, then what purpose does it serve? Several other roles for the Ca^{2+} influx have been suggested, including the replenishment of internal Ca^{2+} stores (13) and the activation of metabolism. By blocking the transsarcolemmal influx of Ca^{2+} in skeletal muscle, Garetto et al. (16) have found evidence that it is this source of calcium that preferentially activates phosphorylase kinase to stimulate glycogenolysis.

Transverse tubule density of dihydropyridine (DHP) binding receptor sites is in excess of 20 pmol•mg sarcolemmal prot^{-1} (calculated from #38) and is more than one order of magnitude higher than any other tissue examined. This has posed some concern because of the relatively small Ca^{2+} current observed; indeed, other tissues, such as heart, have a greater Ca^{2+} current during depolarization, and with a much lower density of dihydropyridine receptors. This has been resolved with the demonstration that less than a few percent of these DHP receptors are functional Ca^{2+} channels (38). Recently, it has been suggested that the ''nonfunctional'' channels may serve as voltage sensors in the T-tubules and play a role in the opening of the ryanodine-sensitive Ca^{2+} channel of the JSR in order to generate contraction (36). This theory does not discount the possibility that a mediator such as IP_3 (44) may be required to link the voltage sensors with the SR Ca^{2+} release. It is also worth noting in this discussion that both the dihydropyridine binding site density and the calcium current are much larger in fast-compared to slow-twitch muscles (27) and skeletal muscle Ca^{2+} channels can be modulated by catecholamines through the production of cAMP (3), resulting in both an increase in I_{Ca} and a positive inotropic response.

Evidence of Sarcolemmal "Failure" in Fatigue

The term *failure* in this heading implies only that fatigue results in changes in physiological parameters that are thought to be regulated by the sarcolemma. The notion that these perturbations serve as possible safety mechanisms to protect the muscle from the potential deleterious effects of maintaining contraction rates has been described in some detail by Edwards (12). The changes that have been observed in fatigue and are associated with sarcolemmal function include alterations in $[K^+]_i$, $[K^+]_o$, $[Na^+]_i$, $[Cl^-]_i$, $[Ca^{2+}]_o$, pH_i, pH_o, E_m, excitability, and coupling. These will be discussed in some detail.

Evidence for disturbances in $[K^+]_i$, $[K^+]_o$, $[Na^+]_i$, and $[Cl^-]_i$ as a consequence of fatigue comes from a variety of experimental approaches. Gonzalez-Serratos et al. (18), using frog semitendinosus, and Sembrowich et al. (39), using rat soleus and gastrocnemius, studied muscle fatigue with electron probe technology. This powerful technique allows for high resolution of tissue analysis, enabling ultrastructural comparisons. The technology, however, reflects elemental content and not ionic activity. Tension produced by electrical stimulation and K^+ contractures were reduced by the fatiguing paradigms, and there was trend for increased intracellular sodium and chlorine and decreased intracellular potassium contents in both studies. Cardiac glycoside treatment did not exacerbate the increase in intracellular sodium produced attendant to fatigue, but resulted in a greater decrease of intracellular potassium (18). Somewhat similar observations were made by Lindinger and Heigenhauser (29) using instrumental neutron activation analysis. The plantaris in a rat hindlimb perfusion model showed significant increases in sodium and chloride and significant decreases in potassium in response to a 5-min period of stimulation in both the red and white portions of the gastrocnemius and plantaris. In addition, they observed increases in intracellular lactate and plasma K^+ and decreases in plasma Cl^-.

Ion-selective electrodes have been used to monitor alterations in the activities of K^+ and Na^+ during fatiguing stimulation. Hnik et al. (20) have demonstrated an increase in $[K^+]_o$ with tetanic contractions in rabbit, cat, and human skeletal muscles. Typical increases were from 5 mM observed at rest to 10 or 15 mM after tetanic stimulation, but no increases were observed in response to single contractions or passive stretch. Juel (25) stimulated both mouse soleus and EDL muscles at 40 Hz for 400 ms of each s for 1 min (960 pulses), resulting in the tension falling to 29% of control. In the EDL, the $[K^+]_i$ fell from 182 to 134 mM, and the E_m dropped from -75 to -57 mV. There was a concomitant increase in $[K^+]_o$. Both $[Na^+]_i$ and $[K^+]_i$ recovered rapidly with time constants around 1.5 min, and the recovery was inhibited in the presence of ouabain. The rate of recovery of $[K^+]_o$ after 20 s of 50 Hz stimulation observed by Hnik et al. (20) was not substantially different from that observed by Juel for $[K^+]_i$ after 1 min of stimulation, as described above. The K^+ loss from the muscle has been estimated to be in the range of 0.3-0.8 nmol per impulse per g (20). The time course of intracellular K^+ recovery after fatiguing stimulation has been calculated by Hansen and Clausen (19) to be consistent with the theoretical value of 16,000 potassium ions transported per Na^+, K^+ pump site per minute; however the stoichiometry of Na^+, K^+ coupling may be altered by the changes in $[K^+]_o$ and $[Na^+]_i$ (31). Although it has been suggested that the Na^+, K^+ pump may be profoundly inhibited during the fatigue process (18), these data suggest that the pump is fully functional during the recovery process.

The degree of loss of K^+ from the intracellular compartment exceeds that of gain of Na^+ by a factor of 3 (25). This has been attributed to an increase in K^+ conductance (gK) attendant to the fatigue process (14, 15). Two factors are thought to contribute to the increase in gK: (a) increase in the Ca^{2+} activation of the K^+ channel due to either a slight increase in $[Ca^{2+}]_i$ or an increased sensitivity of the K^+ channel to $[Ca^{2+}]_i$ or (b) ATP-depletion–dependent activation of gK (40). In vivo these are not necessarily mutually exclusive mechanisms of gK activation, because reduced ATP may lead to elevated $[Ca^{2+}]_i$. In the study on the ATP dependence, however, [ATP] was required to fall to levels around 2 mM to activate K^+ channels. In order to subscribe to the notion that the increase in gK is due to falling [ATP], one would have to argue that either the free ATP near the membrane drops to levels lower than the overall levels observed by NMR or that the patch clamp procedure alters the sensitivity of the channel to ATP. Of course, the decrease in $[K^+]_i$ and increase of $[K^+]_o$ would reduce the magnitude of E_K; the membrane potential, therefore, would also be expected to decrease. Because of the limited volume and restricted diffusion of the T tubules, one might expect $[Na^+]_o$ depletion and $[K^+]_o$ increase to be more severe at this location. Some authors have implicated these changes in ionic concentrations in the etiology of fatigue induced by high-frequency stimulation (24). Simulating these changes in mouse soleus causes slowing of action potential conduction and rapid reduction in force generation. High-intensity fatiguing paradigms have been shown to reduce membrane potentials as well as alter the action potential configuration (32, 46). Although this hypothesis offers an appealing explanation of fatigue mechanisms under certain conditions, one of the main problems is that the recovery of $[K^+]_o$, membrane potential, and action potential configuration is much more rapid than that of tension development (32). The rate of recovery of the normal action potential configuration was similar to that of $[K^+]_o$ (20) and $[K^+]_i$ (25) observed in other studies. It could be argued, however, that the apparent reversal in excitation properties observed across the sarcolemma precedes that in the transverse tubules (28).

Changes in calcium concentrations have also been implicated in the mechanisms of fatigue. Bianchi and Narayan (4) suggested that an efflux of Ca^{2+} from the frog sartorius muscle during stimulation (240 nmol•g^{-1} for 300 twitches) contributed to an accumulation of Ca^{2+} in the T-tubules. At least on theoretical grounds, this could result in failure of T-tubular action potential propagation due to the increased excitation threshold. Howell and Oetliker (21) also suggested that $[Ca^{2+}]$ of the T-tubules of frog semitendinosus increases during fatigue, and they demonstrated failure of action potential propagation in the T tubules under these conditions. The original study by Bianchi's group was done on frog muscle, but the net increase in stimulation-dependent Ca^{2+} efflux was not observed in rat EDL (22) unless the muscle was made hypoxic or EGTA was added. It was concluded that the efflux from the muscle was mediated by Na^+/Ca^{2+} exchange. It has been proposed that stimulation results in a translocation of Ca^{2+} from the SR, resulting in depletion of SR calcium. The electron probe studies of Gonzalez-Serratos et al. (18) and Sembrowich et al. (39), however, have found that SR calcium content increases with stimulation to fatigue. One should bear in mind, however, that this technique quantifies elemental calcium and not Ca^{2+} activity. As a mechansism of fatigue, the notion of depleted SR Ca^{2+} content is beyond the scope of this paper and is discussed in the subsequent article by Dr. Donaldson.

Disturbances in pH_i have long been recognized as a possible mediator of the reduced tension produced by fatigued skeletal muscle. In rat diaphragm preparations stimulated by both high- and low-frequency fatiguing paradigms (33), pH_i, as determined with intracellular pH electrodes, was reduced to 6.3. The recovery of tension was highly correlated with that of pH_i.

Mainwood et al. (30) tested the effect of varying extracellular pH on tension decline and recovery in frog sartorius muscle in response to a wide range of rates of stimulation. This group demonstrated that although the rate of tension decline in response to fatiguing stimulation was not different when the pH_o was increased from 6.4 to 8.0, the rate of tension recovery was significantly improved. Increasing pH_o enhanced the recovery of tension, E_m, action potential configuration, and the rate of lactate efflux. The latter is consistent with the notion of a lactate$^-$/H^+ symport operating to remove lactate from the muscle. Mainwood et al. (30) have argued that the fall of pH_i in response to intense stimulation cannot be entirely responsible for the fall in tension. This assertion arises from the finding that the large suppression of isometric tension observed in fatigue and maintained by low extracellular pH cannot be simulated by intracellular acidification. The experimentally reduced pH_i, however, had a direct and reversible effect on the rate of relaxation.

Juel (26) found that pH_i recovery after 2 min of stimulation of the mouse soleus muscle was more rapid in an external medium of 23 mM HCO_3^-/5% CO_2, compared to 5 mM Tris, when external pH was 7.4 in both cases. However, it should be noted that Tris, with a pK of 8.3, is not an appropriate buffer at this temperature and pH. Recovery of pH_i was slowed in the presence of 0.1 mM amiloride and 4 mM cinnamate, which should block the Na^+/H^+ antiport and lactate$^-$/H^+ symport, respectively. In contrast, SITS (0.5 mM), an inhibitor of the nonspecific anion exchanger, had no effect on the rate of pH_i recovery. As expected, cinnamate also slowed the rate of lactate efflux from the fatigued muscle. It is apparent from several of these studies that pH_i recovers from high-frequency fatiguing stimulation more slowly than does $[K^+]_i$ or $[Na^+]_i$.

In part because the concentration of undissociated lactic acid is an order of magnitude higher at pH_i 6 compared to 7, it has been suggested that under fatigue conditions, efflux of undissociated lactic acid that is not carrier mediated accounts for a substantial component of the total lactate efflux (26, 30). This hypothesis can be challenged on several grounds. First, although the lactic acid concentration is higher at lower pH_i, it still only accounts for no more than 0.7% at pH_i 6 (as opposed to 0.07% at pH_i 7) of the total lactate. Second, at least on theoretical grounds, the lactate symport appears to be capable of transporting at rates consistent with the efflux rates observed in fatigue. With the lactate transporter having an apparent K_m of about 20 mM, being stimulated by high $[lactate^-]_i$ and $[H^+]_i$, and having a V_{max} of transport in cardiac sarcolemmal vesicles (43) that is comparable to the maximum rate of efflux (300 nmol • g^{-1} • min^{-1}) measured by Mainwood et al. (30), carrier-mediated transport of lactate may suffice. However, differences in temperature, tissue, and species make these comparisons tenuous. Characterization of the lactate transporter in skeletal sarcolemmal vesicles and single fibers and the use of more potent inhibitors of the symport (e.g., iBCLA) should resolve this question.

It has been suggested that fatigue induces an uncoupling effect whereby even normal excitation cannot elicit SR Ca^{2+} release and hence contraction (12). Because the mechanism by which transverse tubule excitation is coupled to contraction is not fully understood, it is difficult to propose a fully testable model of uncoupling. However, there are some reasonable candidates. As discussed earlier, the numerous dihydropyridine Ca^{2+} channels in skeletal muscle T tubules may act as voltage sensors that initiate release of Ca^{2+} from the ryanodine-sensitive Ca^{2+} channel of the SR by some undetermined mechanism. One of these may include IP_3 as a mediator; the fatigability of this process is discussed in the subsequent paper. Of interest to the study of fatigue is the recent demonstration that pH can modify the dihydropyridine-sensitive calcium channel (35). Protonation of a single group with a pK in the physiological range serves to reduce the unitary channel conductance 3-fold as the result of a partial block. How this might affect the voltage sensing of the channel or the role it plays in excitation–contraction coupling during fatigue remains to be determined.

Conclusions

Although several aspects of sarcolemmal function appear to be altered under conditions of either high- or low-intensity fatigue, there is some difficulty in causally relating these changes to the etiology of muscle fatigue. In addition to the changes cited in this discussion, several other fatigue-related factors need to be addressed. Low-intensity fatigue, in which the force may be decreased for a prolonged period of time, may be the result of alterations in membrane structure in response to the activation of phospholipases and/or the production of free radicals, which can be produced during exercise (2). The latter can induce lipid peroxidation as well as the direct modification of the transport systems discussed in this article. It could be argued that the sarcolemma is uniquely qualified to contribute to the so-called safety mechanisms because it is responsive to the changes in both extra- and intracellular compartments that are fatigue induced. In recent years, more studies have focused on the role of the sarcolemma in muscle fatigue, and it is hoped that this newfound interest will contribute to the resolution of some of the fundamental issues in muscle fatigue.

Acknowledgments

The author gratefully acknowledges the support of NSERC and discussions with Drs. R. Fitts, M. Jaweed, and M. Thomas that contributed to the preparation of this manuscript.

References

1. Aicken, C.C.; Thomas, R.C. An investigation of the ionic mechanism of intracellular pH regulation in mouse soleus muscle fibers. J. Physiol. (Lond.) 273:295-316; 1977.

2. Alessio, H.M.; Goldfarb, A.H. Lipid perioxidation and scavenger enzymes during exercise: adaptive response to training. J. Appl. Physiol. 64:1333-1336; 1988.

3. Arreola, J.; Calvo, J.; Garcia, M.C.; Sanchez, J.A. Modulation of calcium channels of twitch skeletal muscle fibers of the frog by adrenaline and cyclic adenosine monophosphate. J. Physiol. (Lond.) 393:307-330; 1987.

4. Bianchi, C.P.; Narayan, S. Muscle fatigue and the role of transverse tubules. Science 215:295-296; 1982.

5. Brandt, N.R.; Caswell, A.H.; Brunschwig, J.P. ATP-energized Ca^{2+} pump in isolated transverse tubules of skeletal muscle. J. Biol. Chem. 255:6290-6298; 1980.

6. Brum, G.; Rios, E.; Stefani, E. Effects of extracellular calcium on calcium movements on excitation-contraction coupling in frog skeletal muscle fibres. J. Physiol. (Lond.) 398:441-473; 1988.

7. Brum, G.; Stefani, E.; Rios, E. Simultaneous measurements of Ca^{2+} currents and intracellular Ca^{2+} concentrations in single skeletal muscle fibers of the frog. Can. J. Physiol. Pharmacol. 65:681-685; 1987.

8. Cooper, R.G.; Edwards, R.H.T.; Gibson, H.; Stokes, M.J. Human muscle fatigue: frequency dependence of excitation and force generation. J. Physiol. (Lond.) 397:585-599; 1988.

9. Curtis, B.A.; Eisenberg, R.S. Calcium influx in contracting and paralyzed frog twitch muscle fibers. J. Gen. Physiol. 85:383-408; 1985.

10. Dawson, M.J. Phosphorous metabolites and the control of glycolysis studied by nuclear magnetic resonance. Int. Ser. Sports Sci. 13:116-125; 1983.

11. Donovan, J.A.; Jennings, M.L. Membrane polypeptides in rabbit erythrocytes associated with the inhibition of 1-lactate transport by a synthetic anhydride of lactic acid Biochemistry, 24:561-564; 1985.

12. Edwards, R.H.T. Biochemical bases of fatigue in exercise performance: catastrophe theory of muscular fatigue. Int. Ser. Sport Sci. 13:3-28; 1983.

13. Eisenberg, R.S. Membranes, calcium, and coupling. Can J. Physiol. Pharmacol. 65:686-690; 1987.

14. Fink, R.; Hase, S.; Luttgau, H.C; Wettwer, E. The effect of cellular energy reserves and internal calcium ions on the potassium conductance in skeletal muscle of frog. J. Physiol. (Lond.) 336:211-228; 1983.

15. Fink, R.; Luttgau, H.C. An evaluation of the membrane constants and the potassium conductance in metabolically exhausted muscle fibres. J. Physiol. (Lond.) 263:215-238; 1976.

16. Garetto, L.P.; Carlsen, R.C.; Lee, J.H.; Walsh, D.A. Calcium-dependent regulation of phosphorylase activation in a fast-twitch oxidative-glycolytic skeletal muscle. Mol. Pharmacol. 33:212-217; 1988.

17. Gilbert, J.R.; Meissner, G. Sodium-calcium exchange in skeletal muscle sarcolemma vesicles. J. Membr. Biol. 69:77-84; 1982.

18. Gonzalez-Serratos, H.; Somlyo, A.V.; McClellan, G.; Shuman, H.; Borrero, L.M.; Somlyo, A.P. Composition of vacuoles and sarcoplasmic reticulum in fatigued muscle: electron probe analysis. Proc. Natl. Acad. Sci. USA 75:1329-1333; 1978.

19. Hansen, O.; Clausen, T. Quantitative determination of Na^+-K^+-ATPase and other sarcolemmal components in muscle cells. Am. J. Physiol. 254:C1-C7; 1988.

20. Hnik, P.; Vyskocil, F.; Ujec, E.; Vejsada, R. Work-induced potassium loss from skeletal muscles and its physiological implications. Int. Ser. Sport Sci. 16:345-364; 1986.

21. Howell, J.N. Effects of repetitive activity, ruthenium red, and elevated extracellular calcium on frog skeletal muscle: implications for t-tubule conduction. Can. J. Physiol. Pharmacol. 65:691-696; 1987.

22. Jaweed, M.M.; Bianchi, C.P. Calcium compartments in normal, EGTA-treated and hypoxic rat EDL (abstr.) FASEB J. 2:223; 1988.

23. Johnson, J.H.; Belt, J.A.; Dubinsky, W.P.; Zimniak, A.; Racker, E. Inhibition of lactate transport in Ehlich ascites tumor cells and human erythrocytes by a synthetic anhydride of lactic acid. Biochemistry 19:3836-3840; 1980.

24. Jones, D.A.; Bigland-Ritchie, B. Electrical and contractile changes in muscle fatigue. Int. Ser. Sport Sci. 16:377-392; 1986.

25. Juel, C. Potassium and sodium shifts during in vitro isometric muscle contraction, and the time course of the ion-gradient recovery. Pflügers Arch. 406:458-463; 1986.

26. Juel, C. Intracellular pH recovery and lactate efflux in mouse soleus muscles stimulated in vitro: the involvement of sodium/proton exchange and a lactate carrier. Acta Physiol. Scand. 132:363-371; 1988.

27. Lamb, G.D.; Walsh, T. Calcium currents, charge movement and dihydropyridine binding in fast- and slow-twitch muscles of rat and rabbit. J. Physiol. (Lond.) 393:595-617; 1987.

28. Lännergren, J.; Westerblad, H. Action potential fatigue in single skeletal muscle fibers of Xenopus. Acta Physiol. Scand. 129:311-318; 1986.

29. Lindinger, M.I.; Heigenhauser, G.F. Ion fluxes during tetanic stimulation in isolated perfused rat hindlimb. Am. J. Physiol. 254:R117-R126; 1988.

30. Mainwood, G.W.; Renaud, J.M.; Mason, M.J. The pH dependence of the contractile response of fatigued skeletal muscle. Can. J. Physiol. Pharmacol. 65:648-658; 1987.

31. Marunaka, Y. Effects of internal Na and external K concentrations on Na/K coupling of Na, K-pump in frog skeletal muscle. J. Membr. Biol. 101:19-31; 1988.

32. Metzger, J.M.; Fitts, R.H. Fatigue from high- and low-frequency muscle stimulation: role of sarcolemma action potentials. Exp. Neurol. 93:320-333; 1986.

33. Metzger, J.M.; Fitts, R.H. Role of intracellular pH in muscle fatigue. J. Appl. Physiol. 62:1392-1397; 1987.

34. Pierce, G.N.; Philipson, K.D. Na^+-H^+ exchange in cardiac sarcolemmal vesicles. Biochim. Biophys. Acta 818:109-116; 1985.

35. Prod'hom, B.; Pietrobon, D.; Hess, P. Direct measurement of proton transfer rates to a group controlling the dihydropyridine-sensitive Ca^{2+} channel. Nature 329:243-246; 1987.

36. Rios, E.; Brum, G. Involvement of dihydropyridine receptors in excitation-contraction coupling in skeletal muscle. Nature 325:717-720; 1987.

37. Roos, A.; Boron, W.F. Intracellular pH. Physiol. Rev. 61:296-434; 1981.

38. Schwartz, L.M.; McCleskey, E.W.; Almers, W. Dihydropyridine receptors in muscle are voltage-dependent but most are not functional calcium channels. Nature 314:747-751; 1985.

39. Sembrowich, W.L.; Johnson, D.; Wang, E.; Hutchinson, T.E. Electron microprobe analysis of fatigued fast- and slow-twitch muscle. Int. Ser. Sport Sci. 13:571-576; 1983.

40. Spruce, A.E.; Standen, N.B.; Stanfield, P.R. Voltage-dependent, ATP-sensitive potassium channels of skeletal muscle membrane. Nature 316:736-738; 1985.

41. Stefani, E.; Chiarandini, D. Ionic channels in skeletal muscle. Annu. Rev. Physiol. 44:357-372; 1982.

42. Stewart, P.A. Modern quantitative acid-base chemistry. Can. J. Physiol. Pharmacol. 61:1444-1461; 1983.

43. Trosper, T.L.; Philipson, K.D. Lactate transport by cardiac sarcolemmal vesicles. Am. J. Physiol. 252:C483-C489; 1987.

44. Vergara, J.L.; Tsien, R.Y.; Delay, M. Inositol 1,4,5-triphosphate: a possible chemical link in excitation-contraction coupling in muscle. Proc. Nat. Acad. Sci. USA 82:6352-6356; 1985.

45. Vigne, P.; Brelin, C.; Lazdunski, M. The amiloride-sensitive Na^+/H^+ exchange system in skeletal muscle cells in culture. J. Biol. Chem. 257:9394-9400; 1982.

46. Westerblad, H.; Lännergren, J. Force and membrane potential during and after fatiguing, intermittent and tetanic stimulation of single Xenopus muscle fibres. Acta Physiol. Scand. 128:369-378; 1986.

Fatigue of Sarcoplasmic Reticulum: Failure of Excitation-Contraction Coupling in Skeletal Muscle

Sue K. Donaldson

University of Minnesota, Minneapolis, Minnesota, U.S.A.

The intracellular mechanisms responsible for fatigue of skeletal muscle fibers have not been fully elucidated. There appear to be several forms of fatigue with one type, associated with low-frequency stimulation, involving a failure of excitation-contraction (EC) coupling beyond the step of plasmalemma depolarization (2, 4, 6, 11). Plasmalemma depolarization in the form of an action potential (AP) appears normal, but force generation of the skeletal muscle fiber is diminished or abolished. Insufficient Ca^{2+} is released from the internal stores of sarcoplasmic reticulum (SR), and the contractile apparatus is not activated to shorten and generate normal force levels. Application of caffeine to the low-frequency fatigued fibers causes internal release of Ca^{2+}-activated force generation. Thus, the point of failure is the release of Ca^{2+} from the SR in this one type of fatigue (2, 4, 6, 11).

SR Ca^{2+} release is tightly coupled to plasmalemma depolarization in skeletal muscle fibers (4, 17, 23). Two separate voltage-dependent processes, activation and inactivation (17), appear to be associated with failure of EC coupling in low-frequency fatigue (4). Activation involves gradation of SR Ca^{2+} release as a function of plasmalemma depolarization. However, the steps between transverse tubule (TT) depolarization and opening of the SR Ca^{2+} channel remain a mystery (4, 23). New information is emerging that indicates mechanical-chemical coupling may be involved (9). The chemical step, involving phosphoinositide metabolism (10, 28, 29), has properties that suggest it would be fatigable with repetitive stimulation (1, 18, 21). The voltage-dependent process of inactivation is also poorly understood (4). It may also involve mechanical and chemical steps that contribute to EC coupling in low-frequency fatigue.

EC Coupling in Skeletal Muscle Fibers

Membrane and Molecular Structures

Transmission of the TT voltage signal to the SR occurs at triadic junctions between one transverse tubule and two terminal cisternae (TC) sacs of the SR (4, 23). The sole source of activating Ca^{2+} for the contractile proteins appears to be the SR (3). The SR Ca^{2+} channels are located on the junctional face of the TC (15, 19, 20);

they were termed "feet" processes in morphologic studies and appear to protrude toward the TT (16). Recently, the feet proteins have been isolated and shown to be functional Ca^{2+} channels (19).

The molecular basis of transduction of the voltage signal is also being uncovered. Electrical properties of the TT membrane suggest that a dipole molecule reorients in the membrane with changes in electric field (25). These "voltage-sensing" dipoles appear to be intimately involved in EC coupling because agents that inhibit their movement also inhibit SR Ca^{2+} release despite depolarization of the TT membrane (4, 24). The TT voltage-sensors are hypothesized to be the molecular binding sites for dihydropyridines, a class of Ca^{2+}-antagonist drug that demonstrates voltage-sensitive binding to plasmalemma (24).

The TT and TC membranes are separated by span of approximately 2-15 nm (23). Although physical connections between TT and TC membrane have been postulated, there is no firm evidence that they occur (23). The most plausible link would be between the TT voltage-sensor dipole and the feet processes of the TC (4, 23).

Proposed Mechanisms of EC Coupling

Electrical, chemical, and mechanical TT-to-TC coupling mechanisms have been proposed. All must be voltage regulated, as is EC coupling in intact fibers (4, 17). Voltage-gated ionic channels and ionic currents or conformational change/movement of dipoles might account for this in electrical and mechanical coupling, respectively (4, 23). Chemical coupling requires either voltage-regulated production of substance at the TT, which then diffuses to the SR, and/or voltage-gated affinity of the SR for the chemical (9).

Electrical coupling is unlikely for several reasons. The TT and TC membranes are not in electrical continuity at rest because the capacitance of the SR is not detected along with that of the TTs and sarcolemma; thus, connections would have to occur only during activation (4, 23). The physical basis for TT-TC linkage has yet to be established, and depolarization of the SR prior to Ca^{2+} release has not been detected (22). It appears to be very difficult to ionically depolarize the SR in situ, perhaps because of its high permeability to K^+, Na^+, and Cl^- (8, 30). In studies of single fibers skinned by peeling of the sarcolemma, diffusion potentials could be established across sealed TTs by varying cation/anion composition of the bathing solutions (8); the SR potential appeared to be either unaffected by or unresponsive to depolarizing stimulation (8, 30) via variations in bathing solution composition.

Mechanical coupling involving the TT voltage-sensor dipole has been postulated and remains a viable hypothesis for mechanical transmission (25), although a critical test of it has not been devised. The movement of the voltage-sensor molecules appears essential to TT-TC transmission, but the molecular basis has not been established (4, 24, 25).

Chemical transmission is plausible within certain constraints requiring that certain criteria be met: The chemical signal must be produced at the TT and move to the TC; it must open the TC Ca^{2+} channel; the SR channel stimulation must be turned on and off by TT voltage. Because of the large space between TT and TC, the chemical signal might diffuse away from the junction and become diluted in the cytoplasm;

thus, higher concentrations are required (23). Diffusion from TT to TC is also likely to be slow relative to the millisecond time course of TT to TC communication in vivo (31). Two chemical transmitters that might be physiological have been identified, Ca^{2+} and inositol trisphosphate ($InsP_3$) (4, 23, 28).

Possible Role of Ca^{2+} as a Chemical Signal in EC Coupling

Ca^{2+} was first identified as a stimulus for SR Ca^{2+} release in skinned skeletal muscle fibers (13). Caffeine stimulates SR Ca^{2+} release by lowering the $[Ca^{2+}]$ threshold for this mechanism of Ca^{2+}-induced release (CaIR) (12). CaIR is of questionable physiological significance, however, because agents that block it do not inhibit contraction in intact skeletal fibers. Also, the $[Ca^{2+}]$ threshold is high enough at physiological $[Mg^{2+}]$ ($\geqslant 1$ mM) that Ca^{2+} sufficient to activate the contractile proteins directly would be required (12). In peeled mammalian skeletal muscle fibers, CaIR contributes only a secondary component to SR Ca^{2+} release initiated by ionic depolarization of sealed TTs (8) (Cl^--induced Ca^{2+} release). The $[Ca^{2+}]$ threshold for this secondary component of release is high enough to activate force generation (8). Thus, a substantial source of activating Ca^{2+} would be required to initiate CaIR in skeletal fibers. The only identified TT source of Ca^{2+}, a fast Ca^{2+} current through voltage-gated channels, has been shown to be nonessential to EC coupling (3). Thus, Ca^{2+} appears unlikely to be the chemical signal between TT and TC.

Possible Roles of Phosphoinositide Metabolism and $InsP_3$ in Skeletal Muscle EC Coupling

The role of $InsP_3$ in skeletal muscle EC coupling is still being explored. $InsP_3$ has been shown to elicit Ca^{2+} release from internal membranous stores in a wide variety of cells (1, 18, 21), including skeletal muscle (9, 10, 28, 29, 31). Its production increases with electrically stimulated contraction in intact skeletal muscle (28), although this has not been directly linked to the EC coupling process. Skeletal muscle TT membranes have the requisite PIP_2 and enzymes for $InsP_3$ production (5).

Phosphoinositide metabolism and internal Ca^{2+} release are activated in cells other than skeletal muscle by agonist's binding to plasmalemma receptors, which then stimulates hydrolysis of membrane-bound phosphatidylinositol 4,5-bisphosphate (PIP_2) into 2,3-diacylglycerol (DG) and $InsP_3$. The PIP_2 hydrolysis is catalyzed by phospholipase C, an enzyme that requires membrane-associated Ca^{2+} (1, 18, 21). For skeletal muscle this production of $InsP_3$ might be voltage controlled. A speculative model of voltage control of PIP_2 hydrolysis is shown in Figure 1 where TT depolarization (ΔV) increases hydrolysis of PIP_2 and IP_3 production. Although not shown in Figure 1, in many cells, GTP's binding to G protein molecules regulates the step of agonist/receptor to PIP_2 hydrolysis. There is also evidence for G protein regulation in skeletal muscle (7). $InsP_3$ is quickly degraded by monoesterases (9, 28, 29, 31) in the cytoplasm to $InsP_2$, InsP, and inositol, which is recycled, via an ATP-dependent process, to reform PIP_2 (1, 18, 21). DG has been shown in nonmuscle cell types to "down-regulate" by decreasing the PIP_2 hydrolysis for a given agonist stimulation. Stephenson and Lerner have recently shown that DG may "down-regulate" EC coupling in skeletal muscle (26), perhaps by decreasing the PIP_2 hydrolysis stimulated by TT depolarization (Table 1).

Inositol 1,4,5-trisphosphate is only inositol polyphosphate that causes SR Ca^{2+} release at submicromolar concentrations (10); much of the experimental work characterizing $InsP_3$ stimulation has been conducted using single skeletal fibers (frog, rabbit) skinned (i.e., sarcolemma removed or permeabilized) either mechanically by peeling or chemically (saponin) (10, 28, 29, 31). Exogenous $InsP_3$ causes Ca^{2+} release from internal fiber stores, but it appears to be degraded rapidly by fiber monoesterases (28, 31). We have obtained consistent $InsP_3$-induced Ca^{2+} release and associated force transients by microinjecting 1 nl of $InsP_3$ dissolved in bathing solutions into the myofilament lattice, with the peeled fiber in silicone oil (9, 10). $InsP_3$ appears to stimulate the SR directly because it induces Ca^{2+} release from isolated SR vesicles (29) and opens an SR Ca^{2+} channel (27). It appears to stimulate internal Ca^{2+} release

Table 1 Ionic Constituents in Bathing Solutions Related to Peeled Fiber TT State

TT state	Monovalent ions (mM)					$[K^+] \times [Cl^-]$ (mM²)
	Na^+	$Choline^+$	Cl^-	$Propionate^-$	K^+	
Polarized	4	0	4	+66[a]	66	264
Depolarized	4	62	66	+ 4[a]	4	264

[a]Greater because major anion for all cations in bathing solutions.

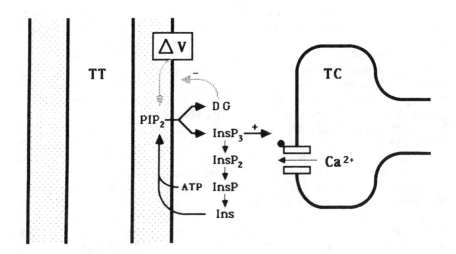

Figure 1. Schematic representation of phosphoinositide metabolism at the TT-TC junction of a skeletal muscle fiber.

in skinned fibers with sealed, polarized TTs (9) as well as those with TTs permeabilized by saponin treatment (28, 29).

Thus, InsP$_3$ appears to fulfill the criteria of being produced at the TT membrane and acting as a stimulus opening the SR Ca^{2+} channel at low concentrations. InsP$_3$ also appears to stimulate independent of Ca^{2+} stimulation of CaIR, in that the InsP$_3$-induced peeled-fiber Ca^{2+} release is unaffected by the presence of 10 mM procaine in the bathing solutions, conditions that block responses to 10 mM caffeine and Ca^{2+} (9, 10). A concentration of 0.5 μM stimulates maximally in the presence of physiological [Mg^{2+}] (1 mM) (9). Ruthenium red, a blocker of the Ca^{2+} channel feet (15), also blocks SR Ca^{2+} release stimulated by InsP$_3$, caffeine/Ca^{2+}, and depolarization of TTs (preliminary data). Thus, all of these stimuli appear to open the same SR Ca^{2+} release channel in peeled skeletal fibers, a preparation that activates and inactivates as a function of graded depolarization similar to intact cells (8, 14).

A major reservation regarding InsP$_3$ as a TT to SR chemical signal is that the time required for InsP$_3$ production, diffusion, and action is anticipated to be too slow to account for EC coupling (31). Lack of restricted diffusion space in the TT-TC junction and rapid degradation of InsP$_3$ add to the problem. However, we have recently established in studies of peeled rabbit skeletal muscle fibers that the SR is sensitized to very low concentrations of InsP$_3$ by depolarization of the TTs (9). Figure 2 illustrates this effect in isometric force traces of a single, peeled, adductor magnus fiber from rabbit (diameter 80μm). The isolated fiber was soaked, prior to peeling, for 3 hours (0°C) in a relaxing solution containing 1mM ouabain to inhibit Na$^+$-K$^+$ ATPase and polarization of the TT membrane (8). After mechanical peeling of the sarcolemma the fiber was mounted in an isometric force transducer and immersed in bathing solutions containing 4 mM Cl$^-$ and 66 mM K$^+$. The peeled fiber was loaded with Ca^{2+} from the bath, rinsed, and then depolarized by raising bath [Cl$^-$] to 66 mM and lowering [K$^+$] to 4 mM (equimolar deletion of propionate and addition of choline$^+$, respectively with 20 μM EGTA); the failure to elicit a Cl$^-$-induced force transient (trace #1) confirms that the TTs in this fiber were not polarized in the resting state, as expected, because of the ouabain presoak. The peeled fiber was then re-equilibrated in the 4 mM Cl$^-$, 66 mM K$^+$ bathing solution at 20 μM EGTA and moved into silicone oil before microinjection of 1 nl, 0.5 μM InsP$_3$ (diluted in 4 mM Cl$^-$, 66 mM K$^+$, 20 μM EGTA bathing solution). The InsP$_3$ elicited SR Ca^{2+} release a maximum force transient for this type of stimulation (trace #2). After rinsing away InsP$_3$ the peeled fiber was next stimulated by 10 mM caffeine (100 μM EGTA) added to the bath; caffeine elicited maximum force generation for this peeled fiber (trace #3). Oligomycin was added to all bathing solutions to block mitochondrial Ca^{2+} cycling; other methods were as published (8,9,10). Thus, following depolarization of TTs with ouabain, 0.5 μM InsP$_3$ (microinjected) stimulated Ca^{2+} release and a force transient that was maximum for InsP$_3$. The same concentration of InsP$_3$ in the same bathing solution but with polarized TTs yields a very small response (not shown, 9). However, concerns remain regarding the ability of InsP$_3$, even when delivered to its binding site (31), to stimulate Ca^{2+} release at a rate consistent with in vivo EC coupling.

The manner in which TT voltage regulates SR sensitivity to InsP$_3$ is unknown but could conceivably involve the TT voltage-sensor as shown in Figure 3. Movement of the dipole could mechanically alter the affinity of the IP$_3$ receptor or the access of InsP$_3$ to the SR binding site. In any event, some TT-TC communication occurs independent of InsP$_3$. We are testing whether InsP$_3$ is an essential chemical cofactor or just modulatory in EC coupling.

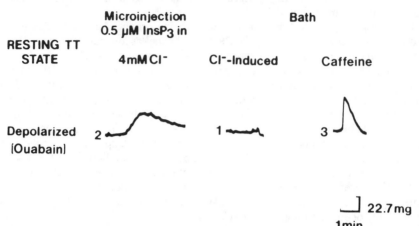

Figure 2. InsP$_3$-induced SR Ca^{2+} release in a peeled rabbit skeletal muscle fiber with depolarized TTs.

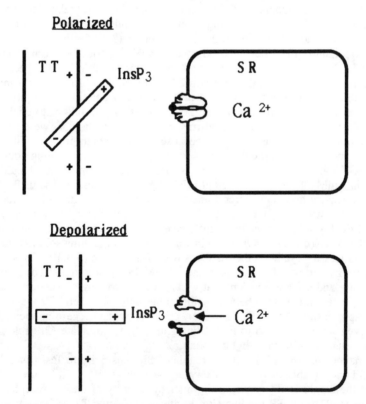

Figure 3. Schematic representation of a possible means for TT voltage control of SR affinity for InsP$_3$.

Fatigue and Skeletal Muscle EC Coupling

Fatigue during low-frequency stimulation appears to be a failure of TT-to-TC transmission. This may involve voltage-dependent TT excitability parameters such as inactivation of the voltage-sensors (4). But there is nothing in the known characteristics of the inactivation process or the behavior of TT voltage-sensors (4) that would explain the long-lasting aspects of fatigue. If $InsP_3$ is an essential component of TT-to-TC communication in skeletal muscle EC coupling, then PIP_2 depletion might contribute to fatigue. If inositol were lost from the cell or degraded, then resynthesis of TT PIP_2 might require considerable time. At this point, the above explanation is purely speculative.

Another critical point that must be explained is why fatigue as result of high-frequency stimulation does not lead to long lasting depression of functional capacity. Perhaps the cellular DG level is higher during high-frequency stimulation because the plasmalemma is depolarized for a longer period per unit of time, compared to low-frequency stimulation. If a threshold DG concentration were required for down-regulation of PIP_2 hydrolysis, then in high-frequency stimulation the PIP_2 pool would be more protected. In this purely speculative view, EC coupling might fail due to PIP_2 depletion in low-frequency fatigue, whereas in high-frequency fatigue $InsP_3$ production would decrease with sparing of the TT PIP_2 pool. Thus, in low-frequency fatigue, a longer recovery time might be required because more PIP_2 must be resynthesized.

Acknowledgments

Appreciation is gratefully expressed to Daniel Huetteman for figure preparation and technical support, and to Gretchen Asmussen for typing the manuscript. Support by NIH grant AR 35132 from USPHS.

References

1. Berridge, M.J. Phosphatidylinositol hydrolysis: a multi-functional transducing mechanism. Mol. Cell. Endocrinol. 24:115-140; 1981.

2. Bigland-Ritchie, B.; Woods, J.J. Changes in muscle contractile properties and neural control during human muscular fatigue. Muscle Nerve 7:691-699; 1984.

3. Brum, G.; Stefani, E.; Rios, E. Simultaneous measurements of Ca^{2+} currents and intracellular Ca^{2+} concentrations in single skeletal muscle fibers of the frog. Can. J. Physiol. Pharmacol. 65:681-685; 1987.

4. Caputo, C. Pharmacological investigations of excitation-contraction coupling. In: Peachey, L.D.; Adrian, R.H.; Geiger, S.R., eds. Handbook of Physiology. Bethesda, MD: American Physiological Society; 1983:381-415.

5. Carrasaco, M.A.; Magendzo, K.; Jaimovich, E.; Hidalgo, C.. Calcium modulation of phosphoinositide kinases in transverse tubule vesicles from frog skeletal muscle. Arch. Biochem. Biophys. 262:360-366; 1988.

6. Cooper, R.G.; Edwards, R.H.T.; Gibson, H.; Stokes, M.J. Human muscle fatigue: frequency dependence of excitation and force generation. J. Physiol. (Lond.) 397:585-599; 1988.

7. Di Virgilio, F.; Salviati, G.; Pozzan, T.; Volpe, P. Is a guanine nucleotide protein involved in excitation-contraction coupling in skeletal muscle? EMBO J. 5:259-262; 1986.

8. Donaldson, S.K. Peeled mammalian skeletal muscle fibers: possible stimulation of Ca^{2+} release via a TT-SR mechanism. J. Gen. Physiol. 86:501-525; 1985.

9. Donaldson, S.K.; Goldberg, N.D.; Walseth, T.F.; Hutteman, D.A. Voltage dependence of inositol trisphosphate-induced calcium released in peeled skeletal muscle fibers. Proc. Natl. Acad. Sci. U.S.A. 85:5799-5753; 1988.

10. Donaldson, S.K.; Goldberg, N.D.; Walseth, T.F.; Huetteman, D.A. Inositol trisphosphate stimulates calcium release from peeled skeletal muscle fibers. Biochim. Biophys. Acta 927:92-99; 1987.

11. Edwards, R.H.T.; Hill, D.K.; Jones, D.A.; Merton, P.A. Fatigue of long duration in human skeletal muscle after exercise. J. Physiol. (Lond.) 272:769-778; 1977.

12. Endo, M. Calcium release from the sarcoplasmic reticulum. Physiol. Rev. 57:71-108; 1977.

13. Endo, M.; Tanaka, M.; Ogawa, Y. Calcium-induced release of calcium from the sarcoplasmic reticulum of skinned skeletal muscle fibres. Nature 228:34-36; 1970.

14. Fill, M.; Best, P. Contractile activation and recovery in skinned frog muscle stimulated by ionic substitution. Am. J. Physiol. 254:C107-C114; 1988.

15. Fleischer, S.; Ogunbunmi, E.M.; Dixon, M.C.; Fleer, E.A. Localization of Ca^{2+} release channels with ryanodine in junctional terminal cisternae of sarcoplasmic reticulum of fast skeletal muscle. Proc. Natl. Acad. Sci. U.S.A. 82:7256-7259; 1985.

16. Franzini-Armstrong, C. Studies of the triad. I. Structure of the junction in frog twitch fibers. J. Cell Biol. 47:488-499; 1970.

17. Hodgkin, A.L.; Horowicz, P. Potassium contractures in single muscle fibers. J. Physiol. (Lond.) 153:386-403; 1960.

18. Hokin, L.E. Receptors and phosphoinositide-generated second messengers. Annu. Rev. Biochem. 54:205-235; 1985.

19. Imagawa, T.; Smith, J.S.; Coronado, R.; Campbell, K.P. Purified ryanodine receptor from skeletal muscle sarcoplasmic reticulum is the Ca^{2+}-permeable pore of the calcium release channel. J. Biol. Chem. 262:16636-16643; 1987.

20. Inui, M.; Saito, A.; Fleischer, S. Purification of the ryanodine receptor and identity with feet structures of junctional terminal cisternae of sarcoplasmic reticulum from fast skeletal muscle. J. Biol. Chem. 262:1740-1747; 1987.

21. Michell, R.H.; Kirk, C.J.; Jones, L.M.; Downes, C.P.; Creba, J.A. The stimulation of inositol lipid metabolism that accompanies calcium mobilization in stimulated cells: defined characteristics and unanswered questions. Philos. Trans. R. Soc. Lond. [Biol.] 296:123-137; 1981.

22. Oetliker, H. An appraisal of the evidence for a sarcoplasmic reticulum membrane potential and its relation to calcium release in skeletal muscle. J. Muscle Res. Cell Motil. 3:247-272; 1982.

23. Peachey, L.D.; Franzini-Armstrong, C. Structure and function of membrane systems of skeletal muscle cells. In: Peachey, L.D.; Adrian, R.H.; Geiger, S.R., eds. Handbook of Physiology. Bethesda, MD: American Physiological Society; 1983:23-71.

24. Rios, E.; Brum, G. Involvement of dihydropyridine receptors in excitation-contraction coupling in skeletal muscle. Nature 325:717-719; 1987.

25. Schneider, M.F.; Chandler, W.K. Voltage-dependent charge movement in skeletal muscle: a possible step in excitation-contraction coupling. Nature 242:244-246; 1973.

26. Stephenson, E.W.; Lerner, S.S. Protein kinase C (PKC) modulators influence E-C coupling steps in skinned muscle fibers (abstr.). Biophys. J. 53:468a; 1988.

27. Suarez-Isla, B.A.; Irribarra, V.; Bull, R.; Oberhauser, A.; Larralde, L.; Jaimovich, E.; Hidalgo, C. Inositol (1, 4, 5)-trisphosphate activates a calcium channel in isolated sarcoplasmic reticulum (SR) membranes (abstr.). Biophys. J. 53:467a; 1988.

28. Vergara, J.; Tsien, R.Y.; Delay, M. Inositol 1, 4, 5-trisphosphate: possible chemical link in excitation-contraction coupling in muscle. Proc. Natl. Acad. Sci. USA 82:6352-6356; 1985.

29. Volpe, P.; Salviati, G.; De Virgilio, F.; Pozzan, T. Inositol 1, 4, 5-trisphosphate induces calcium release from sarcoplasmic reticulum of skeletal muscle. Nature 316:347-349; 1985.

30. Volpe, P.; Stephenson, E.W. Ca^{2+} dependence of transverse tubule-mediated calcium release in skinned skeletal muscle fibers. J. Gen. Physiol. 87:271-288; 1986.

31. Walker, J.W.; Somlyo, A.B.; Goldman, Y.E.; Somlyo, A.V.; Trentham, D.R. Kinetics of smooth and skeletal muscle activation by laser pulse photolysis of caged inositol 1, 4, 5-trisphosphate. Nature 327:249-252; 1987.

The Inhibition of Muscle Contraction by the Products of ATP Hydrolysis

Roger Cooke and Edward Pate

University of California, San Francisco, California and Washington State University, Pullman, Washington, U.S.A.

During fatigue a number of metabolites accumulate within the muscle fiber, and any of these are potential effectors of the actomyosin interaction (39). In particular, inhibition of an enzymatic reaction by the end products of the reaction is a common phenomenon; the actomyosin interaction provides a good example of this type of inhibition. The concentrations of the three direct products of MgATP hydrolysis— MgADP, P_i and H^+—have been examined using NMR and by direct chemical analysis (5, 11, 12, 19, 30, 32, 36, 42). During moderate fatigue all three increase by approximately a factor of 10, while the concentration of substrate remains relatively constant, although exact basal concentrations and observed changes depend upon both muscle type and degree of fatigue. In resting muscle the concentration of MgADP is approximately 10 μM and increases to over 200 μM during long tetanic contractions. The concentration of P_i increases from about 3 mM to over 20 mM, and that of H^+ from 0.1 μM to approximately 1 μM. MgATP levels decrease from 4 mM to only about 3 mM. Thus, we shall consider variations in concentrations in these ranges. Studies of skinned fibers have shown that the actomyosin interaction is affected by changes in the concentrations of all three products of hydrolysis, as well as the substrate. These effects are complex, however, with the different products producing qualitatively different effects on fiber tension, velocity, or ATPase activity.

The skinned fiber preparation, introduced several decades ago by Albert Szent Gyorgi, has provided an excellent method for investigating the mechanical aspects of the contractile interaction. Fibers are most often skinned chemically by immersion in solutions that contain either detergents that solubilize the sarcolemma or high concentrations (50%) of glycerol that disrupt the sarcolemma osmotically. The fibers can then be used immediately or can be stored for several months at $-20°$ C in a solution containing glycerol (50%). The advantage of this preparation is that the experimenter has direct control of the level of activation as well as the composition of the medium that bathes the contractile proteins. Thus, the intracellular conditions associated with unfatigued or fatigued fibers can be mimicked, and their effects on the contractile interaction can be assessed directly. Variations in the concentration of one metabolite can be studied while the concentrations of all other species are held constant. However, several problems are introduced by the use of skinned fibers. The skinned fibers are not as stable as living fibers. Both tension and velocity decrease following activation, accompanied by an increase in compliance and sarcomere heterogeniety. This instability has largely limited the studies of skinned fibers to lower temperatures, 5-15° C, where these processes are relatively slow compared to the time required to measure fiber mechanics.

Methods

In this section we provide a very brief description of the methods used in our laboratory. With relatively modest modifications, similar methods are employed by most other investigators in this field. Thin strips of rabbit psoas muscle were chemically demembranated using a solution containing 50% glycerol, as described in Cooke and Pate (9). Activating solutions for mechanical measurements were obtained by addition of the required concentrations of ATP, ADP, K_2HPO_4, KH_2PO_4, and magnesium acetate to a rigor buffer containing 0.12 M potassium acetate, 5 mM MgAcetate, 1 mM EGTA, 1 mg/ml creatine kinase, 20 mM creatine phosphate, 1 mM $CaCl_2$, and 20 mM TES buffer, pH 7.0, pCa approximately 5. For experiments at pH 6.0 or 6.2, TES buffer was replaced with 20 mM MES buffer. For experiments involving varying concentrations of ADP, creatine phosphate and creatine kinase were omitted. Constant ionic strength was maintained by adjusting the KAcetate concentration.

Single glycerinated fibers were dissected from a small bundle of glycerinated fibers on a cold stage and mounted in a chamber between a solid state force transducer and an arm connected to a rapid motor, as described previously (9). Activation buffer was added to the chamber, and temperature was maintained constant at 10° C. The experimental buffer was stirred by taking up and ejecting 10 μl of solution at a frequency of approximately 2 Hz. Mounted fiber length was approximately 5 mm, and initial sarcomere lengths varied between 2.4 and 2.6 microns, as determined by laser light diffraction. Isometric tension and contraction velocity as a function of release load were determined using protocols described in Cooke et al. (8). In a typical experiment, a fiber was activated by addition of calcium, and two to four load clamps were imposed during the first 30-60 s. The fiber was then discarded. In some cases, more accurate data comparing two conditions were obtained by first measuring two load clamps, then rapidly changing the concentration of a ligand and subsequently measuring two more load clamps. The ATPase activities of psoas fibers were measured using a coupled enzyme system and monitoring the decrease in NADH absorbance as a function of time at 340 nm, as described in Cooke et al. (8).

Force-velocity data from isotonic releases were analyzed by a least-squares, nonlinear fit of the data to an equation derived by A.V. Hill from data on fiber mechanics and energetics, as described in reference 9:

$$V = b(1 - P/P_o) / (a/P_o + P/P_o) \qquad \text{Eq. 1}$$

Here P is the tension at velocity, V; P_o is the isometric tension; and a and b are constants. This equation, termed the Hill equation, has been found to provide reasonable fits to the force-velocity relation of most types of fibers. The maximum velocity of contraction (V_{max}) was determined by extrapolating this equation fit to zero velocity.

The variations of many mechanical properties as a function of substrate and hydrolysis products were analyzed in terms of classical competitive inhibition using the equation

$$T = T_{max} S / [K_m ([1 + C_i]/K_i) + S] \qquad \text{Eq. 2}$$

where T is the parameter in question (e.g., V_{max}, ATPase activity), S is the concentration of substrate, T_{max} is the value extrapolated to infinite substrate concentration, K_m is the Michaelis constant, C_i is the concentration of inhibitor, and K_i is the inhibition constant that describes the strength of inhibition. For both brevity and clarity of presentation, only modeled fits of force-velocity relations are presented in the figures. Standard errors of the mean were approximately 5-10% for all experiments upon which fits were based. For a detailed presentation of original data, readers should consult references 8 and 9.

Results

A number of investigators have studied the effects of variation of substrate, MgATP, and hydrolysis products, MgADP, P_i, and H^+ on the mechanics of contracting, glycerinated muscle fibers. Much of this work has been carried out using glycerinated fast skeletal muscle, although in most cases qualitatively similar results have been obtained with slow skeletal or cardiac muscle. In the results discussed below we will concentrate mainly on those obtained using skinned rabbit psoas fibers.

ATP

A number of studies have considered the effect of variation of MgATP on the mechanics of contracting, glycerinated fibers (7, 18). Data from rabbit psoas muscle suggest that V_{max} is approximately 1.5 muscle lengths per sec at 10° C and exhibits classical saturation behavior with respect to MgATP concentration with a K_m of 180 μM. Above 50 μM MgATP, isometric tension decreases with increasing MgATP concentration, with a total decrease of 25% observed at 4 mM MgATP and K_m for half-maximal decrease of 150 μM. Data from myofibrillar preparations suggest that ATPase also exhibits classical saturation behavior with a K_m of 20 μM, an order of magnitude lower than that observed for V_{max} (37). These data show that the modest changes in substrate that occur during fatigue will cause negligible alterations in fiber function. As MgATP concentration decreases from 4 mM to 3 mM, as might be expected in fatigued muscle, V_{max} will decrease by only 1%; P_o will increase by 1%; and, due to the exceptionally low K_m, ATPase will change by much less than 1%.

ADP

At physiological concentrations of 4 mM MgATP, addition of MgADP results in increasing isometric tension, with a maximal increase of approximately 30% observed at 8 mM MgADP and a K_m for half-maximal increase of 2 mM added MgADP (1, 9). On the other hand, increasing concentrations of MgADP result in a decrease in V_{max}. Analysis of the magnitude of the inhibition in terms of a model for classical, competitive inhibition suggests that MgADP is a somewhat potent inhibitor of

V_{max}, with a K_i of $200-300$ μM (9). This value for K_i is also in the range observed for the inhibition of myofibrillar ATPase by MgADP (37). The effects of MgADP on glycerinated fiber mechanics are summarized in Figure 1, which shows contraction velocity as a function of tension under two different conditions. The upper dashed curve is the fit of the Hill equation (Eq. 1) to the force-velocity data taken at the simulated unfatigued conditions of 4 mM MgATP, 3 mM P_i, pH 7.0 in the presence of creatine phosphate and creatine kinase. The creatine kinase maintains MgADP concentrations at less than 10 μM within the fiber. The lower solid curve is the simulated force-velocity relation using the values of K_m and K_i, given above at 4 mM MgATP, 3 mM P_i, and 500 μM MgADP, a concentration that is probably a little greater than that obtained during moderate fatigue. Tensions are normalized with respect to the isometric tension of the unfatigued fiber; thus, the greater horizontal intercept in the presence of the higher concentration of MgADP. Maximum velocity on the vertical axis corresponds to 1.6 muscle length/sec. The data for the dashed curve were taken from Fig. 4 of reference 8. The solid curve was determined using Eq (1,2). As can be seen in Figure 1, even 500 μM MgADP causes only modest changes in fiber mechanics. Due to the low value of K_m for ATPase activity, 500 μM MgADP causes even less change in fiber ATPase. Summarizing these effects, at a high MgADP concentration appropriate to extreme fatigue, P_o increases by only

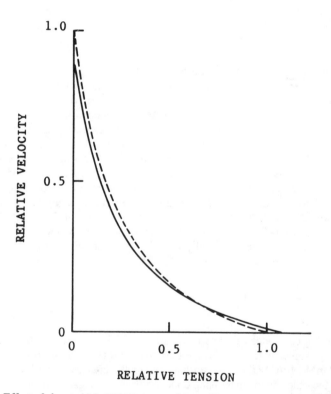

Figure 1.   Effect of elevated MgADP concentration on fiber contraction. Dashed curve gives simulated unfatigued conditions. Solid curve gives simulated fatigue conditions in the presence of high [MgADP].

7%, V_{max} decreases by 9%, and ATPase decreases by 1%. Qualitatively, raising the concentration of MgADP is similar to lowering the concentration of MgATP because both of these changes in ligand concentrations inhibit the same step in the cycle (see Discussion).

Phosphate

The interaction of P_i with actin and myosin has been studied extensively both in skinned fibers and in solution (2, 22, 23, 28, 29, 33, 40). These data have suggested that phosphate release occurs when the myosin head is bound to actin and that it precedes the major force-generating state. The effects of [P_i] on glycerinated fiber mechanics are summarized in Figure 2. The upper dashed curve is a plot of the Hill equation for the assumed unfatigued level of 3 mM P_i concentration; the lower solid curve is the fit to data collected at simulated fatigue levels of 20 mM P_i. Tensions are again normalized with respect to the isometric value at 3 mM P_i. Maximum velocity on the vertical axis again corresponds to 1.6 muscle lengths/sec. The data for the fits was taken from reference 8. As is evident, unlike with MgADP, increasing concentrations of P_i decrease isometric tension while at the same time having

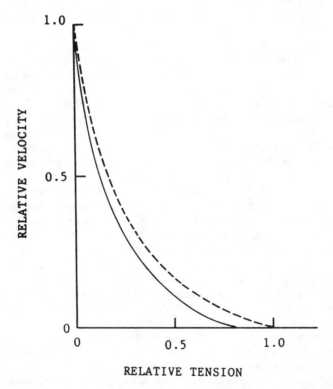

Figure 2.   Effect of elevated [P_i] on fiber contraction. Dashed curve from unfatigued conditions. Solid curve from elevated [P_i] as would be observed in fatigue muscle.

virtually no effect on V_{max}. Measurements of isometric fiber ATPase for this change in P_i concentration suggests that ATPase decreases by 15% at the higher P_i concentration. Qualitatively similar observations have been made by a number of investigators (2, 22, 23, 28, 29, 33, 40).

A number of investigators have suggested that P_i release is involved in the transition from a weakly bound A.M.ADP.P_i state (A and M represent actin and myosin, respectively) to a more strongly bound A.M.ADP state (23, 24). Analysis of models for the cross-bridge cycle suggest that if a transition from a weakly attached state to a strongly bound state is coupled with phosphate release, then isometric tension should decrease linearly with the logarithm of $[P_i]$ (34). This has led us to more carefully examine isometric tension with respect to increases in $[P_i]$ (35). By replacing the principal anion (acetate) in contraction buffers with orthophosphate, and using a sucrose phosphorylase–sucrose enzymatic system to eliminate contaminating phosphate brought into buffers by addition of MgATP and creatine phosphate, we have been able to examine tension over a phosphate range of 0.2 mM to 50 mM (pH 7) and 80 mM (pH 6.2). This represents approximately a 2-1/2 order of magnitude change in the concentration. At pH 7.0 or 6.2, phosphate exists primarily in the $H_2PO_4^-$ and HPO_4^{2-} forms, with more of the diprotonated form at the lower pH. Due to the relationship between the logarithm of products and sums of logarithms, linearity in total P_i implies equivalent linearity in both HPO_4^{2-} and $H_2PO_4^-$. Figure 3 shows isometric tension versus log $[H_2PO_4^-]$ at pH7 (upper curve) and pH 6.2 (lower curve). The data were obtained at 4mM MgATP with creatine kinase and creatine phosphate present to maintain low levels of MgADP. The solid lines are least-squares linear fits to the data and show that tension indeed does appear to be well approximated as linear in the logarithm of phosphate concentration. Error bars show standard error of the mean for 5-8 measurements. Note that in Figure 3 we have chosen to plot the data as a function of $H_2PO_4^-$, not total P_i. This was done, as explained below, to allow us to address the question of which form of phosphate inhibits tension. We point out that other data over more limited ranges of phosphate are also consistent with a linear dependence of tension upon log$[P_i]$. Specifically, the data from Kawai (28) and Kentish (29) give linear plots with log$[P_i]$. One important exception is Nosek et al. (33), who find isometric tension to be linear with absolute concentration. We have no explanation for this difference.

There has been considerable speculation that the inhibition of tension by P_i is due only to the diprotonated form of P_i (13, 33). Our data suggest that this question cannot be answered by measuring the effect of P_i on tension because tension depends on the log$[P_i]$. The effect of increased $[P_i]$ on tension is the same at pH 7 and pH 6.2. An increase in $[P_i]$ by a factor of 10 causes a 30% decrease in tension at both pH 7 and pH 6.2. Kentish (29) and Chase and Kushmerick (4) have also noted that phosphate had a similar effect at two different values of pH. Model simulations show that tension depends linearly on the logarithm of $[P_i]$ and that such a dependence precludes determining which species of phosphate is the active one (34). Although the concentration of the diprotonated species is greater at the lower pH, its concentration will always increase by the same factor as does the total P_i concentration. That is to say, if the total $[P_i]$ is increased by a factor of 10, that of the diprotonated species will also increase by a factor of 10 at any pH. If the data are plotted as a function of the logarithm of the $H_2PO_4^-$ concentration as shown in Figure 3, the data obtained at pH 6.2 still lie below those obtained at pH 7.0,

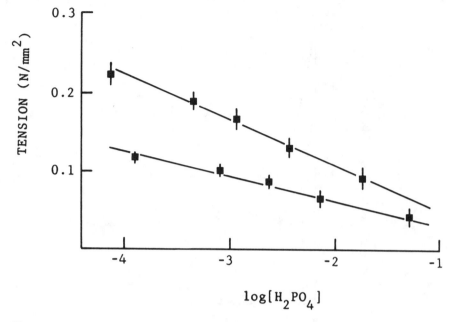

Figure 3. Isometric tension versus $\log[H_2PO_4^-]$ at pH 7.0 (upper curve) and pH 6.2 (lower curve).

eliminating the possibility that the diprotonated form of P_i is the only inhibitor and that the sole effect of pH is to shift more P_i into this form. A determination of the species of P_i involved requires measurement of a parameter that depends directly on $[P_i]$ and not on $\log[P_i]$.

Hydrogen Ions

As in vivo contracting muscle fatigues, pH decreases from 7.0 to levels below 6.5. A number of investigators have studied the effect of changes in pH upon the contraction of skinned fibers (4, 8, 14, 26, 31). The isometric tension is inhibited by about 50% as the pH is lowered from 7 to 6. The maximum velocity of contraction also decreases but to a lesser extent than does tension. The ATPase activity decreases by about the same amount as does the velocity. Figure 4 shows the mechanical response of glycerinated fibers to a decrease in pH, using the data of Cooke et al. (8). The upper dashed curve is the modeled response of unfatigued fibers shown in previous figures, with a pH of 7.0. The lower solid curve is the force-velocity curve obtained at a decreased pH of 6.0 as would be observed in fatigued muscle. Substantial decreases in both V_{max} (27%) and P_o (46%) are observed. Under identical conditions, ATPase decreases by 25% (8).

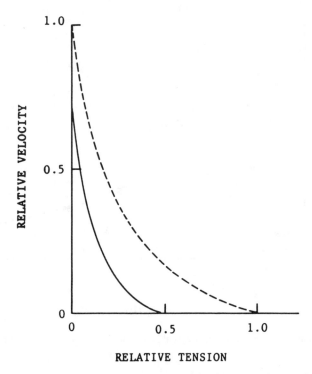

Figure 4.   Effect of elevated H⁺ on fiber contraction. Dashed curve from unfatigued conditions. Solid curve from decreased pH as would be observed in fatigued muscle.

Shape of the Force-Velocity Relation

The curvature of the force-velocity relation is described in the Hill equation (Eq. 1) by the ratio of a/P_o. The ratio of these two parameters is not changed by alterations in the concentrations of P_i or H⁺. However, a greater value of a/P_o, and thus a flatter, less curved force-velocity relation, is obtained when the concentration of MgATP is lowered or that of MgADP is raised. Because the parameter "a" is proportional to the shortening heat, i.e., to the amount of heat released per distance shortened, a lower value should correspond to more efficient contraction. If this interpretation of "a" is valid, it would argue that changes in P_i or H⁺ do not alter the efficiency of the cross-bridge. On the other hand, lowering the concentration of MgATP or raising that of MgADP would decrease efficiency. Because both these changes in nucleotide concentrations decrease the rate of cross-bridge dissociation at the end of the powerstroke, they would in fact decrease the efficiency of contraction.

Other Metabolites

In addition to the direct products of hydrolysis, discussed above, a number of other metabolites increase during fatigue (5,36). A cascade of nucleotides is generated by the degradation of ADP to species in which one or both of the phosphates have been removed. Adenylate kinase generates AMP, which is in turn converted to IMP by AMP deaminase. Essentially, these reactions provide one more available ATP for each monophosphate produced. Although the level of AMP increases very little due to the high activity of AMP deaminase, that of IMP can rise substantially (5,20). Both AMP and IMP can be dephosphorylated, to adenosine and inosine, respectively. Following heavy activity, AMP is regenerated from IMP via an intermediate, adenylosuccinate. Both AMP and IMP are known allosteric effectors of other muscle enzymes, such as phosphorylase, and there has been no systematic study of their effect on the contraction of skinned fibers. A deficiency in AMP deaminase leads to a clinical syndrome characterized by easy fatigability, suggesting that some nucleotides involved in purine nucleotide metabolism may play important roles in skeletal muscle metabolism during fatigue (38).

To explore the possibility that one or more of these nucleotides may have an as-yet-undiscovered allosteric action on the contractile proteins, we tested the effects of all of them on the mechanics of contraction. Single skinned psoas fibers were mounted on the tensiometer and bathed for 5 min in a rigor solution containing 0.1 mM diadenosine pentaphosphate. This molecule is a potent inhibitor of adenylate kinase and thus will prevent the formation of any of the nucleotides discussed above. The fibers were relaxed by addition of 4 mM MgATP, 20 mM creatine phosphate, and 1 mg/ml creatine kinase, then maximally activated by addition of calcium. The pH was 7.0, and the concentration of P_i was 20 mM. Isometric force and the velocity of contraction at 10% of isometric force were measured. The concentration of one of the nucleotides was raised to 2 mM, and both force and velocity were remeasured. None of the nucleotides—AMP, IMP, adenosine, inosine, or adenylosuccinate—altered either force or velocity by more than 5%. In addition to these nucleotides, a number of other molecules also accumulate during fatigue, including ammonia, creatine, pyruvate, and lactate. Addition of these molecules to 10 mM also had no measurable effects on the contraction of skinned fibers. Thus, a variety of metabolites that accumulate during fatigue, some of which are known to affect other muscle enzymes, do not appear to influence the actomyosin interaction. The only known modulators of this interaction are the three direct products of ATP hydrolysis.

Discussion

The data discussed above clearly demonstrate that the accumulation of the products of MgATP hydrolysis affects the contractile interaction. During moderate fatigue the concentration of P_i can increase to 20-30 mM, and the pH can drop to 6.2-6.0. The combined effect of the accumulation of these two products will be to depress isometric tension in skinned fibers by about 60% and to inhibit both the maximum velocity of contraction and the fiber ATPase activity by about 40%. This work suggests that each muscle cross-bridge must function within the constraints imposed by product accumulation. For instance, the model simulations discussed below show that increased levels of P_i must lead to a decrease in tension if P_i is released at the beginning of the powerstroke, as suggested by experiments both on fibers and on proteins in solution. However, the extrapolation of these results to living fibers, where multiple mechanisms determine the final levels of cross-bridge action, may be complex. An additional problem may be introduced because the studies of skinned fibers have been carried out at low temperatures, and it is possible that different results may be obtained at more physiological temperatures.

Fatigue of living muscle fibers is a complex process that undoubtedly involves inhibition of more than one process and that depends upon the protocol used. At least some of the inhibition of function seen in living fibers is accounted for by the inhibition of the actomyosin interaction. Several investigators have examined both intracellular pH and contractile force and found that force is inhibited as H^+ accumulates (15). However, in the period following fatigue, pH has been found to recover significantly, while force remains low (41). Some investigators have found a linear correlation between isometric force and the concentration of diprotonated P_i in living frog muscle (13); however, as discussed both above and in the next section, force depends linearly on $\log[P_i]$, not on $[P_i]$, in glycerinated fibers (34). One difficulty in drawing these correlations is that several variables are changing simultaneously in the living fibers. By using the data discussed in the Results section and measuring the internal concentrations of both H^+ and P_i, one could ask more precisely under what conditions the reduction of muscle force or velocity is accounted for by product inhibition.

In addition to product inhibition, a number of other mechanisms affect muscle function during fatigue. It appears clear that during a lengthy train of intermittent contractions, tension can be depressed by inhibition of the release of calcium from the sarcoplasmic reticulum (21). Product inhibition probably plays a more dominant role in the case of lengthy tetanic contractions, where the activation of the fibers remains fully turned on.

An additional aspect of fatigued fibers seen in vivo is not reproduced by the skinned fibers. During long tetanic contractions, the MgATP hydrolyzed divided by the tension produced (known as the tension cost) decreases by a factor of 2-4. This has been observed in isolated mouse EDL muscle and frog muscle during long tetanic contractions, in isolated frog muscle during intermittent contractions, and in human muscle in situ during intermittent contractions (3, 10, 17). The decrease in tension cost is accompanied by an equivalent decrease in the maximum velocity of contraction, showing that the increased efficiency is due to slower cycling of the cross-bridges (10). The increase in efficiency is seen only in fast skeletal muscle and not in slow skeletal muscle. Thus, when a fast muscle fiber is being used heavily, it becomes more efficient at maintaining tension, probably representing an important mechanism for conserving the remaining supplies of energy. In contrast, the tension cost of the skinned fibers increases by about a factor of 2 when they are transferred into high P_i and H^+ conditions that simulate fatigue. The reason for this discrepancy is not clear. It suggests that some additional mechanisms that affect the contractile interaction remain to be discovered or that product inhibition operates differently under more physiological conditions, such as at higher temperatures.

Models of the Actomyosin Interaction

Data on product inhibition help to define the energetics of the cross-bridge states involved in product release. The disparate effects of the hydrolysis products MgADP,

P_i, and H^+ are somewhat contradictory in terms of general ideas regarding end product inhibition of an enzymatic reaction. We have investigated these differences using mathematical models for cross-bridge function that, following Huxley (25), include both state-transition kinetics and steric constraints imposed by the spatial organization of the fiber. The states involving release of MgADP or P_i have been relatively well characterized in solution (for review, see 6, 16, 24), and these data were used to define the corresponding states in the fiber. In particular we have used a model, similar to that initially proposed by Eisenberg et al. (16), that involves an equilibrium between a weakly attached, low-force A.M.ADP.P_i state at the beginning of a cross-bridge powerstroke and a strongly bound A.M.ADP powerstroke state. Simulations showed that in this case, increased P_i resulted in a decreased isometric force by decreasing the number of bridges attached in the strongly bound state, with little corresponding change in V_{max}. Furthermore, P_o decreases with $\log[P_i]$. The fractional decrease in tension between two different concentrations of P_i is approximately the same at the two values of pH. Even when the data are plotted as a function of $H_2PO_4^-$, the data at pH 6.2 lie below those at pH 7.0, which shows that H^+ must also inhibit tension.

The models suggest that ADP release, on the other hand, occurs at the end of the powerstroke. Increased levels of MgADP result in a slower rate of cross-bridge dissociation by MgATP, with a higher isometric tension resulting from the increased number of attached cross-bridges. The inhibition of velocity arises from heads that are not dissociated by MgATP at the end of the powerstroke but are instead pulled by the relative sliding of the filaments into configurations in which they produce negative work. The effects of the products on fiber tension and velocity appear to be additive. For instance, addition of both P_i and MgADP to fibers produces an effect on velocity or tension that is the sum of that produced by each separately (9). This behavior is also produced by the model, largely because the two products are released at different steps in the cycle. The observed effects of MgADP and P_i could be reproduced by the model, assuming that they are simple competitive inhibitors of the steps in which they are released. However, the effects of H^+ could not be reproduced by changing a single rate constant. Thus, the effects produced by H^+ are probably the result of more complex mechanisms, possibly involving pH-mediated changes at multiple sites on the contractile proteins.

Some investigators have attempted to draw correlations between the mechanics of contraction and the free energy of MgATP hydrolysis (9, 27). The results of both experimental data and theoretical simulations suggest that this is not a simple relationship. The free energy of MgATP hydrolysis depends upon the logarithms of the concentrations of MgATP, MgADP, and P_i. Although raising either MgADP or P_i by a factor of 10 will have the same effect upon the free energy of MgATP hydrolysis, it has very different effects upon fiber velocity or tension: An increase in MgADP increases tension, whereas an increase in P_i decreases tension. Model simulations that reproduce these effects suggest that the two ligands produce different effects because they are released at different steps in the contractile cycle. The release of P_i within the powerstroke leads to an inhibition of tension with an increase in P_i. The release of MgADP at the end of the powerstroke causes an increase in tension because it inhibits the release from actin by MgATP of tension-bearing cross-bridges. A decrease in MgATP concentration also raises tension while decreasing the free energy of hydrolysis of MgATP. Thus, there does not appear to be a simple relation between the free energy of MgATP hydrolysis and either fiber tension, velocity, or ATPase activity.

70   Cooke and Pate

References

1. Abbott, R.H.; Mannherz, H.G. Activation by MgADP and the correlation between tensions and ATPase activity in insect fibrillar muscle. Pflügers Arch. 321:223-232; 1970.
2. Altringham, J.D.; Johnston, I.A. Effects of phosphate on the contractile properties of fast and slow muscle fibers from an Antarctic fish. J. Physiol. (Lond.): 491-500; 1985.
3. Barsotti, R.J.; Butler, T.J. Chemical energy usage and myosin light chain phosphorylation in mammalian skeletal muscle. J. Muscle Res. Cell Motil. 5:45-64; 1984.
4. Chase, P.B.; Kushmerick, M.J. Effects of pH on contraction of rabbit fast and slow skeletal muscle fibers. Biophys. J. 53:935-946; 1988.
5. Chasiotis, D.; Bergstrom, M.; Hultman, E. ATP utilization during intermittent and continuous muscle contractions. Am. J. Physiol. 63:167-174; 1987.
6. Cooke, R. The mechanism of muscle contraction. CRC Crit. Rev. Biochem. 21:53-118; 1986.
7. Cooke, R.; Bialek, W. Contraction of glycerinated muscle fibers as a function of MgATP concentration. Biophys. J. 28:241-258; 1979.
8. Cooke, R.; Franks, K.; Luciani, G.; Pate, E. The inhibition of rabbit skeletal muscle contraction by hydrogen ions and phosphate. J. Physiol. (Lond.) 395:77-97; 1988.
9. Cooke, R.; Pate, E. The effects of ADP and phosphate on the contraction of muscle fibers. Biophys. J. 48:789-798; 1985.
10. Crow, M.T.; Kushmerick, M. Correlated reduction of velocity of shortening and the rate of energy utilization in mouse fast-twitch muscle during a continuous tetanus. J. Gen. Physiol. 82:703-720; 1983.
11. Dawson, M.J.; Gadian, D.G.; Wilkie, D.R. Muscular fatigue investigated by phosphorous nuclear magnetic resonance. Nature 274:861-866; 1978.
12. Dawson, M.J.; Gadian, D.G.; Wilkie, D.R. Mechanical relaxation rate and metabolism studied in fatiguing muscle by phosphorous nuclear magnetic resonance. J. Physiol. (Lond.) 299:465-484; 1980.
13. Dawson, M.J.; Smith, S.; Wilkie, D.R. The [$H_2PO_4^{1-}$] may determine crossbridge cycling rate and force reduction in living fatiguing muscle. Biophys. J. 49:268a; 1986.
14. Donaldson, S.K.B.; Hermansen, L. Differential, direct effects of H^+ on Ca^{2+}-activated force of skinned fibers from the soleus, cardiac, and adductor magnus muscle of rabbits. Pflügers Arch. 376:55-65; 1978.
15. Edman, K.A.P.; Matiazzi, A.R. Effects of fatigue and altered pH on isometric force and velocity of shortening at zero load in frog muscle fibers. J. Muscle Res. Cell Motil. 2:321-334; 1981.
16. Eisenberg, E.; Hill, T.L.; Chen, Y. Cross-bridge model of muscle contraction. Biophys. J. 29:195-227; 1980.

17. Elzinga, G.; Langewouters, G.J.; Westerhof, N.; Wiechmann, A.H.C.A. Oxygen uptake of frog skeletal muscle fibres following tetanic contractions at 18° C. J. Physiol. (Lond.) 346:365-377; 1984.

18. Ferenczi, M.A.; Goldman, Y.E.; Simmons, R.M. The dependence of force and shortening velocity on substrate concentration in skinned muscle fibers from *Rana temporaria*. J. Physiol. (Lond.) 350:519-543; 1984.

19. Fitts, R.H.; Courtwright, J.B.; Kim, D.H.; Witzmann, F.A. Muscle fatigue with prolonged exercise: contractile and biochemical alterations. Am. J. Physiol. 242:C65-C73; 1982.

20. Flanagan, W.; Holmes, E.; Sabina, R.; Swain, J. Importance of purine nucleotide cycle to energy production in skeletal muscle. Am. J. Physiol. (Lond.) 250:C795-C802; 1986.

21. Grabowski, W.; Lobsigee, E.A.; Luttgau, H.C. The effect of repetitive stimulation at low frequencies upon the electrical and mechanical activity of single muscle fibers. Pflügers Arch. 334:222-239; 1972.

22. Herzig, J.W.; Peterson, J.W.; Ruegg, J.C.; Solaro, R.J. Vanadate and phosphate ions reduce tension and increase cross-bridge kinetics in chemically skinned heart muscle. Biochim. Biophys. Acta 672:191-196; 1981.

23. Hibberd, M.G.; Dantzig, J.A.; Trentham, D.R.; Goldman, Y.E. Phosphate release and force generation in skeletal muscle fibers. Science 228:1317-1319; 1985.

24. Hibberd, M.G.; Trentham, D.R. Relationships between chemical and mechanical events during muscular contraction. Annu. Rev. Biophys. 15:119-161; 1986.

25. Huxley, A.F. Muscle structure and theories of contraction. Prog. Biophys. 7:255-318; 1957.

26. Johnston, I.A.; Mutungi, G. Effects of temperature and pH on the contractile properties of skinned fibers isolated from the iliofibularis muscle of the freshwater turtle *Pseudemys scripta elegans*. J. Physiol. (Lond.) 367:79P; 1985.

27. Kammermeier, H.; Schmidt, P.; Jungling, E. Free energy change of ATP-hydrolysis: a causal factor of early hypoxic failure of the myocardium? J. Mol. Cell. Cardiol. 14:267-277; 1982.

28. Kawai, M. The role of inorganic phosphate in crossbridge kinetics in chemically skinned rabbit psoas fibers as detected with sinusoidal and step length alterations. J. Muscle Res. Cell Motil. 7:421-434; 1986.

29. Kentish, J.C. The effects of inorganic phosphate and creatine phosphate in skinned muscles from rat ventricle. J. Physiol. (Lond.) 370:585-604; 1986.

30. Kushmerick, M.J.; Meyer, R.A. Chemical changes in rat leg muscle by phosphorous nuclear magnetic resonance. Am. J. Physiol. 248:C542-549; 1985.

31. Metzger, J.M.; Moss, R.L. Greater H^+-induced depression of tension and velocity in skinned single fibers of rat fast than slow muscles. J. Physiol. (Lond.) 393:727-742; 1987.

32. Meyer, R.A.; Kushmerick, M.J.; Brown, T.R. Application of ^{31}P-NMR spectroscopy to the study of striated muscle metabolism. Am. J. Physiol. 242:C1-C11; 1982.

33. Nosek, T.M.; Fender, K.Y.; Godt, R.E. It is diprotonated inorganic phosphate that depresses force in skinned skeletal muscle fibers. Science 236:191-193; 1987.

34. Pate, E.; Cooke, R. A model of cross-bridge action: the effects of ATP, ADP and P_i. J. Muscle Res. Cell Motil. 10:181-196; 1989.

35. Pate, E.; Cooke, R. Addition of phosphate to active muscle fibers probes actomyosin states within the powerstroke. Pflügers Arch. 414:73-81; 1989.

36. Sahlin, K.; Edstrom, L.; Sjoholm, H.; Hultman, E. Effects of lactic acid accumulation and ATP decrease on muscle tension and relaxation. Am. J. Physiol. 240:C121-C126; 1981.

37. Sleep, J.; Glyn, H. Inhibition of myofibrillar actomyosin subfragment 1 adenosinetriphosphatase by adenosine 5'-diphosphate, pyrophosphate, and adenyl-5'-yl imidodiphosphate. Biochemistry 25:1149-1154; 1986.

38. Swain, J.L.; Sobrina, R.L.; Holmes, E.W. Myoadenylate deaminase deficiency. In: Stanbury, J.B., ed. The metabolic basis of inherited disease. New York: McGraw-Hill; 1983:1184-1191.

39. Vøllestad, N.K.; Sejersted, O.M. Biochemical correlates of fatigue. Eur. J. Appl. Physiol. 57:336-347; 1988.

40. Webb, M.R.; Hibberd, M.G.; Goldman Y.E.; Trentham, D.R. Oxygen exchange between P_i in the medium and water during ATP hydrolysis mediated by skinned fibers from rabbit skeletal muscle. Evidence for P_i binding to a force-generating state. J. Biol. Chem. 261:15557-15564; 1986.

41. Westerblad, H.; Lännergren, J. The relation between force and intracellular pH in fatigued, single Xenopus muscle fibres. Acta Physiol. Scand. 133:83-89; 1988.

42. Wilkie, D.R.; Dawson, M.J.; Edwards, R.H.T.; Gordon, R.E.; Shaw, D. ^{31}P NMR studies of resting muscle in normal human subjects. In Pollack, G.H.; Sugi, H., eds. New York: Plenum Press; 1984:333-347.

Energy Metabolism and Fatigue

Eric Hultman, Mats Bergström, Lawrence L. Spriet, and Karin Söderlund
Huddinge University Hospital, Huddinge, Sweden and University of Guelph, Ontario, Canada

The immediate energy substrate for force production is ATP, and the demand on the energy-delivering processes is to keep the ATP resynthesis at the same rate as the ATP utilization. A constant force generation thus means that both utilization and resynthesis rates are unchanged. Decreasing force generation, that is, fatigue, can be caused primarily by a decreasing rate of ATP utilization by the contractile apparatus or by a decreased rate of ATP resynthesis. The rate of ATP utilization by the muscle varies with the force generation by a factor of several hundred. To meet this requirement of ATP generation, the muscle has evolved three main pathways of ATP resynthesis. The first is by phosphocreatine (PCr), which is only available in small amounts but can buffer against sudden increases in energy demand. At the other extreme, fat has a low capacity to increase ATP formation rate, but its total store of energy is large. Carbohydrate is utilized during all types of muscle contraction, either anaerobically during maximal contraction or aerobically during submaximal force generation.

The estimated theoretical rates of ATP formation from the different substrates are given in Table 1. A limitation of the work output, or fatigue, would occur if the substrate needed for the required force output is exhausted. Theoretically, PCr could be a fatigue factor because the store is small and the maximal rate of energy release is exclusively high. However, glycogen degradation is always initiated simultaneously at high work rates, and isolated PCr utilization will never occur in normal muscle. The resulting combinations of energy-delivering processes will be discussed below. Similarly, as carbohydrate is the most efficient substrate for oxidative phosphorylation, the size of this store could limit submaximal endurance exercise.

The definition of fatigue varies, but the definition given at the Ciba Symposium 1981, "Failure to maintain the required or expected power output," is generally accepted for voluntary exercise. In many experimental studies of electrically stimulated muscles in situ or in isolated muscle, and of muscle preparations, fatigue is defined as "decline in force generation."

Table 1 Maximal Rates of ATP Resynthesis From Different Substrates and Available Amounts

Substrate	Max. ATP formation rate (mmol • s^{-1} • kg^{-1} dry muscle)	Available store (mmol • kg^{-1} dry muscle)
ATP, PCr (ADP, Cr)	11.2	100
Glycogen (lactate)	6.0	~250 (or totally 1,030)
Glycogen (CO_2 + H_2O)	2.2-2.9	13.000
Fatty acids (CO_2 + H_2O)	1.0	Not limiting

Note. For references, see 34.

Energy Metabolism and Fatigue During Endurance Exercise

Endurance exercise, or exercise relying on oxidative production of ATP, is limited to the use of two main substrates, glycogen and fat. Table 1 shows that glycogen degradation gives the highest rate of oxidative ATP production. Already in 1896 it was shown by Chauveau (10) that the respiratory exchange ratio (RQ) increased during exercise when work intensity increased. He suggested that the utilization of carbohydrate was dependent on the work intensity.

Studies by Christensen and Hansen (11) showed that the endurance capacity varied with the food intake, increasing with high carbohydrate intake and decreasing when the diet had a high fat content. Later studies with analyses of glycogen content in muscle (2, 3, 31) showed a direct relation between endurance capacity and the size of the muscle glycogen store and the possibility to vary the store by dietary manipulations. With high carbohydrate intake, the liver glycogen store was also optimized (32), which increased the available store for blood glucose supply during the exercise. It is today generally accepted that lack of available carbohydrate for the working muscle or the central nervous system will result in fatigue, that is, failure to maintain the power output required at a work load of 65-85% of the subject's $\dot{V}O_2$max. Further information of the relation between diet and exercise endurance is presented in a recent review article (37).

Energy Utilization and Fatigue During High-Intensity Contraction

It has been shown in a series of studies with isometric or dynamic exercise (7, 34, 36) that the rate of ATP resynthesis declines at approximately the same rate as the force generation during prolonged contraction. The interpretation of this is either that decreased rate of ATP resynthesis inhibits force development and thus is responsible for fatigue, or that force development decreases due to other factors resulting in a lower rate of ATP hydrolysis. Fatigue, a decrease in force generation, is a reduction of the number of simultaneously attached cross-bridges in the force-generating state. Three different mechanisms could be responsible for a decreased force generation.

1. Lack of available energy for the optimal supply of ATP to actomyosin cross-bridges, or to side reactions such as Na^+/K^+ pumping and Ca^{2+} reuptake by the sarcoplasmic reticulum (SR), which are also ATP dependent
2. Inhibition of any of these processes by products formed in the energy-supplying reactions
3. Alterations of excitation-contraction coupling from the surface action potential to Ca^{2+} release from the SR

Muscle Metabolism During Electrical Stimulation in Normal Muscle

A series of studies utilizing electrical stimulation of the quadriceps femoris muscle will now be described. Electrical stimulation with surface electrodes in combination with the muscle biopsy technique makes it possible to relate contractile and metabolic changes independent of the subject's voluntary effort (33). Tetanic contraction of the quadriceps muscle can be performed continually or intermittently. About 70% of the maximum force is produced at a stimulation frequency of 20 Hz, whereas 90-95% is produced at 50 Hz (56). A typical force registration is shown in Figure 1. The stimulation was intermittent, with 1.6-s contractions and 1.6-s pauses, and was performed with intact or occluded blood circulation to the leg.

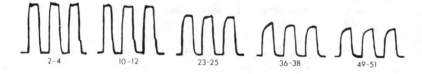

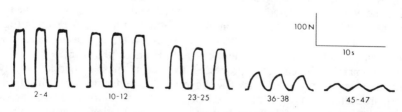

Figure 1.   Force registration during intermittent stimulation with 1.6 s tetanic contractions and 1.6 s rest, stimulation frequency 20 Hz. The figures denote the consecutive numbers of the tetanic stimulations. Upper line denotes open circulation, lower line occluded circulation.

When blood flow is occluded, the force generation decreases rapidly to values corresponding to 10-15% of the initial. The perception of fatigue in the stimulated muscle segment is significant but well tolerated. With intact circulation the force decrease is about 50% of initial during the same stimulation time.

Electrical stimulation of the intact muscle activates the neuromuscular junction, with subsequent release of Ca^{2+} from the SR system. The Ca^{2+} increase initiates cross-bridge turnover and ATP hydrolysis to ADP, with release of inorganic phosphate (P_i) and H^+. ADP is resynthesized to ATP by PCr via the creatine kinase reaction. The Ca^{2+} increase further activates the phosphorylase system, producing hexose-P, which together with ADP and P_i initiate glucolysis (i.e., degradation of glucose-P). The relation between the metabolic processes and the force generation during the stimulation is shown in Figure 2 (58, 59). The electrical stimulation was the same as in Figure 1 and continued for 102 s of contraction (64 contractions). The blood flow to the leg was occluded. Biopsy samples were obtained by percutaneous needle biopsy technique before the start of the stimulation and after 16, 32, 48, and 64 contractions, and analyzed by biochemical methods. Muscle pH was measured in muscle homogenates (60). Force generation by the stimulated knee extensors was measured by a strain gauge connected to a strap fixed to the ankle of the subject.

The results given in Figure 2 show, in the upper panel, the successive decrease in force generation along with a corresponding decrease in ATP resynthesis rate. Initially, about 50% of the ATP resynthesis is derived from PCr degradation and 50% from glucolysis; later on, glucolysis is responsible for most of the ATP resynthesis. The middle panel shows the concentrations of PCr, P_i, and lactate during the stimulation. As lactate is completely dissociated in muscle ($pK_a < 4$), an equimolar amount of H^+ is formed. The creatine kinase reaction—PCr + ADP + $H^+ \rightleftharpoons$ ATP + Cr—will thus be driven to the right by increases in ADP and H^+ resulting from ATP degradation and glucolysis. The increase in H^+ will increase the phosphorylation ratio MgATP/Mg ADP, which is an important determinant for the maximal energy available per mol of ATP hydrolyzed and of the minimum energy necessary to rebuild it. This is a beneficial effect of H^+ accumulation during prolonged contraction, which, however, also means that PCr degradation is related to glucolysis through the H^+ effect. A relation between lactate accumulation and PCr content in muscle has been described earlier in muscle samples obtained after different types and durations of contractile work (26) and also during long-term ischemia (35).

The decreasing PCr content at 16 contractions (Figure 2) will, however, increase ADP in the creatine kinase equilibrium reaction. ADP is also substrate for the adenylate kinase reaction: 2 ADP $\rightleftharpoons$ ATP and AMP. The AMP formed is rapidly deaminated to IMP, with formation of NH_3. Figure 2, lower panel, shows the marked fall in ATP, starting at the point where PCr is essentially depleted and continuing during the contraction period, with equimolar accumulation of IMP. The increase in P_i due to PCr and ATP degradation in the contracting muscle is given in Figure 2 (middle panel), as well as a calculated increase of $H_2PO_4^-$ in muscle water (lower panel). The calculations utilized the measured pH and a pK_a of 6.79 for P_i. The figure summarizes the energetic processes involved in muscle contraction driven by electrical stimulation to fatigue. The suggested fatigue factors are (a) insufficient energy production, (b) depletion of the PCr store, (c) inhibition of energy production or ATP utilization of different levels (by H^+ accumulation), and (d) inhibition of cross-bridge cycling by increased $H_2PO_4^-$.

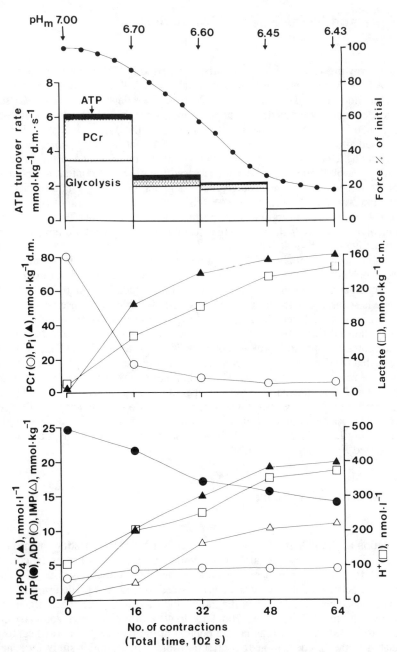

Figure 2. Force generation and energy metabolism in human quadriceps femoris muscle stimulated intermittently at 20 Hz, with 1.6 s tetanus and 1.6 s rest periods. The upper panel shows force, ATP turnover rate, and pH; the middle panel the concentrations of PCr, P_i, and lactate; and the lower panel ATP, ADP, IMP, H^+, and calculated $H_2PO_4^-$.

Fatigue and Total Energy Production

The energy produced during the contraction period in Figure 2 totaled about 300 mmol ATP • kg^{-1} dry muscle (d.m), of which about 210 mmol were derived from anaerobic glucolysis, 70 from PCr, and 20 from ATP degradation. The PCr store is almost completely utilized, and the total energy production by glucolysis seems to be limited at a lactate level of ~ 150 mmol • kg^{-1} (d.m.), a value that is repeatedly observed after exhausting intense exercise of different types (26, 43). The limitation is not due to lack of glycogen, which is about 360 mmol • kg^{-1} (d.m.) in normal muscles. In a preliminary study, we decreased the glycogen content to about 100 mmol by preceding exercise. The glycogen degradation during 1 min of electrical stimulation was still ~65 mmol • kg^{-1} (corresponding to 195 mmol ATP), close to the value observed in muscle with normal glycogen content. The limitation of the glucolytic process is thus due either to inhibition of glucolytic enzymes or to lack of activation of glucolysis.

The ATP decrease of about 50% in fatigued muscle (Figure 2) is repeatedly observed in exhausting voluntary dynamic and isometric exercise and during the electrical stimulation of normal human muscle with occluded blood flow. The same decrease is seen in fatigued frog muscle (48, 49). A further decrease was observed only after caffeine induced contracture of fatigued muscle (48); thus, only after artificially induced Ca^{2+} release in muscle. The ATP content in muscle fatigued by normal contractile stimuli is still well over the K$_m$ for actomyosin ATPase (47). This suggests that the decrease in force generation is not related to a general lack of energy for ATP resynthesis in the muscle but to inhibition of contraction. Recent studies with ATP analyses on separated muscle fibers have also shown that the ATP content is similar in all fiber types without further depletion of any specific fiber type (39, 62). A possible additional explanation for the remaining high ATP would be that a part of the ATP pool in muscle is unavailable for the contractile mechanisms, as suggested by Hohorst et al. (30).

Fatigue and PCr Store

Depletion of the PCr store is observed already after a short-lasting intense contraction. Figure 2 shows that almost the whole store is utilized after 16 contractions, but force is still produced during a further 48 contractions with PCr close to zero. Isometric voluntary contractions sustained to fatigue at predetermined force levels have also been used to study the fatigue mechanism (1, 38). The fatigue point coincided with low PCr at forces from 95% to 40% of the maximal voluntary contraction force (MVC), whereas lactate content at the fatigue point was negatively correlated to the (predetermined) contraction force. In a similar study by Katz et al. (41), the predetermined force was set at 66% MVC. The results showed that the fatigue point coincided with very low levels of PCr (<10 mmol • kg^{-1} d.m.), whereas lactate accumulation varied pronouncedly between subjects. The authors concluded that fatigue was more related to a low PCr content than to a high lactate content.

Maximal bicycle exercise of 2, 6, and 16 min duration was studied by Karlsson and Saltin (40). PCr and ATP were measured after 2-min exercise with the three loads and showed the same low values at all loads, irrespective that one load was exhaustive and the other two could be continued. Another finding speaking against the PCr store as a determinant for fatigue is the observation that recovery of PCr and that of force after contraction are not parallel. Both in isolated frog muscle (21, 22) and in human muscle (33, 43), the recovery of PCr was much faster than the restitution of contraction force (Figure 3), which seemed rather to be related to recovery of the muscle lactate. It is still possible that at critically low levels of PCr, the ATP-ADP buffering and the shuttle function of PCr transporting energy from mitochondria to the contractile system can be disrupted and the rate of ATP resynthesis slowed, resulting in a low available ATP pool at the cross-bridges.

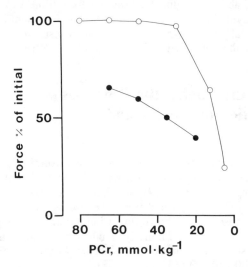

Figure 3.   Force development in relation to PCr content during intermittent stimulation of anoxic muscle (open circle), and in the first 3 min of aerobic recovery (closed circle). In the recovery period, the muscle was stimulated at 20 Hz for 1.6 s at 30 s, and 1, 2, and 3 min after the fatiguing contraction.

Fatigue and Glucolytic Rate

Decreased glucolytic rate as a cause of muscle fatigue has been proposed and related to pH inhibition of glucolytic enzymes. Decreasing pH inhibits both phosphorylase kinase activity and the activity of phosphofructokinase (PFK). This latter enzyme is rate determining for the glucolytic flux and therefore must be precisely matched to the rate of ATP expenditure, which necessitates a both responsive and tight metabolic control. The essential characteristic of PFK control is allosteric inhibition by ATP. This inhibition is increased by H^+ and also augmented by PCr (6, 42, 61). Removal of this inhibition provides the primary mechanism by which PFK responds to increased energy expenditure with the onset of contraction and maintains activity in the face of a decreasing pH. The factors contributing to this are decreased content of inhibitors, that is, ATP and PCr, and increased content of metabolites that either nullify the inhibitory effects of ATP or appear to activate the enzyme directly: ADP, AMP, P_i, fructose-6-P, and hexose bisphosphates. A potent deinhibitor is NH_3 (14), which is produced by deamination of AMP at the latter part of an intensive contraction. As seen in Figure 2, glycolysis continues at a practically unchanged rate during the period of 16-48 contractions, despite the pH drop from 6.70 to 6.45. This means that the pH inhibition of PFK must be nearly completely released. The most important changes during this period (16-48 contractions, Figure 2) are an increase in P_i and an increase in IMP, with equimolar formation of NH_3. It is thus not probable that the glycolytic activity was decreased to an extent that limits ATP generation in the stimulated muscle.

Neither PCr availability nor glycolytic rate seems to limit ATP formation during contraction in a way that can explain fatigue. The ATP content in fatigued muscle is decreased maximally to ∼40-50% of the value at rest, a content that should be sufficiently greater than the K_m for the actomyosin ATPase.

Inhibition of the Contractile Processes by Accumulation of Lactate and P_i

The lactate accumulation during intense anaerobic exercise has been implicated as a possible fatigue agent, suggested as early as the beginning of this century (23). A detailed presentation of the role of H^+ and P_i for the contractile processes is given in this symposium by Cooke and will therefore be discussed only briefly now. Studies of isolated animal muscle have shown direct inhibition of force generation by increased $[H^+]$ (17, 24, 29, 54). Similarly, studies utilizing isolated muscle fiber preparations have shown a decrease of the maximum force generation in the pH interval between 7.0 and 6.0 (15, 16, 18, 52).

In several studies, however, the pH effects seem to give only a partial explanation of fatigue, as in the study by Renaud et al. (51), who observed that the change in tetanic force was much larger in fatigued muscle than could be explained by the change in pH induced experimentally. The authors conclude that a factor other than pH is the limiting factor for force development in fatigued muscles. Similarly, studies of force generation in the recovery phase after fatiguing contraction showed an initial fast recovery of force that could not be explained by pH changes, and thereafter a slower recovery that correlated to $[H^+]$ (22, 44).

Inhibition of force generation by P_i was first observed in insect flight muscle (53, 65) and later also in vertebrate muscle (27). Similar findings have been obtained in skinned psoas fibers from cats (12). They found a decrease in isometric tension by 30%, with a $[P_i]$ increase of 20 mmol • L^{-1}. The effect was augmented by a pH decrease from 7.0 to 6.5. The total decrease was 75% in their preparation. It has recently been suggested that the inhibitor of force generation is the monoionic form HPO_4^{2-}, liberated during ATP hydrolysis (13, 28, 50, 66), whereas HPO_4^{2-} is not an active inhibitor.

A linear relation between force generation and accumulation of lactate and of $H_2PO_4^{-1}$ during the intermittent anaerobic stimulation is presented in Figure 4. The simultaneous formation of P_i from PCr degradation and H^+ from glucolysis makes it difficult to separate these effects from each other or from the effect of the stimulation as such. It is known, however, that PCr is rapidly resynthesized in the recovery period after exercise, whereas lactate disappearance is a slow process (26, 55). Measurements of force recovery were therefore done in this period with analyses of PCr and lactate in biopsy samples (Figure 3). Force in relation to lactate and $H_2PO_4^-$ in the recovery period is plotted together with the results during stimulation in Figure 4.

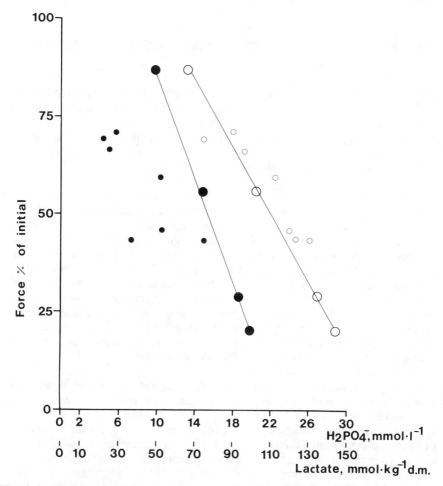

Figure 4.   The relationship between force generation and calculated concentration of $H_2PO_4^-$ (closed circle) and between force and lactate content (open circle) in the stimulated muscle presented in Figure 2. Corresponding relationships are also presented for the muscle during recovery (small closed and open circles) presented in Figure 3.

The results show a tendency to higher force in relation to lactate and a lower force in relation to $H_2PO_4^-$ in the recovery period. This can be interpreted as a positive effect of PCr resynthesis' acting as a P_i acceptor to decrease $H_2PO_4^-$ early in recovery, but also as a depressing effect on force development of the lactate accumulation that remains during the first minutes of recovery. These results bear out the findings by Nosek et al. (50), suggesting that two separate mechanisms are responsible for the development of fatigue—H^+ increase and accumulation of $H_2PO_4^-$—but they also show that none of these factors is solely responsible for fatigue. There is a close negative correlation between force generation and accumulation of H^+ and $H_2PO_4^-$ in contracting anoxic muscle. The correlation is, however, not obvious in muscle during oxidative recovery.

Fatigue Due to Factors Preceding Cross-Bridge Action

In the previous section, fatigue was related to processes directly involved in the cross-bridge action. Factors preceding this state could also be changed during contraction and cause fatigue. Three situations will be described in which the fatigue development is poorly related to availability of energy or changes in intracellular milieu.

In the first study (4), the stimulation protocol was changed as follows: 20 Hz stimulations were done with occluded circulation during 50 s either continuously or intermittently. The intermittent stimulations were 3.2 s stimulation and 3.2 s rest, or 1.6 s/1.6 s and 0.8 s/0.8 s. The stimulation time was equal and the number of stimulation pulses the same in all subjects. Biopsies were obtained before stimulation and after 22 s and 52 s of stimulation. The results (Figure 5) showed a large difference in force generation during the four different stimulations, varying from 90% of initial force after 50 s of continuous stimulation to 32% after 0.8 s of intermittent. The biochemical analyses showed that ATP and PCr levels were similar at the end of the four stimulations and thus unrelated to force generation. The total ATP utilization was highest during the intermittent stimulation with the shortest stimulation periods. The negative correlation between ATP utilization and force indicates that the capability to resynthesize ATP has not reached its limit during the stimulation with longer duration of contractions and, therefore, that energy availability does not generally limit force generation.

There was, however, a correlation between force and lactate concentration and also between force and $H_2PO_4^-$ accumulation at end of contraction. As shown above, these accumulations are directly related to ATP utilization, and it is not possible to decide in this study which, if any, of these factors are significant in reduction of force. During repeated excitation of a muscle, the fatigue may be associated with alterations in Ca^{2+} transport. It has been shown that in fatigue there may be a slowing of Ca^{2+} transport and progressively smaller Ca^{2+} transients. These are possibly due to reduced Ca^{2+} reuptake by the sarcoplasmic reticulum and/or increased binding to Ca^{2+}-binding proteins (5, 46), or to a lack of availability of the "second messenger" for Ca^{2+} release in the inositol triphosphate (63), as discussed by Sue Donaldson at this symposium. Repeated excitations could cause a decline in the resulting force production due to failure of excitation-contraction coupling.

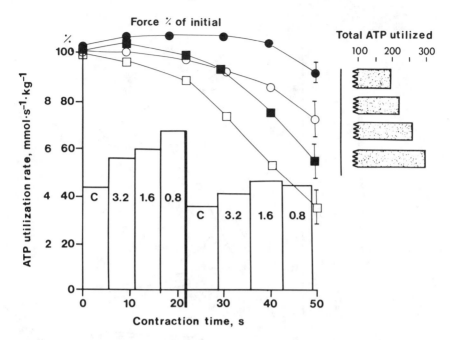

Figure 5. Contraction force, ATP turnover rate, and total ATP utilized during continuous contraction, and during intermittent contractions with stimulation/rest periods of 3.2/3.2, 1.6/1.6, and 0.8/0.8 s. Stimulation frequency 20 Hz. ATP turnover rates are mean values for the time periods 0-20 s and 20-50 s.

In the second study, two different intermittent stimulations were done in the same subject with the same stimulation time, but with different stimulation frequencies: 20 Hz and 50 Hz. The leg blood flow was occluded (Figure 6). The initial force was higher (about 20%), as was the ATP turnover rate at the 50 Hz stimulation. There was a decrease in force along with time, which was most pronounced at 50 Hz stimulation. Thus, after 25 contractions the force was significantly lower after the 50-Hz stimulation compared to force at 20 Hz, but the levels of phosphagens and metabolites were equal, that is, ATP, ADP, PCr, P_i, and lactate showed identical levels. It is thus difficult to relate the larger force decrease at 50 Hz to the energy metabolism or to products formed by the energy-producing processes. Neuromuscular block is not probable because the stimulation was intermittent. The rate of Ca^{2+} transfer is higher during 50-Hz stimulation than during 20 Hz, which may induce an earlier decrease in Ca^{2+} transient during prolonged intermittent 50-Hz stimulation and thus explain the lower force generation.

In the third study, the stimulation protocol was the same as described in Figure 1, utilizing both open and occluded circulation (Figure 7A and 7B). The force decrease was similar during the first 40 s of contraction, as were the changes in energy-rich phosphagens and accumulation of metabolites (34), irrespective of occluded or intact blood supply. After 40 s stimulation, the picture changed in the subjects with

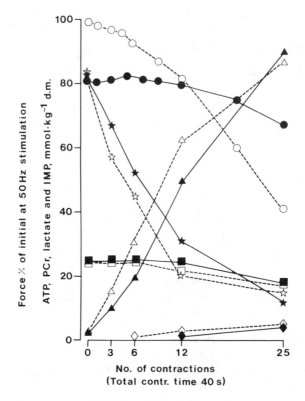

Figure 6.   Force as percentage of initial, and phosphagen and lactate contents, during stimulation with 50 Hz (open symbols) and 20 Hz (closed symbols). Open and closed circles represent force; stars, PCr; squares, ATP; diamonds, IMP; and triangles, lactate.

intact blood flow, due to oxygen supply and transport of lactate. The force decrease was slower, and the lactate accumulation ceased and changed to a decrease at 80 s of contraction. Similarly, both ATP and PCr contents increased.

Still, there was a continued fall in force, which leveled out at about 30% of the initial force after 15 min contraction. At that time, lactate content had decreased by 50% of the value at 60 s contraction and PCr content had increased from 30 to 50 mmol • kg⁻¹ (36). Continuation of the stimulation up to 45 min decreased the force further but only marginally, whereas lactate content approached the level at rest and ATP was normalized while PCr was resynthesized to 80-90% (Figure 8). Apparently, the muscle utilized only oxidative sources for energy production, and the ATP production by the muscle was higher than the utilization, despite continued stimulation with the same frequency. In this type of stimulation, the force decrease cannot be attributed to lack of energy or to accumulation of P_i or lactate. All the described fatigue factors are thus excluded. The dissociation between fatigue factors (ATP decrease, accumulation of P_i, and H^+) and force generation is observed already after 60 s of stimulation.

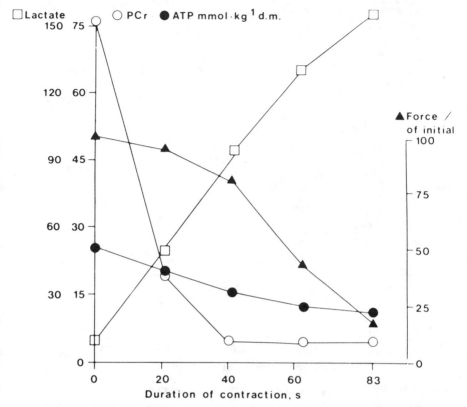

Figure 7A. Force (closed triangle) in percentage of initial, and phosphagen and lactate contents, in the quadriceps femoris muscle during intermittent stimulation of the same type as in Figure 2 with occluded circulation.

In a similar study by Spriet et al. (57), we observed an early decrease of the phosphorylase *a* fraction in the activated muscle, which could explain decreased anaerobic glucolysis. Adrenalin infusion given after 15 min of contraction increased phosphorylase *a* fraction, and the content of hexose-P and lactate in contracting muscle but did not change force generation.

A similar pattern with increased [ATP] and [PCr] with simultaneous decrease in force was observed by Meyer and Terjung (45) in rat muscle stimulated continuously at 5 Hz. The result was interpreted as a lack of force generation by the white fibers in the period between 5 min and 30 min of stimulation. Poor endurance capacity of fast-twitch white fibers from cat gastrocnemius has previously been described by Burke et al. (8), and similar findings in fiber segments of human muscle were reported by Faulkner et al. (19, 20). The decrease in total force development by the mixed quadriceps muscle could thus be explained by a successive decrease in activation of the fast-twitch fibers when the stimulation is prolonged. In these fibers ATP and PCr resynthesis may also occur when other fibers in the same muscle are contracting.

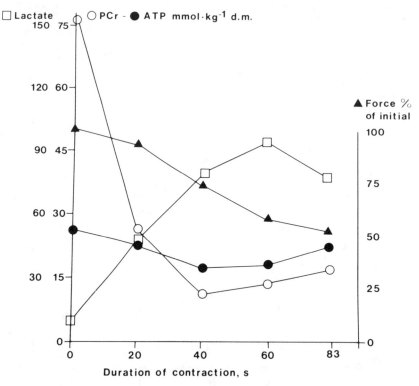

Figure 7B.   The same stimulation with intact blood circulation.

A series of electrical stimulation studies on frog muscle by Westerblad and Lännergren (ref. 64 and personal communications) are also worth commenting on. It was shown that three different fiber types could be isolated from frog muscle, each with clear differences in fatigue resistance, from fast fatiguable to fatigue resistant to very fatigue resistant. After fatiguing contraction with pH decrease, all fiber types regained full tension when treated with caffeine. A depolarizing K^+ solution could also increase tension to 95% in the most fatigue-resistant fibers, but less efficiently in the fast fatigable. It was concluded that the tension reduction induced by intermittent tetanic stimulation was due to activation failure because fatigued fibers produced full tension when caffeine was administered (caffeine is known to release Ca^{2+} from the SR).

The activation failure in the fatigue-resistant fibers, where failure could be completely reversed by K^+, may be due to decreased propagation of the electrically induced depolarization signal via the t tubular system. In the fast-fatiguable fibers that could not be fully activated by K^+, a block in the t tubular–SR communication system seems to be a further effect of the fatiguing stimulation. This block was released by caffeine. The complete recovery of force in fatigued acidotic muscle, which probably also had increased $[P_i]$, speaks against a predominant role for H^+ and/or $H_2PO_4^-$ as fatigue agents in these muscle fibers. If the fiber types in human skeletal muscle function similarly, the results in Figures 7 and 8 could be explained by an early

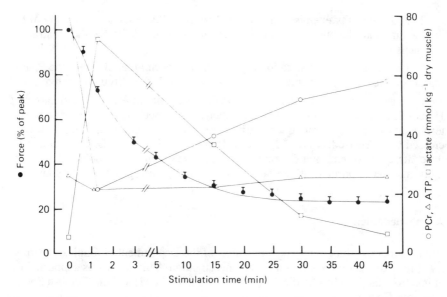

Figure 8.   The same stimulation procedures as in Figure 7B, but continued for 45 min.

failure to activate the fast twitch fibers, leaving the slow twitch fibers as the sole contracting elements during the later part of the contraction. This would explain the low force generation simultaneous with the lack of lactate formation. Resynthesis of ATP and PCr could occur in fatigued nonstimulated fast twitch fibers. This would mean that activation failure could contribute to fatigue already after short-lasting contraction periods in muscle with mixed fiber composition. It could also mean that high-frequency fatigue could partly be explained by rapid-onset activation failure in type 2 glucolytic fibers.

These three experiments (the continuous/intermittent, the 50 Hz/20 Hz, and the oxidative/anoxic) show that neither ADP rephosphorylation capacity nor accumulation of H^+ and/or P_i can explain the decrease in force generation adequately. A factor common to all the experiments is that repeated utilization of the Ca^{2+} transport mechanisms correlates to fatigue. This is obvious in Study 1, showing decreasing force generation when the number of tetani is increased with constant total contraction time. In Study 2 the Ca^{2+} transport at 50 Hz stimulation is quantitatively larger than at 20 Hz stimulation, and the force is lower after the 50 Hz period. In Study 3 the increased number of contractions is the only obvious reason for the force decrease in the aerobic muscle. The mechanism behind the postulated decrease of Ca^{2+} release from the SR cannot, however, be explored in these studies.

Summary

1. Endurance exercise in people is limited to the availability of carbohydrate at submaximal work loads (65-85% of $\dot{V}O_2max$).

2. High-intensity exercise is not limited by the ATP resynthesis capacity of the contracting muscle but by the utilization of available ATP by the contractile mechanism.

3. Decrease in force generation is parallelled by accumulation of H^+ and P_i during anaerobic contraction, but the relation varies with the stimulation frequency.

4. In aerobic muscle the relation between force generation and accumulation of H^+ and P_i exists only initially, whereas other fatigue mechanisms appear to be determinant for force generation when stimulation is prolonged. These factors are decreased Ca^{2+} release from the SR and/or decreased response to the Ca^{2+} release by the contractile proteins in different fiber types. The Ca^{2+} release and the Ca^{2+} sensitivity may be important fatigue factors also initially during muscle stimulation.

Acknowledgment

The authors wish to thank the entire staff of the Department of Clinical Chemistry II for excellent collaboration in this investigation. This work was supported by grants from the Swedish Medical Research Council (02647) and the Swedish Sports Research Council.

References

1. Bergström J.; Harris, R.C.; Hultman, E.; Nordesjö, L.-O. Energy rich phosphagens in dynamic and static work. In: Pernow, B; Saltin, B. Muscle metabolism during exercise. New York–London: Plenum Press; 1971:341-355. (Adv. exp. med. biol.; vol. 11).

2. Bergström, J.; Hermansen, L.; Hultman, E.; Saltin, B. Diet, muscle glycogen and physical performance. Acta Physiol. Scand. 71:140-150; 1967.

3. Bergström, J.; Hultman, E. A study of the glycogen metabolism during exercise in man. Scand. J. Clin. Lab. Invest. 19:218-228; 1967.

4. Bergström, M.; Hultman, E. Energy cost and fatigue during intermittent electrical stimulation of human skeletal muscle. J. Appl. Physiol. (in press).

5. Blinks, J.R.; Rüdel, R.; Taylor, S.R. Calcium transients in isolated amphibian skeletal muscle fibers: detection with aequorin. J. Physiol. (Lond.) 227:291-323; 1978.

6. Bock, P.E.; Frieden, C. Phosphofructokinase: I. Mechanism of pH-dependent inactivation and reactivation of the rabbit muscle enzyme. II. Role of ligands in pH-dependent structural changes of the rabbit muscle enzyme. J. Biol. Chem. 251:5630-5643; 1976.

7. Boobis, L.; Williams, C.; Wootton, S.A. Human muscle metabolism during brief maximal exercise (abstract). J. Physiol. (Lond.) 338:21P-22P; 1982.

8. Burke, R.E.; Levine, D.N.; Tsairis, P.; Zajac, F.E. Physiological types and histochemical profiles in motor units of the cat gastrocnemius. J. Physiol. (Lond.) 234:723-748; 1973.

9. Chasiotis, D.; Bergström, M.; Hultman, E. ATP utilization and force during intermittent and continuous muscle contractions. J. Appl. Physiol. 63:167-171; 1987.

10. Chauveau, A. Source et nature du potential directment utilise dans le travail musculaire d'apres les exchanges respiratoires, chez l'homme en etat d'abstinence. C. R. Acad. Sci. [III] 122:1163-1221; 1896.

11. Christensen, E.H.; Hansen, O. I. Zur metodik der Respiratorischen Quotient-Bestimmung in Ruhe und Arbeit. II. Untersuchungen über die Verbrennungs-Vorgänge bei Landuernder, Schwere Muskel Arbeit. III. Arbeits Fähigkeit und Ehrährung. IV. Hypoglykämie, Arbeitsfähigkeit und Ermüdung. Skand. Arch. Physiol. 81:137-181; 1939.

12. Cooke, R.; Pate, E. The effect of ADP and phosphate on the contraction of muscle fibers. Biophys. J. 48:789-798; 1985.

13. Dawson, M.J.; Smith, S.; Wilkie, D.R. The $[H_2PO_4^{-1}]$ may determine cross-bridge cycling rate and force production in living fatiguing muscle (abstract). Biophys. J. 49:268a; 1986.

14. Dobson, G.P.; Yamamoto, E.; Hochachka, P.W. Phosphofructokinase control in muscle: nature and reversal of pH-dependent ATP inhibition. Am. J. Physiol. 250:R71-R76; 1986.

15. Donaldson, S.; Best, P.; Kerrick, W. Characterization of the effects of Mg^{2+} on Ca^{2+}- and Sr^{2+}-activated tension generated of skinned cat cardiac fibers. J. Gen. Physiol. 71:645-655; 1978.

16. Donaldson, S.K.B. Effect of acidosis on maximum force generation of peeled mammalian skeletal muscle fibers. In: Knuttgen, H.G.; Vogel, J.A.; Poortmans, J., eds. Biochemistry of exercise. Champaign, IL: Human Kinetics Publ., Inc.; 1983:126-133.

17. Edman, K.A.P.; Mattiazzi, A.R. Effects of fatigue and altered pH on isometric force and velocity of shortening at zero load in frog muscle fibres. J. Muscle Res. Cell Motil. 2:321-334; 1981.

18. Fabiato, A.; Fabiato, F. Effects of pH on the myofilaments and the sarcoplasmic reticulum of skinned cells from cardiac and skeletal muscles. J. Physiol. (Lond.) 276:233-255; 1978.

19. Faulkner, J.A.; Claflin, D.R.; McCully, K.K. Power output of fast and slow fibers from human skeletal muscles. In: Jones, N.L.; McCartney, N.; McComas, A.J., eds. Human muscle power. Champaign, IL: Human Kinetics Publ., Inc.; 1986:81-94.

20. Faulkner, J.A.; Jones, D.A.; Round, J.M.; Edwards, R.H.T. Dynamics of energetic processes in human muscle. In: Cerretelli, P.; Whipp, B.J., eds. Proceedings of the international symposium on exercise, bioenergetics and gas exchange. Milan. 1980:81-90.

21. Fitts, F.H.; Holloszy, J.O. Lactate and contractile force in frog muscle during development of fatigue and recovery. Am. J. Physiol. 231:430-433; 1976.

22. Fitts, R.H.; Holloszy, J.O. Effects of fatigue and recovery on contractile properties of frog muscle. J. Appl. Physiol. 45:899-902; 1978.

23. Fletcher, W.M.; Hopkins, F.G. Lactic acid in amphibian muscle. J. Physiol. (Lond.) 35:247-303; 1907.

90 Hultman, Bergström, Spriet, and Söderlund

24. Fretthold, D.W.; Garg, L.C. The effect of acid-base changes on skeletal muscle twitch tension. Can. J. Physiol. Pharmacol. 56:543-549; 1978.

25. Harris, R.C.; Edwards, R.H.T.; Hultman, E.; Nordesjö, L.-O; Nylind, B.; Sahlin, K. The time course of phosphorylcreatine resynthesis during recovery of the quadriceps muscle in man. Pflügers Arch. 367:137-142; 1976.

26. Harris, R.C.; Sahlin, K.; Hultman, E. Phosphagen and lactate contents of m. quadriceps femoris of man after exercise. J. Appl. Physiol. 43:852-857; 1977.

27. Herzig, J.W.; Petersén, J.W.; Ruegg, J.C.; Solaro, R.J. Vandata and phosphate ions reduce tension and increase cross-bridge kinetics in chemically skinned heart muscle. Biochim. Biophys. Acta 672:191-196; 1981.

28. Hibberd, M.G.; Dantzig, J.A.; Trentham, D.R.; Goldman, Y.E. The role of phosphate in cross-bridge kinetics of skinned skeletal muscle fibers. Science 228:1317-1319; 1985.

29. Hill, A.V. The influence of the extended medium on the internal pH of muscle. Proc. R. Soc. Lond. [Biol.] 144:1-22; 1955.

30. Hohorst, H.J.; Reim, M.; Bartels, H. Studies on the creatine kinase equilibrium in muscle and the significance of ATP and ADP levels. Biochem. Biophys. Res. Commun. 7:142-144; 1962.

31. Hultman, E. Studies on muscle metabolism of glycogen and active phosphate in man with special reference to exercise and diet. Scand. J. Clin. Lab. Invest. 19(suppl. 94):1-63; 1967.

32. Hultman, E.; Nilsson, L.H:son. Liver glycogen in man, effect of different diets and muscular exercise. In: Pernow, B.; Saltin, B., eds. Muscle metabolism during exercise. New York–London: Plenum Press; 1971:143-151. (Adv. exp. med. biol.; vol. 11).

33. Hultman, E.; Sjöholm, H. Electromyogram, force and relaxation time during and after continuous electrical stimulation of human skeletal muscle in situ. J. Physiol. (Lond.) 339:33-40; 1983.

34. Hultman, E.; Sjöholm, H. Biochemical causes of fatigue. In: Jones, N.L.; McCartney, N.; McComas, A.J., eds. Human muscle power. Champaign, IL: Human Kinetics Publ., Inc.; 1986:215-238.

35. Hultman, E.; Sjöholm, H.; Sahlin, K.; Edström, L. Glycolytic and oxidative energy metabolism and contraction characteristics of intact human muscle. Human muscle fatigue: physiological mechanisms. Ciba foundation symposium 82. London: Pitman Medical; 1981:19-40.

36. Hultman, E.; Spriet, L.L. Skeletal muscle metabolism, contraction force and glycogen utilization during prolonged electrical stimulation in humans. J. Physiol. (Lond.) 374:493-501; 1986.

37. Hultman, E.; Spriet, L.L. Dietary intake prior to and during exercise. In: Horton, E.S.; Terjung, R.L., eds. Exercise, nutrition and energy metabolism. New York: Macmillan Publ. Co.; 1988:132-149.

38. Hultman, E.; Spriet, L.L.; Söderlund, K. Energy metabolism and fatigue in working muscle. In: Macleod, D.; Maughan, R.; Nimmo, M.; Reilly, T.; Williams, C., eds. Exercise—benefits, limits and adaptations. London: E. & F.N. Spon; 1987:63-84.

39. Jansson, E.; Dudley, G.A., Norman, B.: Tesch, P.A. ATP and IMP in single human muscle fibres after high intensity exercise. Clin. Physiol. 7:337-345; 1987.

40. Karlsson, J.; Saltin, B. Lactate, ATP, and CP in working muscles during exhaustive exercise in man. J. Appl. Physiol. 29:598-602; 1970.

41. Katz, A.; Sahlin, K.; Henriksson, J. Muscle ATP turnover rate during isometric contraction in humans. J. Appl. Physiol. 60:1839-1842; 1986.

42. Lardy, H.A.; Parks, R.E. Phosphofructokinase. In: Gaebler, O.H., ed. Enzymes: units of biological structure and function. New York: Academic Press; 1956:239-278.

43. McCartney, N.; Spriet, L.L.; Heigenhauser, G.J.F.; Kowalchuk, J.M.; Sutton, J.R.; Jones, N.L. Muscle power and metabolism in maximal intermittent exercise. J. Appl. Physiol. 60:1164-1169; 1986.

44. Metzger, J.M.; Fitts, R.H. Role of intracellular pH in muscle fatigue. J. Appl. Physiol. 62:1392-1397; 1987.

45. Meyer, R.A.; Terjung, R.L. AMP deaminase and IMP reamination in working skeletal muscle. Am. J. Physiol. 239:C32-C38; 1980.

46. Nakamura, Y.; Schwartz, A. The influence of hydrogen ion concentration on calcium binding and release by skeletal muscle sarcoplasmic reticulum. J. Gen. Physiol. 59:22-32; 1971.

47. Nanninga, L.B.; Mommaerts, C.R. Studies on the formation of an enzyme-substrate complex between myosin and adenosine-triphosphate. Proc. Natl. Acad. Sci. USA 46:1155-1166; 1960.

48. Nassar-Gentina, V.; Passonneau, J.V.; Rapoport, S.I. Fatigue and metabolism of frog muscle fibers during stimulation and in response to caffeine. Am. J. Physiol. 241:C160-C166; 1981.

49. Nassar-Gentina, V.; Passonneau, J.V.; Vergara, J.L.; Rapoport, S.J. Metabolic correlates of fatigue and of recovery from fatigue in single frog muscle fibers. J. Gen. Physiol. 72:593-606; 1978.

50. Nosek, T.M.; Fender, K.Y.; Godt, R.E. It is diprotonated inorganic phosphate that depresses force in skinned skeletal muscle fibers. Science 236:191-193; 1987.

51. Renaud, J.M.; Allard, Y.; Mainwood, G.W. Is the change in intracellular pH during fatigue large enough to be the main cause of fatigue? Can. J. Physiol. Pharmacol. 64:764-767; 1986.

52. Robertson, S.P.; Kerrick, W.G.L. The effects of pH on Ca^{2+}-activated force in frog skeletal muscle fibers. Pflügers Arch. 380:41-45; 1979.

53. Ruegg, J.C.; Schadler, M.; Steiger, G.J.; Muller, C. Effect of inorganic phosphate on the contractile mechanism. Pflügers Arch. 325:359-364; 1971.

54. Sahlin, K.; Edström, L.; Sjöholm, H.; Hultman, E. Effects of lactic acid accumulation and ATP decrease on muscle tension and relaxation. Am. J. Physiol. 240:C121-C126; 1981.

55. Sahlin, K.; Harris, R.C.; Hultman, E. Resynthesis of creatine phosphate in human muscle after exercise in relation to intramuscular pH and availability of oxygen. Scand. J. Clin. Lab. Invest. 39:551-558; 1979.

56. Sjöholm, H.; Sahlin, K.; Edström, L.; Hultman, E. Quantitative estimation of anaerobic and oxidative energy metabolism and contraction characteristics in intact human skeletal muscle in response to electrical stimulation. Clin. Physiol. 3:227-239; 1983.

57. Spriet, L.L.; Ren, J.M.; Hultman, E. Epinephrine infusion enhances muscle glycogenolysis during prolonged electrical stimulation in humans. J. Appl. Physiol. 64:1439-1444; 1988.

58. Spriet, L.L.; Söderlund, K.; Bergström, M.; Hultman, E. Anaerobic energy release in skeletal muscle during electrical stimulation in man. J. Appl. Physiol. 62:611-615; 1987.

59. Spriet, L.L.; Söderlund, K.; Bergström, M.; Hultman, E. Skeletal muscle glycogenolysis, glycolysis and pH during electrical stimulation in men. J. Appl. Physiol. 62:616-621; 1987.

60. Spriet, L.L.; Söderlund, K.; Thomson, J.A.; Hultman, E. pH measurement in human skeletal muscle samples: effects of phosphagen hydrolysis. J. Appl. Physiol. 61:1949-1954; 1986.

61. Storey, K.B.; Hochachka, P.W. Activation of muscle glycolysis: a role for creatine phosphate in phosphofructokinase regulation. FEBS Lett. 46:337-339; 1974.

62. Söderlund, K.; Hultman, E. The ATP content in single fibers of human skeletal muscle at rest and after exercise. This volume.

63. Vergara, J.; Tsien, R.Y.; Delay, M. Inositol 1,4,5-triphosphate: a possible chemical link in excitation-contraction coupling in muscle. Proc. Natl. Acad. Sci. USA 82:6352-6346; 1985.

64. Westerblad, H.; Lännergren, J. Tension and restoration with caffeine in fatigued Xenopus muscle fibres of various types. Acta Physiol. Scand. 130:357-358; 1987.

65. White, D.C.S.; Thorson, J. Phosphate starvation and the nonlinear dynamics of insect fibrillar flight muscle. J. Gen. Physiol. 60:307-336; 1972.

66. Wilkie, D.R. Muscular fatigue: effect on hydrogen ions and inorganic phosphate. Fed. Proc. 45:2921-2923; 1986.

The Role
of Functional Demand
in Regulating Gene Expression

Species-Specific Responses in Enzyme Activities of Anaerobic and Aerobic Energy Metabolism to Increased Contractile Activity

Jean-Aimé Simoneau, David A. Hood, and Dirk Pette
Universität Konstanz, Konstanz, F.R.G.

Indirect, low-frequency stimulation of skeletal muscle is an experimental model that offers the possibility of investigating effects of short and long periods of sustained contractile activity. An advantage of this model is that the adaptations observed are, most probably, independent of organismic reactions such as central fatigue or changes in the endocrine system. Moreover, maximal intensity can be applied from the beginning of the experiment. On the other hand, exercise training relies on stepwise increases in intensity in order to accustom the animal. This makes it difficult to follow initial training-induced changes.

Stimulation-induced transformation processes at the level of energy metabolism have mostly been investigated in fast-twitch muscles of the rabbit (2, 4, 12-14, 19, 22, 27, 33, 36, 37, 41). The major changes induced by chronic low-frequency stimulation of fast-twitch muscles in this species consisted of substantial decreases in glycolytic enzyme activities together with pronounced increases in enzyme activities involved in aerobic-oxidative pathways. These changes far exceeded those observed in endurance-trained rats or humans (11, 15, 16, 35, 40). The major reason attributed for this discrepancy was the much higher amount of increased contractile activity imposed on the muscle by chronic stimulation. An alternative explanation is the existence of differing species-specific degrees of adaptation. In this regard, we have studied the effects of a standardized stimulation protocol on a fast-twitch muscle in rabbit, rat, guinea pig, and mouse. The tibialis anterior (TA) muscle of the left hindlimb was indirectly stimulated 10 hours/day at 10 Hz via implanted electrodes. To study the time course of the induced changes, animals were killed after different periods of stimulation (38).

Changes in Glycolytic Enzyme Activities

As previously shown (31, 32), chronic stimulation elicits significant decreases in glycolytic enzyme activities of fast-twitch muscle. Our recent comparative study (38) has indicated the existence of differences in the extent of these changes among different species. Thus, the activity of phosphofructokinase (PFK), the chosen reference

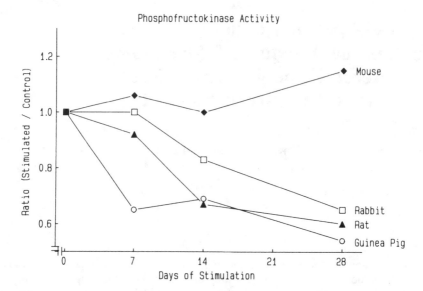

Figure 1.   Time course of changes in phosphofructokinase (PFK) activity in chronically (10 hours/day) stimulated (10 Hz) tibialis anterior muscles of rabbit, rat, guinea pig, and mouse. Values from reference 38 are given as ratios of stimulated versus unstimulated control muscles.

enzyme of glycolysis, decreased after 28 days of stimulation by approximately 40% in rabbit, rat, and guinea pig TA muscles, but was not reduced in mouse TA (Figure 1). In addition, differences existed in the rate of the decays. The decrease in PFK was rapid in guinea pig TA, reaching nearly its lowest value as soon as 7 days after the onset of stimulation. By the same time, PFK activity was almost unaltered in rabbit, rat, and mouse TA (Figure 1). The pattern of changes in the activities of glyceraldehydephosphate dehydrogenase (GAPDH) and lactate dehydrogenase (LDH) was similar to that of PFK in the four mammals under study (38).

Concomitant with a decrease in the total activity of LDH, chronic stimulation resulted in a pronounced rearrangement of its isozyme pattern (13, 18, 31). In rabbit TA, these changes led to a shift of the M-type isozymes toward the H-type isozymes and resulted from an increased fraction of the H-subunit at the expense of the M-subunit (37). Thus, the M-subunit, which amounts to approximately 90% of the total LDH in unstimulated rabbit TA, decreased to about 60% in the 28-day stimulated muscle. The decrease in the amount of the M-subunit was less pronounced in the other species. In the 28-day stimulated muscles, it decreased from 90% to 80% in guinea pig and from 80% to 75% in rat. The percentage of the M-subunit–based isozymes still represented 90% in the 28-day stimulated mouse TA (39).

As previously shown in our laboratory (31, 32, 33), hexokinase (HK) activity responded in a specific manner to chronic stimulation and, instead of decreasing like the other glycolytic enzymes, rose with chronic stimulation. As judged by isozyme electrophoresis, the increase in total HK activity of the stimulated rabbit muscle was mainly due to an increase in the HK-II isozyme (31). Pronounced differences exist between the responses of skeletal muscles in rabbit, rat, guinea pig, and mouse with regard to the extent and time courses of the induced changes in HK activity

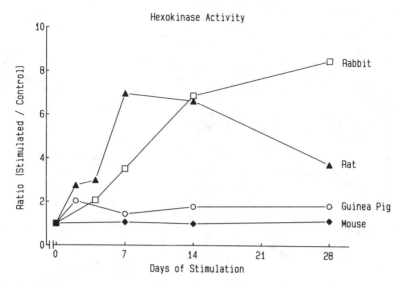

Figure 2. Time course of changes in hexokinase (HK) activity in chronically (10 hours/day) stimulated (10 Hz) tibialis anterior muscles of rabbit, rat, guinea pig, and mouse. Values from reference 38 are given as ratios of stimulated versus unstimulated control muscles.

(38). During the initial phase of adaptation, HK activity increased in the TA muscles of all species. However, maximal increases were about 8-fold in rabbit, 7-fold in rat, 2-fold in guinea pig, and only 1.3-fold in mouse TA. In addition, the increase in HK activity was only transitory in rat and guinea pig (Figure 2).

Changes in Enzyme Activities of Aerobic-Oxidative Metabolism

According to our recent observations (38), increases in enzyme activities of the citric acid cycle and of fatty acid oxidation markedly varied in the TA muscles of the four species investigated. After 28 days of stimulation, citrate synthase (CS), which was used as a marker enzyme of the citric acid cycle, increased 3-fold in rabbit TA, 2.5-fold in rat, 2.3-fold in guinea pig, and only 1.2-fold in mouse (Figure 3). Citrate synthase activities in rabbit TA exhibited the highest increases among the investigated species and responded earlier than in guinea pig and mouse. Similar patterns of increases were recorded in the same animals for another enzyme involved in the citric acid cycle, namely, malate dehydrogenase (MDH), and for 3-hydroxyacyl CoA dehydrogenase (HADH), the chosen reference enzyme of fatty acid oxidation (38).

Morphometric analyses were performed to determine stimulation-induced changes in the mitochondrial volume density of rabbit, rat, and mouse TA muscles. The relative increases in the fractional volume of mitochondria were found to correspond

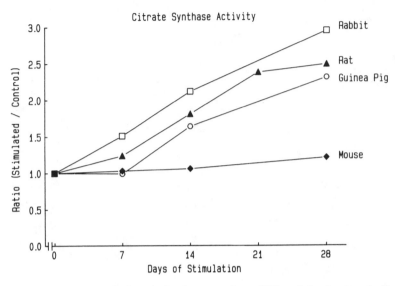

Figure 3. Time course of changes in citrate synthase (CS) activity in chronically (10 hours/day) stimulated (10 Hz) tibialis anterior muscles of rabbit, rat, guinea pig, and mouse. Values from reference 38 are given as ratios of stimulated versus unstimulated control muscles.

to the observed relative increments in CS activity in all three species (Hoppeler, Simoneau, & Pette, unpublished). This close relation supports the notion that CS represents an appropriate marker of the mitochondrially related aerobic-oxidative metabolism.

It is evident from previous (33) and unpublished studies using a 12-hour/day stimulation protocol that the maximal increase in enzyme activities of aerobic oxidative metabolism is not yet reached in the rabbit TA after 28 days of stimulation. Prolonged stimulation in the rabbit revealed that maximal CS activity was attained at a later time. In an experimental series using 10-Hz stimulation during 12 hours/day and stimulation periods up to 120 days, a 5.5-fold increase was reached after 50 days (17). Contrary to results found in the rabbit, CS activity in the rat TA already approached a plateau after 21 days of stimulation (Figure 3). Interestingly enough, this 2.5-fold increase is in the same range of the maximal adaptation of fast-twitch hindlimb muscles observed in long-term endurance training of the rat (11, 15, 16).

Stimulation-Induced Changes in Fatigability

One of the most important functional consequences of chronic stimulation is an increase in the muscle resistance to fatigue. This observation has been reported for various species from several laboratories (1, 5, 6, 7, 10, 21, 23, 25, 30, 34), including for the human (8). The fatigability of muscle fibers has been related to their metabolic profile in such a way that fibers rich in enzyme activities of aerobic-oxidative metabolism are less fatigable than fibers that predominantly base their energy supply on anaerobic carbohydrate catabolism (3, 9). We have addressed this question by following the time courses of the increases both in CS activity and in resistance to fatigue in chronically stimulated rat TA. Our results show that a correlation exists only initially between the induced changes of these two parameters. Thus, the onset of the increase in resistance to fatigue coincided with the beginning in the increase of CS activity. However, CS activity continued to increase with stimulation periods beyond two weeks, whereas resistance to fatigue had reached its maximum by this time (Simoneau & Pette, unpublished).

As follows from the increased resistance to fatigue, the stimulated muscle developed a higher integrated tension output during a 6-min period of repetitive tetanic contractions than the contralateral muscle. Thus, after 2 weeks of stimulation, the integrated tension produced during the 6-min period amounted to 276 kg $\times$ s/g muscle in the stimulated rat TA, and 180 kg $\times$ s/g muscle in the contralateral TA.

Basal Enzyme Activities and Maximal Responses

Differences in basal enzyme activities between the investigated fast-twitch muscles of the different species might be retained as potential factors to explain the various responses observed (Table 1). The notion that the extent of the stimulation-induced changes in enzyme activity is inversely related to their basal levels was previously suggested on the basis of results obtained in chronically stimulated rabbit TA (20). In addition, the fact that chronic low-frequency stimulation failed to increase enzyme activities of aerobic-oxidative metabolism in rabbit soleus, a muscle predominantly composed of type I fibers, also fits with this notion (30). Hoppeler and Lindstedt (18) having morphometrically compared fractional volumes of mitochondria in muscles of a large variety of species, concluded that skeletal muscles of smaller animals are better endowed for aerobic-oxidative metabolism than skeletal muscles of larger animals. Applying this conclusion to our comparative studies, muscles with a high aerobic-oxidative capacity are expected to respond less than muscles with low basal enzyme activities of substrate end-oxidation. This might be due to the fact that the metabolic perturbations induced by a given work load (e.g., 10 Hz stimulation) are less extensive in muscles possessing higher mitochondrial contents (40).

This notion does not appear to be applicable to enzymes representing the glycolytic pathways. For example, in spite of similar absolute (U/g wet weight) and relative HK activity levels (compared to PFK activity) in unstimulated TA muscles of rat and guinea pig (Table 1), great differences were noticed in the response of this enzyme in the two species. Its maximal increase was 7-fold in rat TA but only 2-fold in guinea pig TA (Figure 2, Table 1). Moreover, maximal HK activities were reached after different stimulation periods in the different species (Figure 2).

Similarly, a relation between stimulation-induced decreases in glycolytic enzyme activities and their basal levels does not appear to exist. With regard to the other enzymes, the activities of PFK were similar in mouse, rat, and guinea pig TA muscles

Table 1 Enzyme Activity Values (U/g Wet Weight) in Soleus (SOL) Muscles, Control (TAc), and Stimulated (TAs) Tibialis Anterior Muscles of Rabbit, Rat, Guinea Pig, and Mouse

		Rabbit	Rat	Guinea pig	Mouse
HK	TAc	0.71	1.21	1.22	4.00
	TAs	6.03	8.42	2.48	7.29
	SOL	2.11	2.00	1.25	8.80
PFK	TAc	142	67	78	72
	TAs	82	42	27	71
	SOL	22	18	10	54
CS	TAc	10.5	18.0	23.4	36.0
	TAs	32.0	44.9	57.8	42.4
	SOL	11.8	16.0	14.4	50.2

Note. Values of the stimulated TA muscles (TAs) represent maximal changes. Data are from reference 38.

but decreased to different levels in response to chronic stimulation (Table 1). After 28 days, PFK activity was not reduced in mouse TA but had markedly decreased in rat, guinea pig, and rabbit (Figure 1). However, the final values of PFK were still above those found in normal soleus muscles (Table 1). In contrast, the increases in CS activity in rat, guinea pig, and rabbit exceeded, after long-term stimulation, the respective soleus muscle values. These observations are not unexpected because the predominant response to increased contractile activity consisted—at least in rabbit, rat, and guinea pig—of pronounced increases in the enzyme activities involved in aerobic-oxidative metabolism. In view of this elevation to levels even higher than in soleus, an appropriate glycolytic capacity has to be maintained in order to meet an increased supply of carbohydrate-derived metabolites (i.e., glycogen) in the system of substrate end-oxidation (24).

Conclusion

Our results clearly demonstrate that metabolic adaptations observed in response to a standardized protocol of increased contractile activity in one species may not necessarily reflect the adaptive metabolic responses of another species. The induced increases in enzymes of aerobic-oxidative metabolism seemed to follow a pattern such that the increments observed were inversely related to the basal enzyme activity levels. This rule could explain the absence of noticeable increases in aerobic-oxidative capacity of chronically stimulated mouse TA. It may be speculated that the native aerobic potential of mouse TA is sufficient to meet the metabolic requirement of the imposed increase in contractile activity. This suggests that different metabolic responses of homologous muscles to identical amounts of increased contractile activity are limited by species-specific ranges of adaptation. Chronic low-frequency stimulation of rat fast twitch muscle for 10 hours per day did not induce a higher adaptive increase in the activity of a key enzyme of aerobic-oxidative metabolism (CS) than did a 210-minutes-per-day treadmill running protocol (11). In contrast, a much larger (5.5-fold) increase in CS is induced in rabbit muscle subject to this stimulation protocol. Therefore, it seems that species-related intrinsic properties dictate the degree of adaptation. Also, in view of discrepancies between training studies involving different mammalian species, including humans, we conclude that variable ranges of adaptation represent a major factor in determining the limits of adaptation.

Acknowledgments

This study was supported by the Deutsche Forschungsgemeinschaft, Sonderforschungsbereich 156. J.-A. Simoneau was supported by the Fonds de la Rechereche en Santé du Québec. D.A. Hood was a recipient of stipends from the Muscular Dystrophy Association of America and from the A. von Humboldt-Stiftung. The authors thank Ms. E. Leisner, Ms. S. Krüger, and Ms. I. Traub for excellent technical assistance.

References

1. Brown, M.D.; Cotter, M.; Hudlická, O.; Smith, M.E.; Vrbová, G. The effects of long-term stimulation of fast muscles on their ability to withstand fatigue. J. Physiol. (Lond.) 238:47P-48P; 1973.

2. Buchegger, A.; Nemeth, P.M.; Pette, D.; Reichmann, H. Effects of chronic stimulation on the metabolic heterogeneity of the fibre population in rabbit tibialis anterior muscle. J. Physiol. (Lond.) 350:109-119; 1984.

3. Burke, R.E.; Levine, D.N.; Zajac, F.E. Mammalian motor units: physiological-histochemical correlation in three types in cat gastrocnemius. Science 174:709-712; 1971.

4. Chi, M.M.-Y.; Hintz, C.S.; Henriksson, J.; Salmons, S.; Hellendahl, R.P.; Park, J.L.; Nemeth, P.M.; Lowry, O.H. Chronic stimulation of mammalian muscle: enzyme changes in individual fibers. Am. J. Physiol. 251:C633-C642; 1986.

5. Clark, B.J., III; Acker, M.A.; McKully, K.; Subramanian, H.V.; Hammond, R.L.; Salmons, S.; Chance, B.; Stephenson, L.W. In vivo ^{31}P-NMR spectroscopy of chronically stimulated canine skeletal muscle. Am. J. Physiol. 254:C258-C266; 1988.

6. Cooper, J.; Hudlická, O. Effect on muscle fatigue of the changes in the capillary bed induced by long-term stimulation. J. Physiol. (Lond.) 263:155P-156P; 1976.

7. Cotter, M.; Hudlická, O. Effect of different patterns of long-term stimulation on muscle performance. J. Physiol. (Lond.) 292:20P-21P; 1979.

8. Dubowitz, V.; Hyde, S.A.; Scott, O.M.; Vrbová, G. Effect of long-term electrical stimulation on the fatigue of human muscle. J. Physiol. (Lond.) 328:30P-31P; 1982.

9. Edström, L.; Kugelberg, E. Histochemical composition, distribution of fibres and fatiguability of single motor units. Anterior tibial muscle of the rat. J. Neurol. Neurosurg. Psychiat. 31:424-433; 1968.

10. Eerbeek, O.; Kernell, D.; Verhey, B.A. Effects of fast and slow patterns of tonic long-term stimulation on contractile properties of fast muscle in cat. J. Physiol. (Lond.) 352:73-90; 1984.

11. Green, H.J.; Reichmann, H.; Pette, D. Fibre type specific transformations in the enzyme activity pattern of rat vastus lateralis muscle by prolonged endurance training. Pflügers Arch. 399:216-222; 1983.

12. Harris, B.; Heilig, A.; Hudlická, O.; Leberer, E.; Pette, D.; Tyler, K. Changes in rabbit muscle enzyme activities in response to chronic stimulation with different frequency patterns. In: Semiginovsky, B.; Tuczek, S., eds. Metabolic and functional changes during exercise. Prague: Charles University; 1982:27-31.

13. Heilig, A.; Pette, D. Changes induced in the enzyme activity pattern by electrical stimulation of fast-twitch muscle. In: Pette, D., ed. Plasticity of muscle. Berlin: W. de Gruyter; 1980:409-420.

14. Henriksson, J.; Chi, M.M.-Y.; Hintz, C.S.; Young, D.A.; Kaiser, K.K.; Salmons, S.; Lowry, O.H. Chronic stimulation of mammalian muscle: changes in enzymes of six metabolic pathways. Am. J. Physiol. 251:C614-C632; 1986.

15. Holloszy, J.O. Biochemical adaptations in muscle. Effects of exercise on mitochondrial oxygen uptake and respiratory enzyme activity in skeletal muscle. J. Biol. Chem. 242:2278-2282; 1967.

16. Holloszy, J.O.; Booth, F.W. Biochemical adaptations to endurance exercise in muscle. Annu. Rev. Physiol. 38:273-291; 1976.

17. Hood, D.A.; Pette, D. Chronic long-term electrostimulation creates a unique metabolic enzyme profile in rabbit fast-twitch muscle. FEBS Lett. 247:471-474; 1989.

18. Hoppeler, H.; Lindstedt, S.L. Malleability of skeletal muscle in overcoming limitations: structural elements. J. Exp. Biol. 115:355-364; 1985.

19. Hudlická, O.; Aitman, T.; Heilig, A.; Leberer, E.; Tyler, K.R.; Pette, D. Effects of different patterns of long-term stimulation on blood flow, fuel uptake and enzyme activities in rabbit fast skeletal muscle. Pflügers Arch. 402:306-311; 1984.

20. Hudlická, O.; Tyler, K.R. The effect of long-term high-frequency stimulation on capillary density and fibre type in rabbit fast muscles. J. Physiol. (Lond.) 353:435-445; 1984.

21. Kernell, D.; Donselaar, Y.; Eerbeek, O. Effects of physiological amounts of high- and low-rate chronic stimulation on fast-twitch muscle of the cat hind-limb: II. Endurance-related properties. J. Neurophysiol. 58:614-627; 1987.

22. Klug, G.; Wiehrer, W.; Reichmann, H.; Leberer, E.; Pette, D. Relationships between early alterations in parvalbumin, sarcoplasmic reticulum and metabolic enzymes in chronically stimulated fast-twitch muscle. Pflügers Arch. 399:280-284; 1983.

23. Kwong, W.H.; Vrbová, G. Effects of low-frequency electrical stimulation on fast and slow muscles of the rat. Pflügers Arch. 391:200-207; 1981.

24. Maier, A.; Pette, D. The time course of glycogen depletion in single fibers of chronically stimulated rabbit fast-twitch muscle. Pflügers Arch. 408:338-342; 1987.

25. Mannion, J.D.; Bitto, T.; Hammond, R.L.; Rubinstein, N.A.; Stephenson, L.W. Histochemical and fatigue characteristics of conditioned canine latissimus dorsi muscle. Circ. Res. 58:298-304; 1986.

26. Peckham, P.H.; Mortimer, J.T.; van der Meulen, J.P. Physiologic and metabolic changes in white muscle of cat following induced exercise. Brain Res. 50:424-429; 1973.

27. Pette, D. Activity-induced fast to slow transitions in mammalian muscle. Med. Sci. Sports Exerc. 16:517-528; 1984.

28. Pette, D. Regulation of phenotype expression in skeletal muscle fibers by increased contractile activity. In: Saltin, B., ed. Biochemistry of exercise. Champaign, IL: Human Kinetics Publishers; 1986:3-26.

29. Pette, D.; Müller, W.; Leisner, E.; Vrbová, G. Time dependent effects on contractile properties, fibre population, myosin light chains and enzymes of energy metabolism in intermittently and continuously stimulated fast twitch muscle of the rabbit. Pflügers Arch. 364:103-112; 1976.

30. Pette, D.; Ramirez, B.U.; Müller, W.; Simon, R.; Exner, G.U.; Hildebrand, R. Influence of intermittent long-term stimulation on contractile, histochemical and metabolic properties of fibre populations in fast and slow rabbit muscles. Pflügers Arch. 361:1-7; 1975.

31. Pette, D.; Smith, M.E.; Staudte, H.W.; Vrbová, G. Effects of long-term electrical stimulation on some contractile and metabolic characteristics of fast rabbit muscles. Pflügers Arch. 338:257-272; 1973.

32. Pette, D.; Staudte, H.W.; Vrbová, G. Physiological and biochemical changes induced by long-term stimulation of fast muscle. Naturwissenschaften 8:469-470; 1972.

33. Reichmann, H.; Hoppeler, H.; Mathieu-Costello, O.; Bergen, F. von; Pette, D. Biochemical and ultrastructural changes of skeletal muscle mitochondria after chronic electrical stimulation in rabbits. Pflügers Arch. 404:1-9; 1985.

34. Salmons, S.; Sréter, F.A. Significance of impulse activity in the transformation of skeletal muscle type. Nature 263:30-34; 1976.

35. Saltin, B.; Gollnick, P.D. Skeletal muscle adaptability: significance for metabolism and performance. In: Peachey, L.D.; Adrian, R.H.; Geiger, S.R., eds. Handbook of physiology. Sect. 10: skeletal muscle. Baltimore, MD: Williams and Wilkins; 1983:555-631.

36. Schmitt, T.; Pette, D. Increased mitochondrial creatine kinase in chronically stimulated fast-twitch rabbit muscle. FEBS Lett. 188:341-344; 1985.

37. Seedorf, U.; Leberer, E.; Kirschbaum, B.J.; Pette, D. Neural control of gene expression in skeletal muscle. Effects of chronic stimulation on lactate dehydrogenase isoenzymes and citrate synthase. Biochem. J. 239:115-120; 1986.

38. Simoneau, J.-A.; Pette, D. Species-specific effects of chronic nerve stimulation upon tibialis anterior muscle in mouse, rat, guinea pig, and rabbit. Pflügers Arch. 412:86-92; 1988.

39. Simoneau, J.-A.; Pette, D. Species-specific responses of muscle lactate dehydrogenase isozymes to increased contractile activity. Pflügers Arch. 413:679-681; 1989.

40. Terjung, R.L.; Hood, D.A. Biochemical adaptations in skeletal muscle induced by exercise training. In: Layman, D.K., ed. Nutrition and aerobic exercise. Washington, DC: Am. Chem. Soc.; 1986:8-27.

41. Williams, R.S.; Salmons, S.; Newsholme, E.A.; Kaufman, R.E.; Mellor, J. Regulation of nuclear and mitochondrial gene expression by contractile activity in skeletal muscle. J. Biol. Chem. 261:376-380; 1986.

Purification of the Ryanodine-Sensitive, Calcium-Induced Calcium Release Channel From Canine Cardiac Junctional Sarcoplasmic Reticulum Vesicles

Larry R. Jones, David P. Rardon, Dominic C. Cefali, and Robert D. Mitchell

Indiana University School of Medicine, Indianapolis, Indiana, U.S.A.

The mechanism of Ca release from junctional sarcoplasmic reticulum remains one of the unsolved problems in muscle physiology (4). A Ca release channel activated by micromolar Ca (Ca-induced Ca release channel) has been identified in junctional sarcoplasmic reticulum vesicles isolated from heart (5), but its purification has remained elusive. We observed previously that high concentrations (>100 μM) of the alkaloid ryanodine gives a 10-fold stimulation of ATP-dependent Ca uptake by junctional sarcoplasmic vesicles isolated from heart, and we hypothesized that the agent acts by blocking this Ca release channel (2, 9). In this work, we report purification of the junctional sarcoplasmic reticulum Ca release channel to homogeneity from heart and characterization of its electrical properties after incorporation into planar lipid bilayers. We find that the ryanodine receptor and the Ca release channel are identical proteins.

Purification of Ryanodine Receptor/Ca Release Channel

Canine cardiac junctional sarcoplasmic reticulum vesicles were isolated as previously described (2, 9). The ryanodine receptor was solubilized from junctional sarcoplasmic reticulum vesicles with use of the zwitterionic detergent 3-[(3-cholamido-propyl)-dimethylammonio]-1-propanesulfonate (CHAPS), to be described in detail elsewhere. The solubilized ryanodine receptor in 1% CHAPS was chromatographed on a size-exclusion column in 0.3% CHAPS, and fractions were collected for measurement of [^{3}H]ryanodine binding (1) and protein content (8). Total binding was measured with 20 nM [^{3}H]ryanodine and nonspecific binding in the additional presence of 10 μM nonradioactive ryanodine. The fractions containing the peak of [^{3}H]ryanodine binding activity were pooled, concentrated, and further purified by sucrose density gradient centrifugation employing a linear 9-24% sucrose gradient containing 0.3% CHAPS. Sodium dodecylsulfate polyacrylamide gel electrophoresis (SDS-PAGE) was performed as previously described (3).

Planar Bilayer Studies

Single channel activities were recorded by the Mueller-Rudin lipid bilayer technique (6). A mixture of phosphatidylserine and phosphatidylethanolamine (4:5 weight ratio) in decane was painted over a 0.25-mm-diameter hole in the Lexan partition that separated the cis and trans chambers of the bilayer apparatus. The cis chamber, to which vesicles or purified proteins were added, contained $CaCl_2$, 1 mM; [ethylenebis(oxyethylenenitrilo)]tetracetic acid (EGTA), 1 mM; [tris(hydroxymethyl) aminomethane] (TRIS), 125 mM; N-2-hydroxyethylpiperazine-N'-2-ethanesulfonic acid (HEPES), 250 mM; at pH 7.4. The calculated free Ca concentration in the cis chamber was 1 μM. The trans chamber contained $Ba(OH)_2$, 50 mM; HEPES, 250 mM; at pH 7.4. Under these bi-ionic conditions—where E_{TRIS} is nominally minus infinity, $E_{divalent} = +125$ mV, and $E_{HEPES} = 0$ mV—calcium release channels could be identified as negative current deflections of approximately 4 pA at 0 mV holding potential.

Purification of High Molecular Weight Proteins

We observed that 100% of the [^{3}H]ryanodine binding activity was solubilized from cardiac junctional sarcoplasmic reticulum vesicles with use of the zwitterionic detergent CHAPS. Two peaks of [^{3}H]ryanodine binding activity were recovered when CHAPS-solubilized receptors were fractionated by size-exclusion chromatography (Figure 1A). The first, minor peak of specific binding (fractions 3-11) coincided with the void volume of the column and contained incompletely solubilized receptors. The second, major peak of specific binding (fractions 13-20) contained most of the recovered ryanodine receptors and was enriched in a high molecular weight protein doublet (Figure 1B) (9). The molecular weights of the two proteins comprising the doublet were estimated to be 400,000 and 350,000. Nonspecific [^{3}H]ryanodine binding measured in the column fractions was negligible (Figure 1A).

The major peak of [^{3}H]ryanodine binding recovered from the size exclusion column was further fractionated by sucrose density gradient centrifugation. Sucrose gradient fractions were then assayed for protein contents and [^{3}H]ryanodine binding. Fractions recovered toward the top of the gradient (fractions 2-19) showed no [^{3}H]ryanodine binding (Figure 2A) and contained mostly contaminant proteins (Figure 2B). A large peak of [^{3}H]ryanodine binding and a small peak of protein were recovered near the bottom of the sucrose gradient (Figure 2A, fractions 23-26); the high molecular weight proteins, purified to homogeneity as assessed by SDS-PAGE (Figure 2B), were localized to these fractions. The recovery of purified high molecular weight proteins/ryanodine receptor complex by this method was routinely 200 μg from 40 mg of junctional sarcoplasmic reticulum protein. Scatchard analysis of purified receptors (data not shown) revealed a homogeneous population of binding sites, with a $K_d = 4.4$ nM; the B_{max} from multiple preparations ranged between 175 and 280 pmol [^{3}H]ryanodine bound/mg of protein. Receptors were purified 20- to 30-fold relative to specific binding activity detected in the parent junctional sarcoplasmic reticulum vesicles (10 pmol/mg protein).

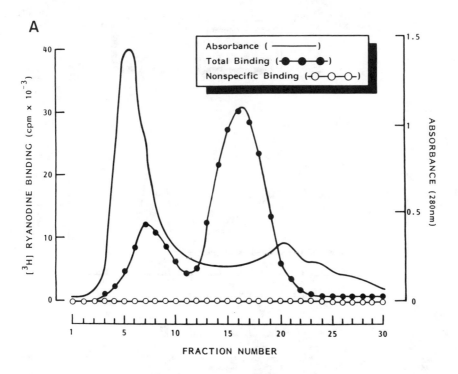

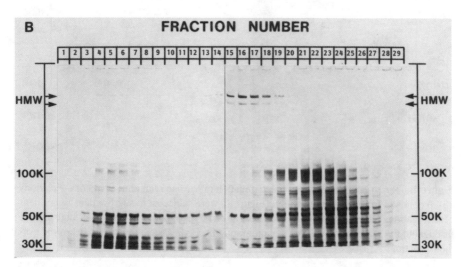

Figure 1. Size exclusion chromatography of CHAPS-solubilized cardiac ryanodine receptors. Panel A depicts results of [³H]ryanodine binding assay conducted on column fractions. Plain line depicts absorbance at 280 nm; line with closed circles, total binding measured with 20 nM [³H]ryanodine; line with open circles, nonspecific binding measured in the additional presence of 10 μM nonradioactive ryanodine. Panel B is a photograph of an SDS-gel stained with Coomassie blue of the column fractions. HMW designates high molecular weight protein.

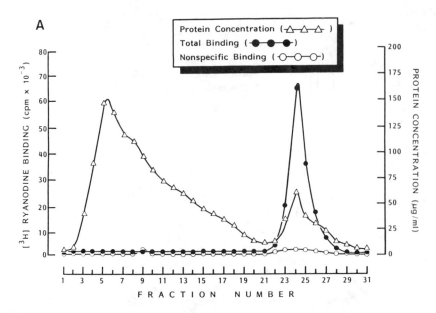

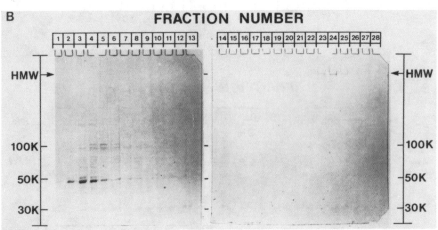

Figure 2. Sucrose density gradient centrifugation of cardiac ryanodine receptors. Fractions 13-20 obtained from the sizing column (Figure 1) were subjected to sucrose density gradient centrifugation. Panel A shows the distribution of [³H]ryanodine binding and total protein throughout the gradient. Panel B is a photograph of a Coomassie blue-stained gel of the gradient fractions.

The high-molecular-weight proteins/ryanodine receptor exhibited single channel activity similar to that detected with native sarcoplasmic reticulum vesicles. Typical channel activity recorded from purified high molecular weight proteins is depicted in Figure 3A. Two channels of different conductances were apparent. The large conductance channel in the purified preparation appeared identical to the large conductance channel exhibited by native cardiac sarcoplasmic reticulum vesicles (7) (Rardon

& Jones, unpublished data). Openings, however, were less frequent, and the open state amplitudes were less well resolved than those obtained with native vesicles. Nevertheless, the large conductance channel often exhibited prolonged openings with well-resolved amplitudes (Figure 3A, bottom panel). From such well-resolved openings, the mean slope conductance was determined to be 96 ± 13 pS (Figure 3B). The slope conductance of the purified high-molecular-weight proteins was therefore similar to that of the Ca channel measured in native junctional sarcoplasmic reticulum vesicles (7). A second, small conductance channel (slope conductance ~5.5 pS) was also frequently observed (Figure 3A). In other experiments, we observed that Ca channel openings required micromolar Ca on the cis side of the bilayer. Millimolar ATP on the cis side greatly increased Ca channel open time, as did nanomolar concentrations of ryanodine. Concentrations of ryanodine greater than 100 micromolar on the cis side of the bilayer tended to close the Ca channel.

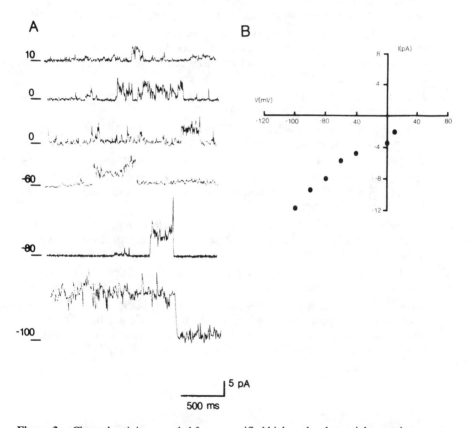

Figure 3. Channel activity recorded from a purified high-molecular-weight protein preparation. In Panel A the closed state of the channel is noted by the solid dark line to the left of each current record. The opening of the channel is an upward deflection, which represents negative current flow. Panel B is the I-V relationship of the large conductance channel depicted in Panel A.

Our results strongly suggest that the high-molecular-weight proteins, the junctional sarcoplasmic reticulum feet structures, the ryanodine receptor, and the Ca-induced Ca release channel are all the same protein. The availability of a purified Ca release channel from cardiac junctional sarcoplasmic reticulum vesicles, which is electrically active, should allow more discerning experiments on basic mechanisms regulating excitation-contraction coupling and Ca release from junctional sarcoplasmic reticulum in heart.

References

1. Glossman, H.; Ferry, D.R. Assay for calcium channels. Methods Enzymol. 109:573-50; 1985.

2. Jones, L.R.; Cala, S.E. Biochemical evidence for functional heterogeneity of cardiac sarcoplasmic reticulum vesicles. J. Biol. Chem. 256:11807-11818; 1981.

3. Jones, L.R.; Maddock, S.W.; Besch, H.R., Jr. Unmasking effect of alamethicin on the (Na+, K+)-ATPase, beta-adrenergic receptor-coupled adenylate cylcase, and cAMP-dependent protein kinase activities of cardiac sarcolemmal vesicles. J. Biol. Chem. 225:9971-9980; 1980.

4. Martonosi, A.N. Mechanisms of Ca^{2+} release from sarcoplasmic reticulum of skeletal muscle. Physiol. Rev. 64:1240-1320; 1984.

5. Meissner, G. Ryanodine activation and inhibition of the Ca^{2+} release channel of sarcoplasmic reticulum. J. Biol. Chem. 261:6300-6306; 1986.

6. Mueller, P.; Rudin, D.O. Bimolecular lipid membranes. Techniques of formation, study of electrical properties, and induction of gating phenomena. In: Passow, H.; Stampfl, R. eds. Laboratory techniques in membrane biophysics. New York: Springer-Verlag; 1969:141-156.

7. Rousseau, E.; Smith, J.S.; Hederson, J.S. Single channel and $^{45}Ca^{2+}$ flux measurements of the cardiac sarcoplasmic reticulum calcium channel. Biophys. J. 50:1009-1014; 1986.

8. Schaffner, W.; Weissman, C. A rapid, sensitive, and specific method for determination of protein in a dilute solution. Anal. Biochem. 56:502-514; 1983.

9. Seiler, S.; Wegener, A.D.; Whang, D.D.; Hathaway, D.R.; Jones, L.R. High molecular weight proteins in cardiac and skeletal muscle junctional sarcoplasmic reticulum vesicles bind calmodulin, are phosphorylated and are degraded by Ca^{2+}-activated protease. J. Biol. Chem. 257:8550-8557; 1984.

PART III

Determinants of Compensatory Muscular Growth: A Biochemical Perspective

Cardiac Growth Response to Chronic Exercise

Karel Rakusan

University of Ottawa, Ottawa, Ontario, Canada

Biochemistry of exercise cannot be fully understood without consideration of the related functional and morphological events. Some biochemical processes precede functional and morphological changes, whereas others are the direct consequences of such changes. Compensatory growth is a frequent but not obligatory finding in adaptations to physical training. The so-called athlete heart is characterized by increased cardiac dimensions and mass as well as by an increased volume of individual myocytes. The degree of organ and cell hypertrophy is usually small in comparison to cardiac hypertrophy observed in clinical medicine or in experimental animals with chronic pressure or volume overload. Similarly, the degree of hypertrophy of myocytes from various skeletal muscles subjected to chronic isometric exercise is much higher than an increased size of cardiac muscle cells.

In this review, we plan to summarize the cardiac growth response to chronic exercise at the organ and tissue level. In the latter case, two main tissue components, namely, cardiac myocytes and coronary capillaries, will be considered. Most of the examples presented are derived from the experimental studies utilizing rats, but some results and their possible implications to the response of the human heart will also be discussed.

Cardiac Size and Mass

Cardiac size and mass can be easily determined at the end of chronic exercise in experimental animals. On the other hand, similar measurements in the autopsy material are influenced by the causes of death and rarely coincide with the peak training period. Nevertheless, Harvey is credited with the following observation in 1628: "Hence for all animals, and for man also, the thicker, harder and more solid they are in fleshy build, and the more fleshy and muscular their hands and feet and the greater their distance from the heart, so are their hearts more fibrous, thick, robust and muscular. And this is an obvious necessity. On the other hand, the more finely-textured they are, the softer in build and the slenderer, so do they have a heart that is more flaccid and softer, less fibrous inside or not at all fibrous, and weak.

Until recently, the choice of in vivo methods for cardiac size and mass determinations was limited. Phonocardiography, X-ray examination, ECG, and vectocardiography yield some information concerning cardiac size that is only semi-quantitative at best. On the other hand, modern echocardiography permits relatively accurate measurement of the ventricular wall thickness and cavity diameter, from which reasonable estimates of the left ventricular mass may be obtained.

A recent review of Schaible and Scheuer (20) summarizes several selected cross-sectional studies that have used echocardiography to measure cardiac dimension and mass in well-trained endurance athletes. In all cases, significant hypertrophy of the left ventricles has been observed (39-80% increase when compared to sedentary controls). The type of hypertrophy observed in these endurance-trained athletes was an eccentric hypertrophy, characterized by increases both in chamber dimensions and in wall thickness. A certain degree of right ventricular hypertrophy has also been observed. The results were independent of gender (i.e., they were similar in both male and female subjects). In contrast, in longitudinal studies on previously sedentary populations, no changes or rather moderate increases in left ventricular mass have been observed in spite of significant improvement of the subjects' performance.

The difference between the longitudinal and cross-sectional studies is striking. There are several possible explanations. The cross-sectional studies examined cardiac dimensions in competitive athletes, presumably with long histories of training. In the case of previously sedentary subjects, the length of exercise varied from 2-6 months, with the training intensity adjusted to 70-80% of the maximum oxygen consumption. On the other hand, it is known from observations on both human subjects and experimental animals that increases in cardiac mass and size may develop rapidly and also may reverse rapidly after cessation of training. An alternative explanation would be that genetic differences led to the natural selection of subjects with larger cardiac mass to the group of high-performance athletes. This may also be indirectly supported by the observation that cardiac hypertrophy is normally reversible after cessation of training, except in the case of top athletes (9). Thus, the differences may be the result of genetic endowment, of long-term and strenuous training, or of a combination of both.

The effect of age on cardiac response to exercise has been studied by Perrault and coworkers (10, 11). A 20-week endurance program resulted in a similar increase in maximal working capacity in both young (approximately 19 years old) and middle-aged (approximately 40 years old) subjects. Left ventricular and septal wall thickness did not change following training either in young or in middle-aged subjects. On the other hand, a small but significant increase in left ventricular end-diastolic diameter was observed following training in young, but not in middle-aged, subjects. No significant differences were found between groups of young (average age 23 years) and master (average age 62 years) cyclists when examined echocardiographically for left ventricular dimensions, in spite of lower $\dot{V}O_2$max observed in master cyclists.

In contrast to athletes adapted to long-term dynamic exercise, athletes who perform static or strength exercises appear to have thicker walls but unchanged dimensions of ventricular cavity (9). Thus, this type of response may be qualified as concentric hypertrophy. Obviously, few physical activities can be described as purely dynamic or static. Nevertheless, one can summarize that dynamic types of exercise result in a moderate degree of eccentric hypertrophy, whereas predominantly static exercises are associated with moderate concentric hypertrophy.

As we mentioned in the Introduction, cardiac mass determination is much easier in experimental animals. The only potential problem is the usage of relative heart weight. The relative cardiac weight simply means the absolute cardiac weight expressed as a fraction of body weight. It is a useful index for comparing cardiac growth response in subjects or experimental animals of similar body weights. It may be misleading, however, when the body weights of the experimental and control groups differ significantly, as is often the case. For instance, when the body weight is significantly reduced because of the exercise, an increased relative cardiac weight is partly a reflection of a decrease in body weight per se because the relative cardiac weight even in normal animals is higher in low-body-weight groups and decreases with growth. The proper comparison should be made using body weight controls obtained either directly or by using expected cardiac weights calculated from data collected in a large sample of the normal population.

Similar to cardiac growth response to exercise in humans, various exercise programs in experimental animals result in moderate or no increase in cardiac mass. This is well illustrated by the comprehensive review of Harpur (4), which analyzes various exercise programs in rats. Out of 24 studies in the literature in which treadmill running was applied, 58% reported increase in cardiac mass. Swimming exercise, especially programs using 2 hours of swimming or more, resulted more often in cardiac hypertrophy, and its degree was usually higher than after treadmill running. Harpur (4) collected from the literature 36 reports on the effect of swimming in rats, out of which 68% reported an increase in cardiac mass.

Finally, the degree of physical activity influences cardiac muscle growth if one compares the ratio of heart weight to body weight in various species. For instance, if 42 species of fish are classified according to their motility, it appears that the most mobile species have the relatively largest hearts (12). Relative heart weights are invariably lower in the domesticated form than in the wild form of the same species (12, 25). To what extent active movement is the causal factor cannot be decided. The differences are becoming even larger when one compares "athletic" and "nonathletic" animals of analogous species, such as mouse and bat or rabbit and hare, in which the heart weights differ 3-fold in animals of similar body weights (23-25).

Cardiac Myocytes—Number and Volume

Proliferation of cardiac myocytes in mammalian hearts stops in the early postnatal period, and further growth is realized by an increase in size of the muscle cells. It is not clear, however, exactly when or why the proliferation stops. Adult values of muscle cell numbers are reached during the first few postnatal months in human hearts and the first few postnatal weeks in rat hearts (16). The type of cardiac response to a growth stimulus is dependent on the developmental stage of the organism. If the stimulus is applied in the early developmental stage, both hyperplasia and hypertrophy of cardiac myocytes may be detected, whereas later on hypertrophy of cardiac muscle cells is the typical response (18). Therefore, the typical response to chronic exercise is characterized by hypertrophy of myocytes exclusively. The only exception may be the case of comparing wild to domesticated animals, which seems to indicate the presence of hyperplasia as well (12, 25). In this case, however, the influence of a genetic component to the hyperplastic response is highly probable. The typical response to chronic exercise therefore is a moderate increase in cardiac mass due to an increase in volume of the individual cardiac muscle cells. At the present time, we do not know whether the increase is similar in various regions of the heart and whether the shape of cardiac myocytes remains unaltered.

Coronary Capillaries

The effect of chronic exercise on coronary vasculature has been investigated quite extensively. The results are variable, partly due to poor understanding of quantitative morphology and the interpretation of data. The total and relative volume of the coronary vascular bed may be estimated by using corrosive casts or radioactive tracers (15). The utilization of corrosive casts is quite instructive in description of vascular geometry, including branching, but it is unreliable for quantitative data. Chances of imperfect filling, especially of the terminal vascular bed, and the possibility of bubbles in larger vessels are too high. Their effect on the total weight of the corrosive cast can mask actual changes in capillarization. The use of radioactive tracers appears to be more appropriate. Even in this case, however, only average values of vascular capacity may be obtained, which is inferior to the information obtained from the morphometric methods.

Various morphometric methods have been applied in studies of cardiac capillarization (for their review, see ref. 15). Histoautoradiographic methods have been used in several exercise studies. This method reveals, however, only formation of DNA in endothelial nuclei. We are not sure whether this is accompanied by an increased number of endothelial cells. An increased number of endothelial cells may result in an increased capillary surface. We still do not know whether the increased surface is a sign of an increased number of capillaries or an increase in the length of individual vessels (tortuosity). Similarly, an increased fiber:capillary ratio does not necessarily mean an improved capillarization, if it is accompanied by an increased size of cardiac myocyte, as is often the case in hearts from exercising animals.

A more suitable index of capillarization, introduced by Krogh (6), is the radius of the tissue cylinder supplied by a single capillary. The radius is defined as the mean half-distance between adjacent capillaries on cross-section and may be computed from the capillary density (N/mm²). Tissue oxygenation, however, is influenced not only by the mean values of the Krogh cylinder but also by its variability, that is, by the heterogeneity of the capillary spacing. Estimates of the heterogeneity index may be complemented by modern stereological parameters, which include measurements of capillary surface density, length density, and degree of anisotropy (7, 19).

Most of the reviews of the literature emphasize the beneficial effect of exercise on the coronary vascular bed. Several of them report exclusively or predominantly increased vascularization of the hearts from exercised animals. In contrast, in our own recent review, we tabled 14 studies, of which 7 reported no change, 4 a decrease, and 3 an increase in capillary density in hearts from animals subjected to chronic exercise (17). What is a possible source of this discrepancy? Wyatt's review "Physical Conditioning and the Coronary-Artery Vasculature" (26) can serve as an example. Table 2 of his review contains 15 studies on myocardial capillary density. Thirteen reported an increase and only 2 old studies found a decrease in myocardial capillary density after physical conditioning. Close examination of Wyatt's table, however, leads to a different conclusion. Three papers deal with autoradiography only, with no data on capillary density. Capillary density was also not investigated in the studies of Bloor and Leon (3), Bell and Rasmussen (fiber-capillary ratio only) (2), and Thorner (density of nonmuscle nuclei) (21). None of the above methods yields reliable information on myocardial capillarization. Papers by Wyatt and Mitchell (27) as well as by Bloor and Leon (3) are listed as reporting increased capillary density, although in the original articles no statistical significance was found. Thus, the only two remaining studies reporting an increased capillary density are those of Poupa et al. (12) and Tomanek (22). In the first case, it is a comparison of various species according to their physical activity, and Tomanek reported significant increase after chronic running in young but not in old rats.

To summarize the data, no conclusive evidence can be found for a general statement that chronic exercise increases the capillarization of mammalian hearts. Relatively small changes in capillary density due to chronic exercise will be influenced by additional modifiers such as the age of the organism (the younger the organism, the more likely that the exercise will elicit capillary growth) (22), and the type and intensity of exercise (a possibility of optimal schedule) (1).

Similar to the case of cardiac hypertrophy, special attention should be paid to the comparison of athletic to nonathletic animals, the former being characterized not only by substantially larger hearts but also by higher capillary density. This is true even in the case of wild and laboratory variants of the same species, Rattus Norvegicus, that differ in their mode of life and activity patterns (25). Even in this case, possible reasons for the difference are more complex and include genetic, nutritional, and environmental aspects, in addition to the obvious differences in the motor activity.

Exercise and Heart Pathology

Failure of chronic exercise to substantially increase myocardial capillarization is not surprising. A shorter diffusion distance as a result of a higher capillary density has no significant effect on the myocardial PO_2, though it lessens its dependence on myocardial oxygen consumption (14). More important may be an improvement in myocardial capillarization in various pathological situations. There are some reports in the literature indicating that chronic exercise may improve capillarization and eventually influence the size of myocardial infarction (8, 13). Eventually, even more important may be a restoration of capillary density in situations like cardiac hypertrophy, in which decreased capillarization is one of the major features. Therefore, we attempted to influence, by exercise capillarization, cardiac hypertrophy in renal hypertensive rats. The experiments have been described extensively in our recent publication (19). The following is only a brief summary.

Female Sprague-Dawley rats were made hypertensive by the two kidney/one clip Goldblatt procedure, whereas control animals were sham-operated. One week later, half of the animals were subjected to moderate swimming exercise (2 hours/day for a period of 6 weeks, with a preceding acclimation period). The other half remained sedentary. Thus, 4 experimental groups were formed: control rats that were exercised or kept sedentary, and corresponding renal hypertensive animals either exercised or sedentary. In hypertensive rats, significantly increased left ventricular weights and reduced coronary reserves were found. Cardiac hypertrophy in hypertensive rats was characterized by lower capillary density, larger heterogeneity of the capillary net, and a less uniform orientation of capillaries in space (see Figures 1-3).

CAPILLARY DENSITY

	SED	SWIM	
SHAM	E: 4765 ± 165 M: 4553 ± 157	4592 ± 165 4779 ± 123	⎤
RHR	E: 4033 ± 127 M: 3959 ± 158	3995 ± 100 3994 ± 133	⎦ p < .01
	NS		

E: ENDOMYOCARDIUM, M: MIDSECTION

Figure 1.   Capillary density in 4 experimental groups: SED, sedentary; swim, swimming; sham, sham-operated; RHR, renal hypertensive rats. Number of capillaries per mm² of cross-section, average values ± SEM.

HETEROGENEITY OF CAPILLARY SPACING
(Log SD x 100)

	SED	SWIM	
SHAM	E: 64 ± 2 M: 64 ± 2	58 ± 2 62 ± 2	⎤
RHR	E: 65 ± 2 M: 68 ± 3	65 ± 2 66 ± 3	⎦ p < .05
	NS		

E: ENDOMYOCARDIUM   M: MIDSECTION

Figure 2.   Heterogeneity of capillary spacing expressed as log SD in the 4 experimental groups described in Figure 1. The higher the log SD, the larger the variability of capillary spacing, and vice versa. Average values ± SEM.

Chronic swimming did not significantly influence any of the investigated indexes of capillaries from hypertrophic hearts. In the normotensive rats, chronic swimming resulted in only a moderate increase in total capillary length, associated with a small increase in the left ventricular weight of similar degree. Thus, chronic exercise in normotensive rats induced a moderate increase in total capillary length per left ventricle, whereas it did not alleviate impaired capillarization of hypertrophic hearts from hypertensive rats.

ANISOTROPY CONSTANT (K)
AND CORRECTION FACTOR (cKo)

	SED	SWIM	
SHAM	E: 5.3 ± 0.4 (1.07) M: 4.3± 0.4 (1.09)	4.2 ± 0.4 (1.09) 4.2 ± 0.3 (1.09)	]
RHR	E: 4.0 ± 0.3 (1.09) M: 3.6 ± 0.2 (1.10)	3.9 ± 0.2 (1.09) 3.4 ± 0.2 (1.12)	] <.01
	NS		

ALSO E: M <.05
E: ENDOMYOCARDIUM, M: MIDSECTION

Figure 3. Anisotropy constant K and correction factor cKo in the 4 experimental groups described in Figure 1. The higher the constant K, the more the capillaries are aligned according to their preferential axis, and vice versa. Correction factor in brackets is used for calculating capillary length density (numerical density × correction factor). Average values ± SEM.

Conclusion

The cardiac growth response to chronic exercise is relatively small. Moderate increase in cardiac mass due to increase in the size of myocytes may or may not be accompanied by proportional changes in vascular growth. Reports on the effect of exercise are not uniform, mainly due to various mixtures of known modifiers of the cardiac response. The most important of these are the age of the organism (younger animals responding more than older ones), sex, genetic influences, type, and intensity and duration of exercise.

References

1. Anversa, P.; Ricci, R.; Olivetti, G. Effects of exercise on the capillary vasculature of the rat heart. Circulation 75(Suppl. 1):1-12; 1987.
2. Bell, R.D.; Rasmussen, R.L. Exercise and the myocardial capillary-fiber ratio during growth. Growth 38:237-244; 1974.
3. Bloor, C.M.; Leon, A.S. Interaction of age and exercise on the heart and its blood supply. Lab. Invest. 22:160-165; 1970.
4. Harpur, R.P. The rat as a model for physical fitness studies. Comp. Biochem. Physiol. 66A:553-574; 1980.

5. Harvey, W. An anatomical disputation concerning the movement of the heart and blood in living creatures. Whitteridge, G., translator. Oxford, England: Blackwell Scientific Publ.; 1976.

6. Krogh, A. The number and distribution of capillaries in muscles with calculations of the oxygen pressure head necessary for supplying the tissue. J. Physiol. (Lond.) 52:409-415; 1919.

7. Mathieu, O.; Cruz-Orive, L.M.; Hoppeler, H.; Weibel, E.R. Estimating length density and quantifying anisotropy in skeletal muscle capillaries. J. Microscopy 131:131-146; 1983.

8. McElroy, C.L.; Gissen, S.A.; Fishbein, M.C. Exercise-induced reduction in myocardial infarct size after coronary artery occlusion in the rat. Circulation 57:958-961; 1978.

9. Morganroth, J.B.; Marion, B.J.; Henry, W.L. Comparative left ventricular dimensions in trained athletes. Ann. Intern. Med. 82:521-524; 1975.

10. Perrault, H.; Lajoie, D.; Peronnet, F.; Nadeau, R.; Tremblay, G.; Lebeau, R. Left ventricular dimensions following training in young and middle-aged men. Int. J. Sports Med. 3:141-144; 1982.

11. Perrault, H.; Peronnet, F.; Ferguson, R.J.; Ricci, G.; Lebeau, R.; Nadeau, R.A. Left-ventricular dimensions and maximal oxygen uptake in young and master cyclists. Can. J. Sport Sci. 12:219-224; 1987.

12. Poupa, O.; Rakusan, K.; Ostadal, B. The effect of physical activity upon the heart of vertebrates. Medicine and Sport 4:202-233; 1970.

13. Przyklenk, K.; Groom, A.C. Can exercise promote revascularization in the transition zone of infarcted rat hearts? Can. J. Physiol. Pharmacol. 62:630-641; 1984.

14. Rakusan, K. Oxygen in the heart muscle. Springfield, IL: Thomas; 1971.

15. Rakusan, K. Assessment of cardiac growth. In: Zak, R., ed. Growth of the heart in health and disease. New York: Raven Press; 1984:25-40.

16. Rakusan, K. Cardiac growth, maturation and aging. In: Zak, R., ed. Growth of the heart in health and disease. New York: Raven Press; 1984:131-164.

17. Rakusan, K. Microcirculation in the stressed heart. In: Legato, M.J., ed. The stressed heart. Boston: M. Nijhoff Publ.; 1987:107-123.

18. Rakusan, K.; Korecky, B. Regression of cardiomegaly induced in newborn rats. Can. J. Cardiol. 1:217-222; 1985.

19. Rakusan, K.; Wicker, P.; Abdul-Samad, M.; Healy, B.; Turek, Z. Failure of swimming exercise to improve capillarization in cardiac hypertrophy of renal hypertensive rats. Circ. Res. 61:641-647; 1987.

20. Schaible, T.F.; Scheuer, J. Cardiac adaptations to chronic exercise. Prog. Cardiovasc. Dis. 27:297-324; 1985.

21. Thorner, W. Trainingversuche an Hunden. Arb. Physiol. 8:359-370; 1935.

22. Tomanek, R.J. Effects of age and exercise on the extent of the myocardial capillary bed. Anat. Rec. 167:55-62; 1970.

23. Wachtlova, M.; Poupa, O.; Rakusan, K. Quantitative differences in the terminal vascular bed of the myocardium in the brown bat and the laboratory mouse. Physiol. Bohemoslov. 19:491-495; 1970.

24. Wachtlova, M.; Rakusan, K.; Poupa, O. The terminal vascular bed in the heart of the hare and the rabbit. Physiol. Bohemoslov. 14:328-331; 1965.

25. Wachtlova, M.; Rakusan, K.; Roth, Z.; Poupa, O. The terminal vascular bed of the myocardium in the wild rat and the laboratory rat. Physiol. Bohemoslov. 16:548-554; 1967.

26. Wyatt, H.L. Physical conditioning and the coronary-artery vasculature. In: Kalsner, S., ed. The coronary artery. London: Groom Helm; 1982.

27. Wyatt, H.L.; Mitchell, J. Influences of physical conditioning and deconditioning on coronary vasculature of dogs. J. Appl. Physiol. 45:619-625; 1978.

Acceleration of Myosin Heavy Chain Isoform Transitions During Compensatory Hypertrophy of Developing Avian Muscles

David A. Essig, Suzanne Kamel-Reid, David L. DeVol, Peter J. Bechtel, Radovan Zak, and Patrick K. Umeda
University of Illinois at Chicago and University of Illinois at Urbana-Champaign, Illinois, U.S.A

In response to increased tension demands created by addition of a weight, passive stretch, or removal of a synergist, skeletal muscle fibers undergo compensatory hypertrophy. This phenomenon has been well studied in the chicken due to the relative ease by which hypertrophy can be induced in wing musculature by noninvasive methods. Besides an increase in muscle fiber cross-sectional area, a change in histochemical fiber type is also observed in these models of hypertrophy (14, 25). For example, hypertrophy of the slow tonic anterior latissimus dorsi (ALD) muscle is accompanied by a loss of the B' fiber population (nomenclature of Ashmore; 1, 2). On the other hand, with compensatory growth of the patagialis (PAT) muscle, a fast-twitch muscle, the nonoxidative fibers (α white) are transformed into highly oxidative alpha red fibers. The molecular basis for these changes in fiber type are in part the result of specific alterations in the distribution of slow and fast myosin isoforms.

In the past few years, our group has been investigating the changes in the expression of myosin isoforms in chicken fast and slow skeletal muscle in response to overload hypertrophy. Our approach has been to analyze the expression of the native myosin molecule as well as the heavy chain (HC) subunit at the protein and mRNA levels. The present paper focuses upon the changes in expression that occur in hypertrophied chicken fast and slow skeletal muscle, and on the relationship of these changes to ongoing developmentally regulated myosin isoform transitions. The control of myosin HC gene expression during hypertrophy-induced isoform transitions will also be addressed.

Muscle Development and Myosin HC Expression

In fast and slow muscles, there are distinct forms of the myosin protein that possess different ATPase activities. These differences result from the expression of distinct polymorphic forms of the HC subunit (24, 28). Furthermore, in skeletal muscle the expression of these HCs varies during development (28). These changes probably reflect a type of functional adaptation of the muscle because ATPase activity (5) and the distribution of fast and slow HCs (20) are directly correlated with contractile velocity.

In vertebrate fast skeletal muscle, there are four or more fast myosin HC isoforms expressed sequentially during the embryonic, neonatal, and adult periods (4, 27, 28). The genetic basis for the multiplicity of fast myosin HC isoform resides in a family of distinct genes (21) that are transcribed in response to developmentally regulated signals. In contrast to the diversity of fast myosin HCs, only one (mammalian) and two (avian) slow HC isoforms have been identified in developing slow muscle fibers. In mammals the slow skeletal and beta cardiac myosin HCs are encoded by the same gene (22, 23), which in slow skeletal muscle is expressed throughout development (18). On the other hand, in chicken slow tonic muscles such as the ALD, two slow HCs, SM-1 and SM-2, have been identified (16, 17). The SM-1 HC is the major isoform in the embryonic ALD, accounting for 80% of the myosin HC. During development there is a shift toward replacement of the SM-1 by SM-2 HC such that it accounts for 75-85% of the slow myosin in the adult chicken ALD (16, 17). The transition toward expression of the SM-2 HC is functionally significant because the slowing of the fiber contractile velocity with age is highly correlated with the content of the SM-2 HC (20A).

The developmental changes in myosin HC isoform expression in the chicken fast and slow muscles occur over an extended time frame. For example, the transition from SM-1 to a predominantly SM-2 HC profile is not complete until 8-10 weeks after hatching (16). Because we (16) and others (14) have utilized young (5- to 6-week-old chickens) to study compensatory hypertrophy, the ongoing developmental changes must be considered when examining the effects of compensatory hypertrophy on myosin HC expression in the avian model.

Hypertrophy Models

The slow tonic ALD muscle rapidly enlarges by the addition of an extra load to the wing (16). A lead weight covered with soft gauze is wrapped around one wing of each experimental chicken just above the radioulnar joint. Each chicken serves as an internal control because only one wing is weighted. Chickens are weighed daily, and the mass of the lead weight is maintained at 10% of body weight. The growth stimulus in this model has been postulated to be the result of both passive stretch and increased isometric tension. The patagialis (PAT), a fast-twitch muscle, can be induced to hypertrophy by using a model of continuous passive stretch (3). The musculature of one wing is stretched by stapling a rigid cardboard sleeve over the wing to fully extend the elbow joint. The contralateral wing serves as the control.

Masses of the ALD and PAT muscles with 12-14 days' overload are increased significantly ($p < 0.05$) to 260% and 150% of the contralateral control value (6, 16). The relatively larger increase in ALD mass is probably due to the continued maintenance of the wing weight at 10% of body mass. The extent of this hypertrophy can be maintained for up to 28 days (6). By contrast, the growth of PAT peaks after 14 days of passive stretch (unpublished observations), likely due to release of stretch by addition of sarcomeres to the ends of the fibers.

Native Isomyosins

As an initial step in our analysis, the effects of hypertrophy on the distribution of native myosin isoforms were examined. Total myosin was extracted from minced muscle samples with Guba/Straub buffer (7); electrophoresis was performed under nondenaturing conditions, as described by Hoh (12). The relative proportions of the isomyosins in the gels were measured with a densitometer equipped with an integrator. In the ALD there are two slow isomyosins, SM-1 and SM-2, which are homodimers of SM-1 and SM-2 HCs, respectively (17). Each native slow myosin contains predominantly $LC1_s$ and $LC2_s$ subunits (11). The effect of 12 days of hypertrophy in the ALD is to greatly decrease the relative amount of the SM-1 isomyosin from approximately 35% to 10% (16). During normal muscle development the percentage of SM-1 decreases to about 20% of total myosin by about 10 weeks and remains constant through adulthood (11, 16). Thus, the data indicated that 14 days' hypertrophy enhances both the rate and the extent of this process.

The corresponding changes in the distribution of fast isomyosins in the hypertrophied PAT have been investigated in a recent experiment (8). In avian fast muscles, there are typically three isomyosins—FM-1, FM-2, and FM-3—that can be distinguished under nondissociating gel conditions (13). The basis for the differences in migration has been attributed to myosin light chain (LC) subunit composition. All three fast isomyosins possess a pair of $LC2_f$ subunits but differ in the distribution of $LC1_f$ and $LC3_f$. FM-1 and FM-3 contain a homodimer of $LC3_f$ and $LC1_f$, respectively, whereas FM-2 is a heterodimer of $LC3_f$ and $LC1_f$. The effect of hypertrophy was to decrease the relative amounts of FM-1 while increasing the amount of FM-3. No changes in the relative proportion of the FM-2 isomyosin have been noted. During normal development, the FM-3 isomyosin is the major isomyosin prior to hatching, whereas FM-2 and FM-3 represent only 20% of total myosin. However, by 1 week posthatching, there are roughly equal proportions of all 3 isomyosins, which are maintained through to adulthood (11). Thus, in the PAT the effect of hypertrophy at the level of the native myosin molecule was to reverse normal developmental trends. However, it has not been directly investigated whether these observed effects are reflected by a corresponding change in the ratio of $LC1_f$ to $LC3_f$. In addition, a shift in the developmentally regulated myosin HC isoform distribution could also change the ratio of native isomyosins.

Analysis of Myosin HC Isoforms

The goal of these experiments was to investigate whether the expression of the HC mRNAs encoding fast and slow isoforms were changed by compensatory hypertrophy. These data were important for at least two reasons. For one, it allowed us to assign the level (i.e., pretranslational or translational) at which the expression of the protein HC isoforms are regulated. The data fulfilled another purpose with regard to fast myosin isoform expression. At present, there appears to be a large number of highly homologous but distinct fast HC isoforms identified at the mRNA level (21, 27), but they cannot be distinguished by techniques at the protein level.

Thus, to identify possible changes in fast HC isoform expression that would not be detected with native myosin analysis, we analyzed fast HC isoform expression in PAT at the mRNA level.

The technique of S1 nuclease mapping was used to measure relative amounts of slow and fast HC mRNA isoforms in hypertrophied ALD and PAT. A detailed description of the procedure as applied to myosin HC isoforms is found in Umeda et al. (27). The PAT muscle was relatively uncharacterized in terms of its developmental pattern of myosin HC expression. Thus, RNA was isolated from the PAT at selected stages of development as well as from chickens in which the wing was passively stretched for 2 weeks, starting at 5 and 36 weeks of age (8). In the embryonic PAT, two fast embryonic myosin HC mRNAs were expressed, a pattern similar to the pectoralis muscle (27). One week following hatching, the relative amounts of the two embryonic HC mRNAs declined and were replaced by a myosin HC mRNA tentatively identified as a neonatal isoform. Six weeks later, in PAT differentiation another HC mRNA corresponding to an adult HC is coexpressed with the neonatal myosin HC mRNA. By 38 weeks of age, the adult isoform predominates over the neonatal HC. In 52-week-old adult chickens, the adult isoform is exclusively expressed. Hypertrophy in 7-week-old birds was associated with such a dramatic decrease in the amount of the neonatal isoform relative to the adult that only the adult isoform remains (8). With hypertrophy of the PAT muscle of 38-week-old birds, a similar result was also observed. The relative amounts of the neonatal and adult mRNA levels were quantified by densitometry, and results showed that in 5-week-old birds, the ratio increased from 0.8 to 14.2, whereas in 38-week-old chickens, the ratio increased from 2.8 to 16.4. Thus, in terms of HC expression, the hypertrophy in fast as well as slow musculature of the chicken produces an accelerated appearance of the adult myosin HC isoform profile.

Regulation of Myosin HC Expression by Hypertrophy

The ALD muscle was selected over the PAT to study this question because only two HC isoforms are expressed (SM-1 and SM-2) and the ratio of the two HC proteins can be easily estimated by electrophoresis of myosin under native (16) or denaturing conditions (17). In addition, specific monoclonal antibodies are available to each HC and have been used to determine the individual synthesis rates of the HC isoforms during ALD hypertrophy (Gregory et al., this volume).

An experiment was undertaken in which the expression of SM-1 and SM-2 HC protein and mRNA was measured during overload-induced hypertrophy at selected time points (15). Expression of the HC protein was estimated in four individual muscles, and RNA was extracted from pooled muscle samples at 1, 2, 3, 7, and 14 days following addition of the wing weight. To estimate the expression of the slow HC mRNAs, a cDNA clone for the SM-1 HC mRNA was used. The characterization of this clone (15/2) and another (6/1) that codes for SM-2 are described in detail in a forthcoming manuscript (Essig et al., submitted for publication).

On the control side, the age-related decline in percentage of SM-1 HC protein was matched closely by a parallel decline in the percentage of SM-1 HC mRNA. Similarly, during compensatory growth, the relatively greater rate of decline in the percentage of SM-1 HC correlated with the decrease in relative expression of SM-1 HC mRNA. When the results from control and hypertrophied ALD are combined, the relationship between HC protein and mRNA is highly significant (r = 0.88, $p < 0.05$). The data are consistent with the notion that the relative amounts of SM-1 and SM-2 HC during normal and compensatory growth are controlled by the steady state levels of the individual mRNAs. This would correspond to regulation of gene expression at the pretranslational level. Whether actual control occurs at the site of transcriptional initiation or in post-transcriptional processes cannot be distinguished with our data. However, in general, myosin HC mRNA expression appears to be regulated by transcriptional control mechanisms. Thus, future efforts will be directed at testing whether compensatory growth mediates differential expression of slow myosin HC mRNAs at the level of transcription.

Stimulus

Our results in avian slow and fast skeletal muscle suggest that the growth produced in these models as a result of stretch/overload accelerates the rate of normal developmentally regulated HC isoform transitions. In other studies the physiological factors that might be critically necessary to produce the effects of compensatory growth on HC isoform distribution were determined. We considered whether the absolute size of the muscle, the increased tension demands, or the rate of growth would determine the ratio of SM-1 to SM-2 during ALD muscle growth. The first of these variables regarding size seemed not important because there was no relationship between the percentage SM-1 in normal muscles of a given mass and the percentage of SM-1 in hypertrophied muscle of the same mass (see ref. 16).

The role of tension was examined in a recent study (15) using denervation hypertrophy. In this model, originally devised by Feng (9), the brachial plexus innervating the entire wing musculature (including the ALD) is severed in 1-week-old chickens. Regrowth of the nerve is prevented by sealing the stump with rubber tubing. In addition, the feathers of the wing are glued to the rib cage to alleviate wing droop and resultant stretch of the ALD. The results of this study indicated that 1 month following denervation, there was a 2-fold decrease in the percentage of SM-1 myosin (30% to 15%), associated with a moderate hypertrophy of the ALD. Thus, despite the absence of nerve-mediated active tension and passive tension (prevention of wing droop), the increased growth with denervation was accompanied by a shift toward elimination of the SM-1 isoform. It could be suggested, therefore, that the increased tension demands associated with weight-induced hypertrophy of the ALD, although certainly a stimulus for growth, may not in fact determine the shift in slow myosin HC isoform distribution. This led us to the tentative conclusion that some variable associated with the *rate* of growth may be important in determining myosin HC isoform transitions.

To confirm this suggestion, we tested the hypothesis that slowing the rate of ALD muscle growth would inhibit the normal rate of SM-1 myosin decline during development. This was accomplished by reducing the weight experienced by the ALD (15). Approximately two-thirds of the radius, ulna, and humerus were surgically removed, being careful not to disturb the tendon insertion of the ALD and its nerve and blood supply. This procedure was observed to slow the rate of ALD growth significantly over a 2-month period following surgery. In the growth-retarded ALD, the percentage of SM-1 28 days following amputation was 2-fold higher than in controls. These data, in conjunction with the denervation-induced hypertrophy experiment, suggest that factors associated with the rate of growth may modulate the rate of slow myosin HC isoform switching. Exactly what this (these) factor(s) might be was not clear from our experiments. We predict, however, that there could be one or more types of "autocrine" factors because compensatory growth occurred in the same external hormonal milieu as for control muscles. A suitable cell culture model of compensatory muscle growth (see below) may be one approach to examining the factors involved in myosin HC isoform gene expression.

Relationship of Chicken and Rat Models of Compensatory Hypertrophy

The overall findings of our work in chickens indicates a relationship between compensatory and developmental growth regulation of myosin HC isoforms. Our results, however, are somewhat difficult to directly compare with recent data from hypertrophied rat muscles, where, depending upon the muscle studied, there are qualitative alterations in the distribution of fast and slow myosin isoforms (19A). For example, in rat plantaris, a fast-twitch muscle, hypertrophy causes an increased expression of slow and Type IIa myosin HC mRNAs and a decrease in the relative amount of the IIb HC mRNA. On the other hand, in the slow-twitch soleus muscle, Type IIa myosin HC expression declines as it is replaced by slow myosin HC. Thus, in the rat the enlarged muscle acquires a qualitatively different myosin phenotype and does not involve an apparent redistribution of developmental isoforms.

There are several reasons why there may be apparent differences between these two models. First, the chicken expresses a greater variety of fast and slow myosin HC isoforms than the rat (21). Second, the expression of myosin HC isoforms in the rat during development occurs at a more accelerated rate than in the chicken. For example, the transition from neonatal to adult fast myosin HC expression is complete in the rat hindlimb by 4 weeks of age (19). Because most studies in the rat have initiated hypertrophy at 4-5 weeks of age, the muscle is fully differentiated in terms of its myosin HC phenotype. This contrasts with the chicken, in which muscles are overloaded at 5 weeks of age but myosin HC isoform transitions continue to occur for up to 8 weeks in the ALD (16) and as long as 36-52 weeks in the PAT (8). Finally, the models of hypertrophy in the rat and chicken probably involve different stimuli. After synergist ablation (removal of the gastrocnemius muscle) in the rat, the plantaris muscle shows an increased expression of slow myosin HC. It is possible that this is the result of altered biomechanics and recruitment patterns created by synergist removal such that the plantaris is beginning to acquire the properties of a postural muscle such as the soleus. This is especially true in the plantaris when both the soleus and gastrocnemius muscles are removed (26). Thus, the adaptations caused by synergist ablation appear to include not only a growth response but also a phenotypic change associated with a new functional role. In the chicken models of hypertrophy, the functional demands created by the overload may be similar to those experienced later in adulthood because there are not any "new" isoforms synthesized; rather, the compensatory hypertrophy only hastens the appearance of the adult myosin phenotype. This suggests that the changes in myosin HC isoform expressions are due to a change in the rate of growth and are not complicated by a new functional role, as may be the case in the rat synergist ablation models.

Summary

Overall, our data indicate there may be a link between compensatory growth and the expression of developmentally regulated myosin HC isoform transitions. This appears to be true in developing fast as well as slow skeletal muscles. In the case of the slow myosin HC isoforms, the control of this accelerated HC isoform distribution with compensatory growth is regulated at the pretranslational level.

Our future efforts will be to continue to determine the exact mechanism involved in the growth regulation of developmentally expressed isoforms of myosin HC. To facilitate progress in this area, we are currently using a cell culture model of stretch-induced hypertrophy (10). Preliminary data indicate that repetitive mechanical stretching of cultured myotubes results in a complete disappearance of embyronic and neonatal fast HC isoform mRNAs and a corresponding increase in adult HC mRNA expression (Essig & Vandenburgh, unpublished results). Thus, it should be possible to examine whether these observed changes in culture can be localized to specific gene sequences using DNA-mediated gene transfer experiments. The results of this strategy could eventually lead to the isolation of specific protein-binding factors involved in regulation of myosin HC isoform switching.

Acknowledgments

This work was supported in part by grants from NIH (HL09172, HL16637, and HL20592) and the Muscular Dystrophy Association. A portion of this work was funded by an NIH postdoctoral fellowship (AM07482) at The University of Chicago and later by a grant from the Campus Research Board at The University of Illinois at Chicago. Partial support for this work was also provided by The University of Illinois Agricultural Station.

References

1. Ashmore, C.R.; Doerr, L. Comparative aspects of muscle fiber types in different species. Exp. Neurol. 31:408-418; 1971.
2. Ashmore, C.R.; Kikuchi, T.; Doerr, L. Some observations on the innervation patterns of different fiber types of chick muscle. Exp. Neurol. 58:272-284; 1978.

3. Ashmore, C.R. Stretch-induced growth in chicken wing muscles: effects on hereditary muscular dystrophy. Am. J. Physiol. 242:C178-183; 1982.

4. Bandman, E.; Matsuda, R.; Strohman, R.C. Developmental appearance of myosin heavy and light chain isoforms in vivo and in vitro in chicken skeletal muscle. Dev. Biol. 93:508-518; 1982.

5. Barany, M. ATPase activity of myosin correlated with speed of muscle shortening. J. Gen. Physiol. 50:197-218; 1967.

6. Brown, C.R.; Palmer, W.K.; Bechtel, P.J. Effects of passive stretch on growth and regression of muscle from chickens of various ages. Comp. Biochem. Physiol. 86A:443-448; 1987.

7. d'Albis, A.; Pantaloni, C.; Bechtel, P.J. An electrophoretic study of native myosin isozymes and of their subunit content. Eur. J. Biochem. 99:261-272; 1979.

8. Essig, D.A.; Devol, D.L.; Bechtel, P.J. Fast myosin expression during developmental and compensatory growth of avian patagialis skeletal muscle. Can. J. Sport Sci. 13:11P; 1988.

9. Feng, T.P.; Jung, H.W.; Wu, W.Y. The contrasting trophic changes of the anterior and posterior latissimus dorsi of the chick following denervation. Acta Physiol. Sin. 25:431-444; 1962.

10. Hatfaludy, S.J.; Shansky; Vandenburgh. Metabolic alterations induced in cultured muscle by stretch/relaxation activity. Am. J. Physiol. 25:C175-C181; 1989.

11. Hoh, J.F.Y. Developmental changes in chicken skeletal myosin isoenzymes. FEBS Lett. 98:267-270; 1979.

12. Hoh, J.F.Y.; McGrath, P.A.; Hale, P.T. Electrophoretic analysis of multiple forms of cardiac myosin: effect of hypophysectomy and thyroxine replacement. J. Mol. Cell. Cardiol. 10:1053-1076; 1978.

13. Hoh, F.Y.H. Light chain distribution of chicken skeletal muscle myosin isozymes. FEBS Lett. 90:297-300; 1978.

14. Holly, R.G.; Barnett, J.G.; Ashmore, C.R.; Taylor, R.G.; Mole, P.A. Stretch-induced growth in chicken wing muscles: a new model of stretch hypertrophy. Am. J. Physiol. 238(Cell Physiology 7):C62-C71; 1980.

15. Kamel-Reid, S. The expression and regulation of myosin heavy chain isoform genes in chicken slow muscle. Chicago: University of Chicago; 1987. Dissertation.

16. Kennedy, J.M.; Kamel, S.; Tambone, W.W.; Vrbova, G.; Zak, R. The expression of myosin heavy chain isoforms in normal and hypertrophied chicken slow muscle. J. Cell Biol. 103:977-983; 1986.

17. Matsuda, R.; Bandman, E.; Strohman, R.C. The two myosin isoenzymes of chicken anterior latissimus dorsi muscle contain different myosin heavy chains encoded by separate mRNAs. Differentiation 23:36-42; 1982.

18. Narusawa, M.; Fitzsimons, R.B.; Izumo, S.; Nadal-Ginard, B.; Rubinstein, N.A.; Kelly, A.M. Slow myosin in developing rat skeletal muscle. J. Cell Biol. 104:447-459; 1987.

19.   Periasamy, M.; Wieczorek, D.F.; Nadal-Ginard, B. Characterization of a developmentally regulated perinatal myosin heavy-chain gene expressed in skeletal muscle. J. Biol. Chem. 259:13573-13578; 1984.

19A. Periasamy, M.; Gregory, P.; Martin, B.J.; Stirewalt, W.S. Regulation of myosin heavy-chain gene expression during skeletal-muscle hypertrophy. J. Biol. Chem. 257:691-698; 1989.

20A. Reiser, P.J.; Greaser, M.L.; Moss, R.L. Myosin heavy chain composition of single cells is strongly correlated with velocity of shortening during development. Devel. Biol. 129:400-407; 1988.

20.   Reiser, P.J.; Moss, R.L.; Guilian, G.G.; Greaser, M.L. Shortening velocity in single fibers from adult rabbit soleus muscles is correlated with myosin heavy chain composition. J. Biol. Chem. 260:9077-9080; 1985.

21.   Robbins, J.; Horan, T.; Gulick, J.; Kropp, K. The chicken myosin heavy chain family. J. Biol. Chem. 261:6606-6612; 1986.

22.   Saez, L.; Leinwand, L.A. Characterization of diverse forms of myosin heavy chain expressed in adult human skeletal muscle. Nucleic Acids Res. 14: 2951-7969; 1986.

23.   Sinha, A.M.; Friedman, D.J.; Nigro, J.M.; Jakovcic, S.; Rabinowitz, M.; Umeda, P.K. Expression of rabbit ventricular alpha-myosin heavy chain messenger RNA sequences in atrial muscle. J. Biol. Chem. 259: 6674-6680; 1984.

24.   Sivaramakrishnan, M.; Burke, M. The free heavy chain of vertebrate skeletal myosin subfragment 1 shows full enzymatic activity. J. Biol. Chem. 257:1102-1105; 1982.

25.   Sola, O.M.; Christensen, D.L.; Martin, A.W. Hypertrophy and hyperplasia in adult chicken anterior latissimus dorsi muscle following stretch with and without denervation. Exp. Neurol. 41:76-100; 1973.

26.   Tsika, R.W.; Herrick, R.E.; Baldwin, K.M. Interaction of compensatory overload and hindlimb suspension on myosin isoform expression. J. Appl. Physiol. 62:2180-2186; 1987.

27.   Umeda, P.K.; Kavinsky, C.J.; Sinha, A.M.; Hsu, H.J.; Jakovcic, S.; Rabinowitz, M. Cloned mRNA sequences for two types of embryonic myosin heavy chains from chick skeletal muscle. J. Biol. Chem. 258:5206-5214; 1983.

28.   Whalan, R.G.; Sell, S.M.; Butler-Browne, G.S.; Schwartz, K.; Bouveret, P.; Harstrom, I.P. Three myosin heavy chain isozymes appear sequentially in rat muscle development. Nature 292:805-809; 1981.

Molecular Basis
of Myosin Heavy Chain Isozyme Transitions
in Skeletal Muscle Hypertrophy

Patricia Gregory, Gwen Prior, Muthu Periasamy, Jacques Gagnon, and Radovan Zak

University of Chicago, Chicago, Illinois and University of Vermont, Burlington, Vermont, U.S.A.

The ability of contractile activity to influence the mechanical performance and biochemical composition of muscle has been recognized for some time. Fast-twitch muscles, for example, can be converted to slow-twitch muscles if their nerves are surgically crossed, thus revealing the importance of the type of innervation in determining the phenotype of a muscle (5). Chronic artificial electrical stimulation of fast muscles with a low frequency characteristic of a slow nerve also leads to a fast-to-slow transformation, indicating that the pattern of electrical activity is an important determinant of the characteristics of a muscle (25). However, even phasic stimulation with bursts of a high-frequency (60-Hz) stimulus results in fast-to-slow transformation, leading some authors to believe that the total amount of contractile activity produced in the muscle is more important than the pattern of stimulation (29). Although there are limits to the extent of such transformations (30), the remarkable plasticity of fully differentiated adult skeletal muscle has been clearly established (14, 23, 24, 27).

Our goal was to determine the nature and extent of changes in myosin isozymes that occur with normal physiological increases in contractile activity, where the innervation remains intact and the pattern of stimulation is not externally imposed. We used animal models of skeletal muscle hypertrophy induced by work overload and stretch, as well as a model of spontaneous running exercise. The experimental strategy was to induce a change in protein expression and measure the changes in the content of specific proteins and their rates of synthesis, as well as the messenger RNA content and changes in the levels of specific mRNAs, in order to study the regulation of the protein changes.

The first experiments were carried out in rats, where hypertrophy was induced by surgical removal of the gastrocnemius muscle, leaving the remaining synergists—the fast plantaris and the slow soleus—to take over the work load of the excised muscle (2, 15). We studied the changes in myosin isozymes in the plantaris and soleus after 4 and 11 weeks of hypertrophy (11). Myosin is a major contractile protein consisting of heavy and light chain subunits that exist in several different isoforms and that are members of a tissue-specific, developmentally regulated multigene family (18). These isozymes can be separated in their native state by nondenaturing pyrophosphate polyacrylamide gel electrophoresis (7, 13), and their relative amounts

134   Gregory, Prior, Periasamy, Gagnon, and Zak

can be quantitated by scanning densitometry. Normal control plantaris (Figure 1a) contains primarily fast myosins (FM1, FM2, and FM3), about 20% intermediate myosin (IM), an isozyme characteristic of fast Type IIa fibers, and a very small amount of slow myosin (SM; 5.3% ± 0.2). After 11 weeks of hypertrophy (Figure 1b), there was 3 times as much slow myosin (16% ± 1; $p < 0.001$), and 2 times the amount of IM (39% ± 1) as in control plantaris (23% ± 1; $p < 0.001$). These increases were balanced by losses of fast myosin, particularly of FM1, which was greatly reduced at 4 weeks and had completely disappeared by 11 weeks (11). Because the hypertrophied muscles were about 50% larger than controls, the relative increases in SM and IM also represent absolute increases in the amounts of SM and IM in hypertrophied plantaris.

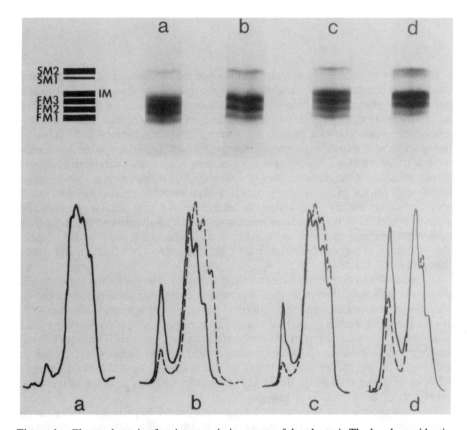

Figure 1.   Electrophoresis of native myosin isozymes of the plantaris The bands are identified in the schematic at the right. Densitometric scans of experimental groups (b) and (c) are superimposed on scans of normal plantaris. Scan (d) (hypertrophy plus exercise) is superimposed on scan (b) (hypertrophy) to illustrate alterations in the myosin isozyme profile. *Note.* From "Changes in Skeletal Muscle Myosin Isoenzymes With Hypertrophy and Exercise" by P. Gregory, R.B. Low, and W.S. Stirewalt, 1986, *Biochemistry Journal,* Vol. 245. Copyright 1986 by The Biochemical Society, London. Reprinted by permission.

We also employed a model of spontaneous running exercise, where the rats lived in exercise wheels (20) in which they ran voluntarily as much as 18 km/day (11). With running exercise, the changes in the plantaris (Figure 1c) were similar to those observed with hypertrophy in that there was a doubling of the amount of SM (12% ± 1; $p < 0.01$). However, the two stimuli are clearly different because, unlike hypertrophy, there was no increase in the size of the plantaris with exercise, the FM1 isozyme was still present at control levels at 11 weeks, and the isozyme changes were complete at 4 weeks. When both stimuli were present in the same muscle, by combining synergist removal and running exercise, the stimulus to hypertrophy appeared to override that of exercise, with a disappearance of FM1 and a doubling of the proportion of IM (Figure 1d). Furthermore, the nearly 6-fold increase in the proportion of slow myosin (29% ± 3; $p < 0.001$) in the combined hypertrophy-plus-exercise group was equal to the sum of the increases found with either treatment alone, indicating that the two stimuli were additive with respect to the accumulation of slow myosin. Thus, an increase in contractile activity induces different myosin isozyme changes depending on the nature of the stimulus, and the extent of change is affected by the intensity of the increase in contractile activity.

To determine whether the changes in myosin isozymes were due to changes in gene expression, as the protein data implied, we analyzed the changes in specific myosin heavy chain (MHC) messenger RNAs in the plantaris after 11 weeks of hypertrophy and exercise, using the technique of S-1 nuclease mapping analysis (4, 31). Figure 2 shows the results obtained with a probe derived from pMHC40, a cDNA specific for the fast Type IIa MHC mRNA (18). There was an increase in both the slow MHC mRNA and the fast IIa MHC mRNA, and a corresponding decrease in the fast Type IIb mRNA. It appears, therefore, that the increase in SM with hypertrophy was due to an increase in the slow MHC mRNA, and that the increase in IM was accompanied by an increase in the fast IIa MHC mRNA.

We also looked at the changes in native myosin isozymes in the slow soleus with hypertrophy and found that in contrast to the fast plantaris, there was a loss of intermediate and fast myosins (11), which was accompanied by a corresponding decrease in the mRNA for the fast Type IIa MHC (Figure 2). The slow MHC mRNA, however, was increased, as in the plantaris. Thus, the fast IIa myosin heavy chain gene was regulated in opposite directions in fast and slow muscles, whereas the slow myosin heavy chain was up-regulated in both muscle types, suggesting that individual muscles respond differently to a common signal.

Changes in the myosin isozyme profile on pyrophosphate gels can be due either to changes in myosin heavy chain or myosin light chain (LC) subunits because both influence the electrophoretic mobility of the native myosin. We therefore examined the light chain composition of 11-week control and hypertrophied plantaris and soleus muscles. With hypertrophy, there was a slight decrease in the fast myosin light chains LC1f, LC2f, and LC3f in the plantaris, which was balanced by increases in slow light chains LC1s and LC2s, and little or no change in the soleus, when analyzed by two-dimensional polyacrylamide gel electrophoresis (not shown). These light chain alterations are consistent with what might be predicted on the basis of the changes observed in the native myosin isozymes and our knowledge of their light chain composition (7). When we examined the expression of myosin light chain genes (21) using northern (RNA) blot hybridization techniques (22), we found an expected decrease in LC2f mRNA in the plantaris but no change in the LC1f:LC3f ratio, indicating that the changes in native myosin could not be attributed solely to changes

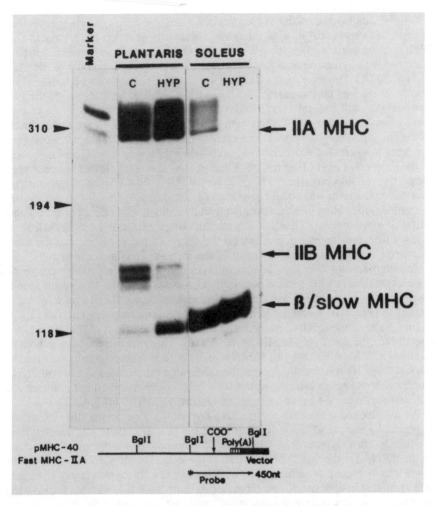

Figure 2. S-1 nuclease mapping analysis of MHC gene transcripts from 11-week control (C) and hypertrophied (HYP) plantaris and soleus muscles The broad band approximately 300 nt long indicates full protection of the probe (fast IIa MHC mRNA). Partially protected fragments 150 nt and 125 nt long represent fast IIb and B/slow skeletal MHC mRNAs, respectively. Numbers at the left indicate size markers.

in light chain composition. In addition, there was a substantial amount of the fast LC3f mRNA in both control and hypertrophied soleus (Figure 3). This unusual finding of a high level of fast LC mRNA in a predominantly slow muscle indicates that there may be translational control of the synthesis of this light chain because the LC3f protein was present only in trace amounts, whereas the level of LC3f mRNA expression was approximately equal to its expression in the fast plantaris (Figure 3). The presence of untranslated or undertranslated LC3f has also been reported for mouse soleus (3).

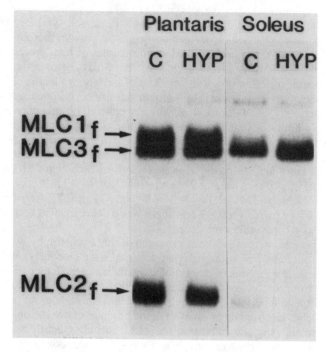

Figure 3. Northern blot hybridization of myosin light chain mRNAs from 11-week control (C) and hypertrophied (HYP) plantaris and soleus muscles Each lane contains 10 μg of RNA. Blots were hybridized (22) with [32P]-labeled probes (21) for MLC1f/MLC3f (top) and MLC2f (bottom).

We concluded that normal physiological increases in muscle activity, such as work overload and running exercise, can induce myosin transformation in a fast-to-slow direction and that these changes are due to alterations in both myosin heavy chain and light chain gene expression. Furthermore, the fast Type IIa gene is regulated in opposite directions in fast and slow muscles with the same stimulus, corroborating the tissue-specific regulation of the MHC gene family by thyroid hormone demonstrated by Izumo et al. (16). Finally, the changes induced depend on the nature of the increased contractile activity, as well as on the intensity.

We turned then to another model of work overload hypertrophy in which the changes in myosin isozymes occur more rapidly, so that we could measure the transient alterations in protein turnover and mRNA content that underlie the changes in protein composition. This model consists of hypertrophy of the chicken slow anterior latissimus dorsi (ALD) muscle that results from the attachment of a lead weight to the wing (28). The ALD of a 5-week-old chicken normally contains two myosin isozymes, SM1 and SM2 (Figure 4), but undergoes a gradual developmental decrease in the proportion of the SM1 isozyme over a period of many weeks (17). This developmentally regulated loss can be greatly accelerated by the overload hypertrophy stimulus, which induces a loss of almost 50% of the SM1: protein within the first 3 days (Figure 4).

We wanted to know whether the loss of SM1 that occurred with overload hypertrophy was due to increased degradation of SM1, decreased synthesis of SM1, or increased synthesis of the SM2 isozyme during muscle growth, thereby diluting out the existing pool of SM1. The fractional synthesis rates of total protein and of the individual SM1 and SM2 isozymes during the first 3 days of overload were measured in vivo after injection of a flooding dose of [^{3}H]phenylalanine (10, 12). The MHC isozymes were separated by immunoadsorbent chromatography using monoclonal antibody CCM-52 (6, 17), which specifically binds only to the SM1 isozyme. At 24 hours, when the muscle weight had already increased by 38%, the synthesis rate of total protein was doubled (24.7 ± 1.6%/day vs. 14.0 ± 1.1%/day for contralateral controls, $n = 8$, $p < 0.05$ by paired t test) and continued to increase further at 48 and 72 hours. However, both myosin heavy chain isozymes showed a drop in synthesis rate at 24 hours (SM2: 8.4 ± 1.3%/day vs. 11.9 ± 1.6%/day for controls; SM1: 2.1 ± 0.5%/day vs. 7.4 ± 0.7%/day for controls; $n = 6$, $p < 0.05$ by paired t test). Thus, there was a delay in switching on the synthesis of a major contractile protein.

The initial drop in myosin synthesis observed during hypertrophy was surprising in light of the increase in muscle size that occurred simultaneously. We therefore sought an independent means of determining synthesis rates. Intact polyribosomes were isolated from control and overloaded ALD, then translated in vitro in the presence of [^{35}S]methionine (9). Figure 5 shows an autoradiogram of an SDS-polyacrylamide gel electrophoretic analysis of the products of translation. At 24 hours the overall protein synthetic activity in the ALD, including actin, was increased, whereas the synthesis of myosin heavy chain was depressed, confirming the results obtained in vivo. The delay in stimulation of myosin synthesis in the ALD therefore appears to be real.

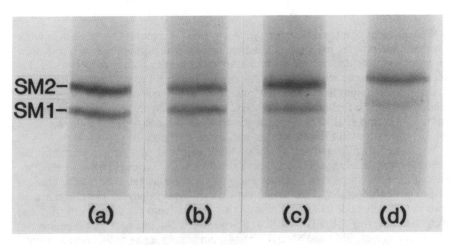

Figure 4.   Native gel electrophoresis of myosin from control and overloaded ALD muscles Pyrophosphate polyacrylamide gel electrophoresis was carried out as described in (11). Typical gels are shown from (a) control, and (b) 24-hour, (c) 48-hour, (d) 72-hour overloaded ALD muscles. Bands are identified in the schematic at left.

We next wanted to know whether the alterations observed in SM1 and SM2 synthesis could fully account for the rapid disappearance of SM1 from the ALD or whether the SM1 was specifically degraded. The absolute amount of SM1 protein in control and overloaded muscles can be calculated from several measured values: the weight of the muscle, the protein concentration, the percentage of protein that is MHC, and the proportion of MHC that is SM1. At 72 hours the control ALD had lost almost half of the SM1 protein despite a 50% increase in muscle size over the same time period. This suggests that degradation of the SM1 isozyme occurred and that increased degradation of specific proteins may play a key role in muscle adaptation to functional overload.

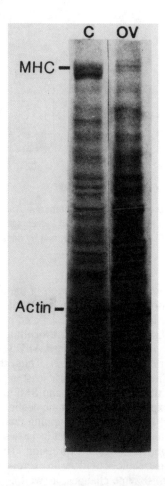

Figure 5.   In vitro translation of polyribosomes from 24-hour Control (C) and overloaded (OV) ALD muscles Figure is an autoradiogram of a gradient SDS-PAGE of [35S]-labeled products of translation. The position of the MHC and actin bands are indicated at the left.

By 72 hours the synthesis rate of SM1 had recovered from the drop at 24 hours, but at 48 hours some individual overloaded muscles still had a depressed SM1 synthesis rate (Figure 6). Surprisingly, those muscles that had lost the greatest amount of SM1 protein by 48 hours had the highest SM1 synthesis rate. This inverse relationship of SM1 synthesis rate and content may indicate that a feedback stimulation of SM1 synthesis occurred in response to the SM1 degradation. In any case, the implication is that rapid turnover of individual proteins results in a faster transition in muscle phenotype.

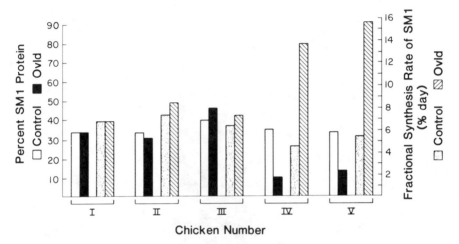

Figure 6.   Comparison of percentage of SM1 content and fractional synthesis rate of SM1 in individual ALD muscles after 48 hours of overload Percentage of SM1 refers to the percentage of total myosin that is the SM1 isozyme, determined by densitometric scanning of native gels (11).

Finally, we turned to the question of regulation of the altered patterns of protein turnover we observed with overload hypertrophy. We looked first at total poly-A containing messenger RNA levels using a radiolabeled poly-U probe hybridized to known amounts of total RNA immobilized on nitrocellulose filters. At 72 hours the percentage of RNA that was mRNA in overloaded ALD was greatly increased when compared to the contralateral control (Figure 7). Thus, the increased protein synthetic activity of overloaded muscles is regulated at least in part by increases in mRNA content. Furthermore, the alterations in SM1 and SM2 synthesis rates are consistent with differential gene expression, based on the decline in the proportion of SM1 mRNA with time observed in S1-nuclease mapping analyses (8).

In summary, we have found that physiological increases in contractile activity can cause dramatic alterations in muscle gene expression. These alterations depend on the nature of the increased contractile activity, with exercise and overload hypertrophy producing different myosin isozyme changes, as well as on the intensity, because these two stimuli are additive with respect to accumulation of slow myosin. The

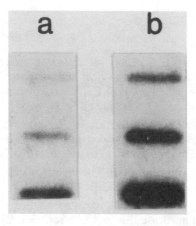

Figure 7.   Total poly-A containing messenger RNA levels in control and overloaded ALD muscles The three bands in each sample contain 2 (top), 4 (middle), and 8 μg (bottom) of total RNA.

fast IIa MHC gene is regulated in opposite directions in different muscle types with the same stimulus, whereas the slow MHC gene is up-regulated in both fast and slow muscles, indicating that the changes are tissue-specific and that individual muscles respond differently to common signals. Furthermore, the MHC transitions with hypertrophy involve a delayed stimulation of myosin synthesis and increased degradation of one MHC isozyme. Finally, rapid turnover of individual proteins results in a faster transition in muscle phenotype.

The functional significance of myosin isozyme changes in unknown. However, some of the functional consequences can be inferred from studies in which cardiac ventricular muscle composed of only the V-1 isomyosin was compared with muscle containing only the V-3 isozyme (1). The speed of contraction was slower, and the thermomechanical efficiency was higher, in hearts composed of V-3, whereas the opposite was true for V-1. Thus, a heart composed of the V-1 isozyme, such as occurs in thyrotoxicosis, would be energetically wasteful, whereas a heart that has hypertrophied due to pressure overload and switched to the V-3 isozyme, has compensated not only in terms of increased muscle mass but also in terms of the improved economy of force production and muscle relaxation. Because fibers of the ALD containing SM2 have been shown to have a slower speed of contraction than SM1 fibers (26), the transition from SM1 to SM2 that we observed with overload hypertrophy may confer a functional advantage over and above the increased capacity for force production due to the increased size.

Acknowledgments

We are grateful to Dr. Bernardo Nadal-Ginard for providing the rat myosin heavy chain cDNA probe. This work was supported by PHS DK28480, NIH-PO HL 28001-05, HL 20592, and HL 16637 from the National Institutes of Health.

References

1. Alpert, N.R.; Mulieri, L.A.; Litten, R.Z. Isoenzyme contribution to economy of contraction and relaxation in normal and hypertrophied hearts. In: Jacob, R.; Gulch, R.W.; Kissling, G. eds. Cardiac adaptation to hemodynamic overload, training and stress. Darmstadt, FRG: Steinkopff Verlag; 1983:147-157.

2. Baldwin, K.M.; Valdez, V.; Herrick, R.E.; MacIntosh, A.M.; Roy, R.R. Biochemical properties of overloaded fast-twitch skeletal muscle. J. Appl. Physiol.: Respir. Environ. Exerc. Physiol. 52:467-472; 1982.

3. Barton, P.J.R.; Buckingham, M.E. The myosin alkali light chain proteins and their genes. Biochem. J. 231:249-261; 1985.

4. Berk, A.J.; Sharp, P.A. Sizing of early adenovirus mRNAs by gel electrophoresis of S1 endonuclease digested hybrids. Cell 21:721-732; 1977.

5. Buller, A.J.; Eccles, J.C.; Eccles, R.M. Interactions between motoneurons and muscles in respect of the characteristic speeds of their responses. J. Physiol. (Lond.) 150:417-439; 1960.

6. Clark, W.A.; Chizzonite, R.A.; Everett, A.W.; Rabinowitz, M.; Zak, R. Species correlations between cardiac isomyosins: a comparison of electrophoretic and immunological properties. J. Biol. Chem. 257:5449-5454; 1982.

7. d'Albis, A.; Pantaloni, C.; Bechet, J.-J. An electrophoretic study of native myosin isozymes and their subunit content. Eur. J. Biochem. 99:261-272; 1979.

8. Essig, D.A.; DeVol, D.L.; Reid, S.K.; Bechtel, P.J.; Zak, R.; Umeda, P.K. Acceleration of myosin heavy chain isoform transitions during compensatory hypertrophy of developing avian muscles. This volume.

9. Gagnon, J.; Tremblay, R.; Rogers, P.A. Protein phenotype and gene expression in the rat perineal levator ani muscle. Comp. Biochem. Physiol. 80B:279-286; 1985.

10. Garlick, P.J.; McNurlan, M.A.; Preedy, V.R. A rapid and convenient technique for measuring the rate of protein synthesis in tissues by injection of [^{3}H]phenylalanine. Biochem. J. 192:719-723; 1980.

11. Gregory, P.; Low, R.B.; Stirewalt, W.S. Changes in skeletal muscle myosin isoenzymes with hypertrophy and exercise. Biochem. J. 238:55-63; 1986.

12. Gregory, P.; Low, R.B.; Stirewalt, W.S. Fractional synthesis rates in vivo of skeletal-muscle myosin isoenzymes. Biochem. J. 245:133-137; 1987.

13. Hoh, J.F.Y.; McGrath, P.A.; White, R.I. Electrophoretic analysis of multiple forms of myosin in fast-twitch and slow-twitch muscles of the chick. Biochem. J. 157:87-95; 1976.

14. Holloszy, J.O.; Coyle, E.F. Adaptations of skeletal muscle to endurance exercise and their metabolic consequences. J. Appl. Physiol.: Respir. Environ. Exerc. Physiol. 56:831-838; 1984.

15. Ianuzzo, C.D.; Gollnick, P.D.; Armstrong, R.B. Compensatory adaptations of skeletal muscle fiber types to a long-term functional overload. Life Sci. 19:1517-1524; 1976.

16. Izumo, S.; Nadal-Ginard, B.; Mahdavi, V. All members of the MHC multigene family respond to thyroid hormone in a highly tissue-specific manner. Science 231:597-600; 1986.

17. Kennedy, J.M.; Kamel, S.; Tambone, W.W.; Vrbova, G.; Zak, R. The expression of myosin heavy chain isoforms in normal and hypertrophied chicken slow muscle. J. Cell. Biol. 103:977-983; 1986.

18. Mahdavi, V.; Strehler, E.E.; Periasamy, M.; Wieczorek, D.; Izumo, S.; Grund, S.; Strehler, M.A.; Nadal-Ginard, B. Sarcomeric myosin heavy chain gene family: organization and pattern of expression. In: Emerson, C.; Fischman, D.A.; Nadal-Ginard, B.; Siddiqui, M.A.Q., eds. Molecular biology of muscle development. New York: Alan R. Liss; 1986:345-361. (UCLA symp. mol. cell biol. new series; vol. 29).

19. Maniatis, T.; Fritsch, E.F.; Sambrook, J. Molecular cloning: a laboratory manual. New York: Cold Spring Harbor Laboratory; 1982.

20. Mondon, C.E.; Doklas, B.; Reaven, G.M. Site of enhanced insulin sensitivity in exercise-trained rats. Am. J. Physiol. 239:E169-E177; 1980.

21. Periasamy, M.; Strehler, E.E.; Garfinkel, L.I.; Gubits, R.M.; Ruiz-Opazo, N.; Nadal-Ginard, B. Fast skeletal muscle light chains 1 and 3 are produced from a single gene by a combined process of differential RNA transcription and splicing. J. Biol. Chem. 259:13595-13604; 1984.

22. Periasamy, M.; Wieczorek, D.F.; Nadal-Ginard, B. Characterization of a developmentally regulated perinatal myosin heavy-chain gene expressed in skeletal muscle. J. Biol. Chem. 259:13573-13578; 1984.

23. Pette, D., ed. Plasticity of muscle. New York: de Gruyter; 1980.

24. Pette, D. Activity-induced fast to slow transitions in mammalian muscle. Med. Sci. Sports Exerc. 16:517-528; 1984.

25. Pette, D.; Muller, W.; Leisner, E.; Vrbova, G. Time dependent effects on contractile properties, fibre population, myosin light chains and enzymes of energy metabolism in intermittently and continuously stimulated fast twitch muscles of the rabbit. Pflügers Arch. 364:103-112; 1976.

26. Reiser, P.J.; Greaser, M.L.; Moss, R.L. Myosin heavy chain composition of single cells from avian slow skeletal muscle is strongly correlated with velocity of shortening during development. Dev. Biol. (in press).

27. Salmons, S.; Henriksson, J. The adaptive response of skeletal muscle to increased use. Muscle Nerve 4:94-105; 1981.

28. Sola, O.M.; Christenson, D.L.; Martin, A.W. Hypertrophy and hyperplasia of adult chicken anterior lattisimus dorsi muscles following stretch with and without denervation. Exp. Neurol. 41:76-100; 1973.

29. Sreter, F.A.; Pinter, K.; Jolesz, F.; Mabuchi, K. Fast to slow transformation of fast musles in response to long-term phasic stimulation. Exp. Neurol. 75:95-102; 1982.

30. Staron, R.S.; Gohlsch, B.; Pette, D. Myosin polymorphism in single fibers of chronically stimulated rabbit fast-twitch muscle. Pflügers Arch. 408:444-450; 1987.

31. Wieczorek, D.F.; Periasamy, M.; Butler-Browne, G.S.; Whalen, R.G.; Nadal-Ginard, B. Co-expression of multiple myosin heavy chain genes, in addition to a tissue-specific one, in extraocular musculature. J. Cell Biol. 101:618-629; 1985.

The Relationship of Myocardial Chronotropism to the Biochemical Capacities of Mammalian Hearts

C.D. Ianuzzo, S. Blank, N. Hamilton, P. O'Brien, V. Chen, S. Brotherton, and T.A. Salerno

York University, North York; Guelph University, Guelph; and the University of Toronto, Toronto, Ontario, Canada and Yale University, New Haven, Connecticut, U.S.A.

A muscle cell contains three major biochemical systems that confer physiological expressions to muscle (Figure 1): (a) the metabolic system, which transduces substrate-derived energy into ATP; (b) the calcium-regulating system, which times the contraction-relaxation cycle; and (c) the contractile system, which produces muscular force. It is well known that each of these biochemical systems has the inherent property of plasticity, or malleability. The specific physiological and biochemical signals that activate the remodeling of muscle cell biochemistry have been given considerable scientific attention, but at present they are still only partially understood. Two of the major regulatory determinants of these three biochemical systems in cardiac muscle are physiological demands imposed upon the muscle and the systematic thyroid status.

To gain insight into the role of physiological demand in regulating these biochemical systems, we used a comparative biological approach. Among the different-sized mammals studied, there was a 25,000-fold difference in heart mass and 10-fold differences in metabolic rates and resting heart rates (14, 46). In order to maintain their higher metabolic rates, the hearts of smaller mammals must pump relatively more blood per unit of time than larger mammals. Therefore, it is logical that the malleable biochemical systems of cardiac muscle would adjust to accommodate the differences in physiological demands of different-sized mammals. The physiological demand, as expressed by the cardiac minute work rate of a mammal's heart, is the mathematical product of stroke work times the frequency of contractions per minute (i.e., heart rate). Among the different-sized mammals compared, a number of hemodynamic parameters remain constant, including oxygen transport capacity per volume of blood, arterial blood pressure, stroke work index, and ventricular wall stress per unit mass of tissue (14, 20, 24). Therefore, the primary determinant of cardiac minute work among different mammals is heart rate.

The other well-known determinant of the biochemical character of cardiac muscle, besides physiological demand, is the thyroidal trophic influence (30, 47). The thyroidal influence on different mammalian hearts was assumed to be constant because the plasma thyroid hormone concentrations among mammals has been reported to

THREE BIOCHEMICAL SYSTEMS

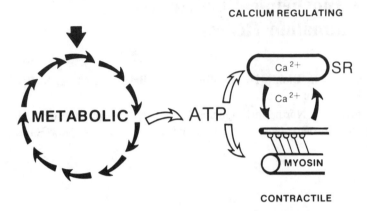

Figure 1.   Three major biochemical systems that determine physiological expression of muscle. Substrate-derived energy is transduced by the metabolic system into ATP, which is required by the calcium-regulating and contractile systems to perform their respective functions in the muscle cell.

be similar (26, 37). The overall purpose of the studies described in this paper has been to determine whether the functional demand associated with myocardial contraction frequency is significantly related to the capacities of the three central biochemical systems (Figure 1) that bestow physiological expression to cardiac muscle.

Another study summarized in this paper tested the hypothesis that heart rate is the hemodynamic correlate of these three central biochemical systems (Figure 1). A chronic perturbation in heart rate was imposed on the hearts of large mammals. To accomplish this, cardiac pacemakers were surgically implanted in Yorkshire pigs, with the pulse generators set at about twice the normal resting heart rate for 5-6 weeks. The adaptations in the biochemical character were then determined and compared with predicted results from the allometric equations of the comparative heart study.

The specific purposes of these studies were (a) to determine the correlative and proportional relationships between heart rate and heart mass and the capacity of these three biochemical systems, (b) to determine to what extent the capacities of these systems exist in normal mammalian hearts, and (c) to determine whether experimentally imposed tachycardia on the heart of a large mammal will result in the biochemical adaptations predicted from the allometric equations derived from the comparative mammalian heart data.

Methods

Biochemical parameters of the ventricular myocardium were compared among animals from 7 mammalian orders: C.D.-1 mouse, $n = 4$-6; Sprague Dawley rat,

n = 4-5; Hartley guinea pig, n = 4-5; New Zealand white rabbit, n = 4-6; mongrel dog, n = 4-9; Yorkshire swine, n = 5-9; Hereford cattle, n = 4-6. With the exception of cattle, hearts were removed following anesthesia of the animals with sodium pentobarbitol (60 mg/kg, ip). Cattle hearts were removed following exsanguination of the animals. Ventricular myocardial tissue was either quickly frozen in liquid nitrogen and stored at $-70°$ C or immediately processed for enzymatic analyses.

Chronic tachycardia was experimentally imposed for 35-42 days on hearts of 9 Yorkshire pigs with initial weights of 25 kg by surgically implanting cardiac pacemakers (Medtronics of Canada Ltd.). The pacemaker lead was attached to the left atrium, and the pulse generator was set at 180 pulses per minute, which is approximately twice the normal adult pig's resting heart rate. Control pigs were sham operated and had a suture placed in the left atrium instead of the pacemaker lead. Following 5-6 weeks of pacing, the pigs were sacrificed by exsanguination while under anesthesia, and the hearts were excised from the animals.

Maximal enzymatic activities of citrate synthase (CS) and oxoglutarate dehydrogenase (ODH) were determined according to Srere (42) and Cooney et al. (13), respectively. The capacity of myocardial beta-oxidation of fatty acids was assessed using maximal 3-hydroxyacyl-CoA dehydrogenase activity (HADH) (5). Myocardial glycogenolytic and glycolytic capacities were determined from maximal activities of total phosphorylase (PHOS), (32), phosphofructokinase (PFK), (40) and hexokinase (HK) (5). Substrate utilization was measured from the production of radioactively labeled $^{14}CO_2$ from [U-^{14}C]-glucose (GLU) or [1-^{14}C]-palmitate (PAL) in the incubation media, as described by others (3, 6, 7). The microsomal fraction of myocardial sarcoplasmic reticulum (SR) was isolated by differential centrifugation according to the procedures of Harigya and Schwartz (19), using the modifications of O'Brien et al. (33). The SR-Ca^{2+} ATPase activity was determined as described by O'Brien (34).

Cardiac myofibrils were isolated from muscle homogenates as previously reported by Solaro et al. (41). Myofibrillar-ATPase (MF-ATPase) and myosin ATPase (M-ATPase) activities (pH 7.0) were measured according to Baldwin et al. (2) and Pagani and Solaro (35), respectively. M-ATPase activity was assayed from the purified myofibrils and calculated assuming that myosin constitutes 42% of the myofibrillar protein (31). Total protein was determined following the procedures of Lowry et al. (29), using bovine serum albumin as the standard. Isozymes of myosin were electrophoretically separated from crude homogenates as described by Hoh et al. (22).

Myocardial tissue was fixed for electron microscopy as described by Lee et al. (27). Transverse and longitudinal sections were mounted in single-slot formvar-coated grids and examined with a Philips EM200 or EM201. Mitochondrial and myofibrillar areas from composite electron micrographs (8,000× magnification) were digitized from tracings on acetate sheets using a Numonics Corp. Electronic Graphics Calculator. Digitized data were confirmed from weighed acetate tracings of cells that were partitioned into myofibrillar, mitochondrial, and residual cellular areas.

One-way analysis of variance and Duncan's Multiple Range Test were used to determine statistical differences between biochemical parameters (p < .05). The degree of association between two average values was determined by the Pearson product moment correlation coefficient. Statistically significant correlation coefficients are identified with an asterisk (*). Linear regression analysis of log-log data was used for estimation of the equation of the line of best fit for related variables. Confidence intervals were calculated for the estimate of the slope of the regression line. Homogeneity of independent regressions was tested to determine whether two independent slope estimates could be considered to be estimates of a common slope (44). Slopes of the power equations are statistically different when exponents are different by 0.05.

Results and Discussion

The allometric relationship between body mass and heart mass among the 7 different mammals used in this study is shown in Figure 2. This proportional relationship has been well established (24, 25, 43) and is in agreement with the data from this study. The percentage of heart mass relative to body mass ranged from 0.15% to 0.85%. Heart mass also had a significant relationship with the established resting heart rates of these 7 mammals (8, 11) (Figure 3). The exponent for the power equation was similar to that of Holt et al. (24). In this study the biochemical parameters are compared to heart mass. The reader, in order to make the association between physiological demand and biochemical capacities, will therefore need to keep in mind that heart mass is significantly correlated with the hemodynamic parameter of heart rate.

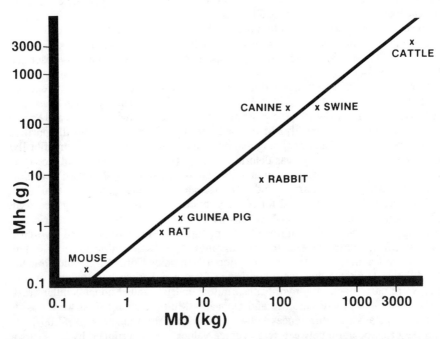

Figure 2.   Scaling of heart mass to body mass. Ranges of mammalian heart and body masses exceed 5 orders of magnitude between mice and cattle. A positive linear relationship exists between these two physiological parameters when the data are transformed into base 10 log and graphed as log-log plots.

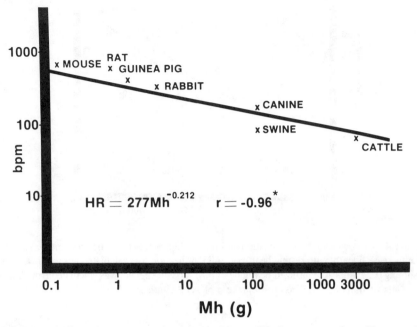

Figure 3. Scaling of heart rate to heart mass. Mammalian heart rate scales with a negative slope to heart mass and is significantly correlated to heart mass of the animal.

As indicated above, heart rate is the primary determinant of the energetic requirements of the myocardium. To illustrate this, estimates of ATP utilization and oxygen consumption for the heart rates of these 7 mammals are shown in Figure 4. The value of 0.21 μmol ATP utilized per beat per gram of heart (48) was used in these calculations, with the assumption that this remained constant among the different mammals. These basic underlying relationships shown in Figures 2, 3, and 4 provide a basis on which the correlative association between physiological function and the comparative biochemical findings of this study can be related.

Allometric Scaling of Metabolism

The glycogenolytic and glycolytic capacities were estimated by determining the maximal enzyme activities of PHOS and PFK, respectively. The average activity for PHOS for all the mammalian hearts was 18 μmol per gram per minute. The enzyme activities among the hearts were not proportional to heart size or heart rate. This was also the case for the glycolytic enzyme, PFK, which had an average activity of 39 μmol per gram per minute. The log-log plots of the allometric power equations do not show a proportional relationship between heart mass and glycogenolytic and glycolytic capacities (Figure 5). These findings show that the myocardial glycogenolytic/glycolytic capacities are constant among the mammals' hearts and are not related to heart mass or heart rate. This is different than skeletal muscle glycolytic capacity, which has been shown to scale positively with mammal size (16).

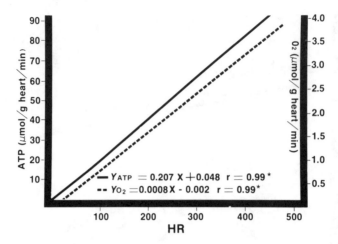

Figure 4. Myocardial ATP utilization and oxygen uptake. ATP utilization and oxygen uptake increase linearly with resting heart rate. ATP utilization was calculated per g of heart/min, assuming 0.21 μmol ATP utilized/beat/g heart (48). Oxygen uptake was calculated from known constants of mitochondrial oxygen uptake/mol ATP synthesized.

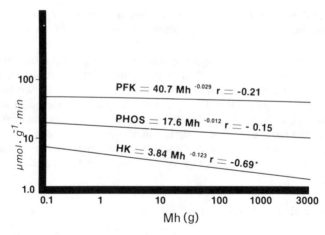

Figure 5. Glycolytic capacity of mammalian myocardia. Glycolytic capacity is represented by maximal activities of phosphorylase (PHOS), phosphofructokinase (PFK), and hexokinase (HK).

However, the activity of hexokinase, an enzyme classically categorized as glycolytic, scales proportionately to heart mass (Figure 5), with a negative slope comparable to those of the mitochondrial enzymes (Figure 6). This finding is consistent with hexokinase being an adaptable enzyme that responds in a similar way to the mitochondrial enzymes with exercise training (23) and chronic electrical stimulation of skeletal muscle (21).

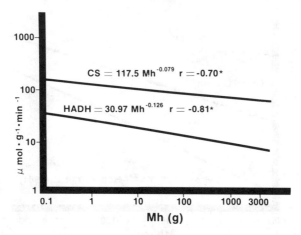

Figure 6. Oxidative capacity of mammalian myocardia. The oxidative capacity was assessed from maximal citrate synthase (CS) and 3-hydroxyacyl-CoA dehydrogenase (HADH) activities.

Our interpretation of these findings is that the differences in the energetic requirements of mammalian hearts are not reflected in proportional differences in the glycolytic potential. Therefore, myocardial glycolytic capacity is not apparently regulated by function but by either intrinsic myogenic or other epigenetic factors.

The capacities of the Krebs cycle and the beta-oxidation of fatty acids were estimated using CS and HADH activities, respectively. CS activities in cattle hearts averaged 73 μmol per gram per minute, compared to 181 in mice. This 2.5-fold difference had a significant negative correlation with heart mass (Figure 6) and a positive correlation with heart rate ($r = 0.86*$). Because CS has been questioned as being a good marker for aerobic potential (13), we compared CS activity to that of ODH in the hearts of 4 different mammals. CS activities were highly correlated with ODH activities ($r = 0.98*$), with comparable incremental differences between the hearts. Total CS activity per heart was calculated in order to compare the scaling relationship with the total mitochondrial volume per heart as reported by Hoppeler et al. (25), as shown in Figure 7. The scaling exponents, as would be expected, were similar (i.e., 0.92 for CS and 0.96 for mitochondrial volume). The correlative relationship between total CS activity and the estimated cardiac work rate (CWR) per minute per heart (24) is shown in Figure 8. This emphasizes that there is significant and proportional association ($r = 0.99*$) between the aerobic potential and cardiac minute work. HADH had a 3-fold range in activity from the cow to the mouse, with a scaling exponent to heart mass similar to that of CS (Figure 6). HADH activity was also significantly correlated with resting heart rate ($r = 0.93*$).

As an added confirmation of the relationships among aerobic metabolic potential, heart size, and heart rate, ^{14}C-glucose and ^{14}C-palmitate oxidation rates were determined. The oxidation rates of these substrates were inversely related to heart mass (Figure 9) and directly related to heart rate (i.e., $r_{GLU} = 0.88*$, $r_{PAL} = 0.94*$). The rates of substrate oxidation were also highly correlated with the activities of the two mitochondrial enzymes, CS ($r_{GLU} = 0.86*$), and HADH ($r_{PAL} = 0.98*$). These comparative differences in aerobic potential were also observed morphologically from

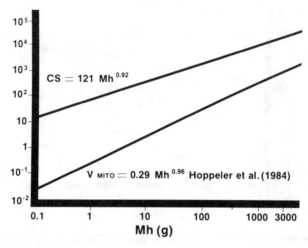

Figure 7. Myocardial mitochondrial density and total citrate synthase activity. Total CS activity scales similarly to the mitochondrial density of mammalian hearts (25) relative to heart mass. Total CS activity is expressed as μmol • min^{-1} • gram^{-1}.

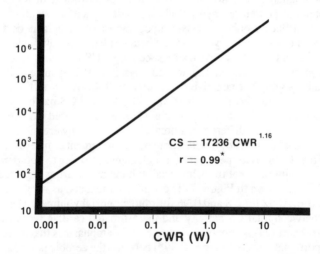

Figure 8. Relationship between myocardial total citrate synthase activity. Total CS activity is significantly correlated with cardiac work rate (CWR) of mammalian hearts.

electron micrographs of heart tissue from cattle ($n = 2$) and mice ($n = 2$) (Figure 10). The percentage of mitochondrial area in longitudinal sections was 19% and 38% for cattle and mice, respectively.

In summary, the major point of these findings is that the aerobic potential of the myocardia from different-sized mammals is highly correlated with heart mass and, therefore, the hemodynamic parameter of heart rate. This suggests that a causal relationship may exist between the frequency of myocardial contractions and the level of myocardial aerobic capacity, at least, when stroke work remains constant.

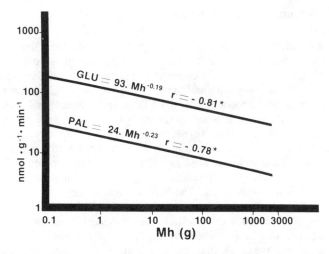

Figure 9. Myocardial substrate oxidation capacity and ^{14}C-glucose and ^{14}C-palmitate oxidation rates are inversely correlated with heart mass. Myocardial substrate oxidation rates were 10-fold higher in smaller than in larger animals.

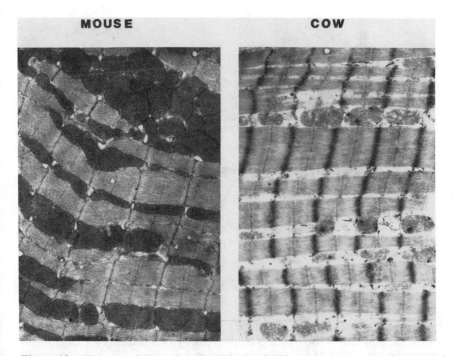

Figure 10. Electron micrographs (magnification 8,000×) of mouse and cattle ventricular myocardial tissue. Comparisons of mitochondrial area are presented in the text.

Scaling of Calcium Regulatory Capacity

The sarcoplasmic reticulum (SR) is the organelle that controls the timing of the contraction-relaxation cycle by its fine and rapid regulation of sarcoplasmic calcium (12). SR-Ca^{2+} ATPase activity, the enzymatic expression of the Ca^{2+} pump, is correlated with Ca^{2+} uptake capacity and the rate of myocardial relaxation (38); it has been estimated to consume about 30% of the ATP in active cardiac and skeletal muscle (1, 36). In this study and in another recent study (33), we hypothesized heart rate to be a hemodynamic correlate of SR calcium uptake capacity. Knowing that myocardial SR-Ca^{2+} uptake capacity was adaptable and correlated with the diastolic period, it seems logical it would alter its calcium-sequestering capacity to accommodate inherent chronotropic differences in rate. These comparative heart data are in agreement with this hypothesis. The SR-Ca^{2+} uptake capacity, as indicated by the SR-Ca^{2+} ATPase in the microsomal fraction, was highly correlated both with heart mass (Figure 11) and with the differences in resting heart rates (r = 0.98*). These findings are also in agreement with a recent morphological study showing a greater relative volume of SR in hearts with high beating rates compared to those with slower beating rates (17). We found a 30% smaller cross-sectional area of myofibrils in the mouse compared to the cow, which is consistent with the increased calcium flux in and out of myofibrils in mammal hearts with high contraction frequencies. These results are consistent with the above hypothesis that the differences in contraction-relaxation times associated with different heart rates is a determinant of myocardial calcium uptake capacity.

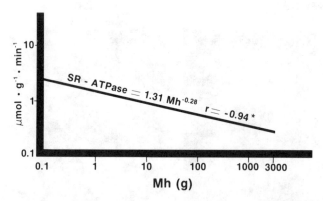

Figure 11. Ca^{2+} regulation capacity of mammalian myocardia. SR-ATPase activity decreases significantly as heart mass increases. SR-ATPase activities were approximately 13-fold higher in mouse than cattle hearts.

Scaling of the Contractile System

The myosin ATPase activity of different skeletal and cardiac muscles has been shown to have a positive correlation with the velocity of shortening (4, 15, 18) and an inverse relationship with the economy of maintaining force (36, 39). From these studies and that of Lompre et al. (28)—which showed that hearts of smaller mammals expressed the V_1 myosin (high ATPase activity) phenotype, whereas larger mammals expressed the V_3 (low ATPase activity) isoform—we postulated that myosin and myofibrillar ATPase activities would be congruent with the frequency of myocardial contractions. We did, however, modify this postulate to take into consideration that the ATPases are determined primarily by the ventricular myosin isoforms, of which there are only three. Therefore, if heart rate is the hemodynamic correlate with myosin types, there may be threshold frequencies that result in stepwise increments in the myosin and myofibrillar ATPase activities, instead of a smooth gradation across these different mammalian hearts.

The myosin (M) and myofibrillar (MF) ATPase activities are presented in Figure 12. The M-ATPase activities ranged from 0.21 to 1.40 μmol P_i per mg protein per min. The largest incremental change in activity, which was 4-fold, occurred between the guinea pig and the rat. These M-ATPase activities are comparable to those summarized by Swynghedauw (45). The MF-ATPase activities ranged from 0.17 to 0.40 μmol per mg protein per min, with a 2.4-fold incremental step in the level of activity between the guinea pig and the rat (Figure 12). The differences in the proportions of myosin isoforms are consistent with the differences in M- and MF-ATPase activities between the guinea pig and the rat (Figure 13). These data show

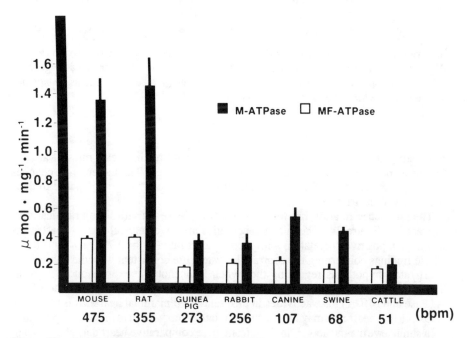

Figure 12.   Myosin (M-) and myofibrillar (MR-) ATPase activities in mammalian myocardia. M- and MF-ATPase activities display a stepwise increment in hearts of mammals having resting heart rates greater than 300 bpm. The histogram illustrates average activity and standard deviation for species. MF-ATPase activity and M-ATPase activity are represented by open and solid bars, respectively.

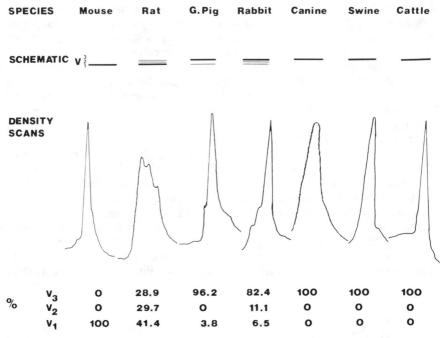

SPECIES	Mouse	Rat	G.Pig	Rabbit	Canine	Swine	Cattle

Figure 13. Native myosin isoforms. The proportions of ventricular native myosin (V_1, V_2, V_3) from mammalian hearts are illustrated schematically as isoforms separated by gel electrophoresis (top row), as densiometric scans of the gels (middle row), and as quantitation of the integrated tracings of the gels (bottom).

that mammal heart mass of 1 gram or less, and with resting heart rates of at least 300 beats per min, express primarily the V_1 myosin type. The incremental changes observed between these 2 mammals are disproportionately large compared to their difference in heart rates.

The allometric relationship for M- and MF-ATPase activities are graphically illustrated in Figure 14. The ATPase activities are inversely related to heart mass and have a positive correlation with resting heart rate ($r_M = 0.77*$, $r_{MF} = 0.81*$). These findings concerning the contractile system are consistent with the "threshold heart rate" hypothesis regarding the switch in phenotypic expression of myosin. These findings also agree with heart rate being the physiological correlate of M-ATPase and MF-ATPase activities in different-sized mammal hearts. It is therefore plausible that heart rate may have a causal relationship with myosin gene expression.

In summary, the metabolic findings from these comparative heart data show strong correlative relationships between heart mass and heart rate with each of the three major biochemical systems studied. The only exception was the glycolytic component of the metabolic system.

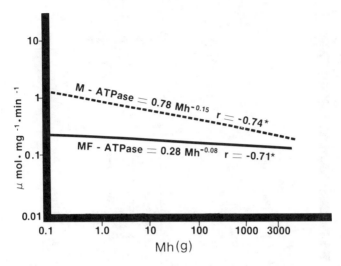

Figure 14.   Scaling of myosin (M-) and myofibrillar (MF-) ATPase activities to heart mass. M- and MF-ATPase activities scale inversely with base 10 log of heart mass and with resting heart rate. M- and MF-ATPase were approximately 7- and 2.5-fold higher in mouse than cattle hearts, respectively.

Range of Capacities of These Myocardial Biochemical Systems

It was also the purpose of this comparative heart study to gain insight into the extent to which these major biochemical systems exist in normal mammalian hearts. The range of capacities of these systems in the mouse compared to the cow, as indicated by the marker enzyme activities for the respective systems, are illustrated in Figure 15.

The Krebs cycle and β-oxidative components of the metabolic system had a 2.5- to 3.2-fold range in their capacities among these different orders of mammalian hearts, whereas the glycolytic component had a range that differed between some mammals by 30-50%, which was independent of heart mass and heart rate among the different-sized hearts. The Ca^{2+}-regulating capacity had a 13-fold difference among these hearts, with a significant allometric relationship with heart mass and resting heart rate. The differences in the contractile system enzyme activities were 6.4-fold for M-ATPase and 2.4-fold for the MF-ATPase.

The range of capacities observed among hearts from these different orders of mammals provides a framework from which myocardial biochemical adaptations can be considered and provides an understanding of the extent to which the proportional relationships of these systems can exist without pathological consequences. Disruption of the proportionate relationships of these biochemical systems may confer physiological myocardial failure, as may a pathological influence on a single biochemical system.

158   Ianuzzo et al.

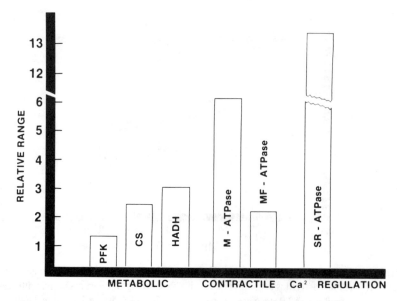

METABOLIC   CONTRACTILE   Ca² REGULATION

Figure 15. Extent of myocardial biochemical capacities. This figure represents the percentage of difference in biochemical capacities between the mouse (RHR = 475) and cattle (RHR = 51).

Biochemical Adaptations With Chronic Tachycardia

To further test whether our underlying hypothesis from the comparative heart data was correct (i.e., whether comparative myocardial chronotropism is the physiological parameter that sets the biochemical capacities of cardiac muscle), we experimentally imposed chronic tachycardia on the hearts of mammals and compared the empirical adaptations of these biochemical systems with the predicted outcomes using the allometric relationships. We expected that chronic tachycardia imposed on the heart of a large mammal would result in biochemical adaptations that would cause it to resemble the heart of a smaller mammal. In these experiments chronic tachycardia at 180 bpm was imposed on hearts of pigs for 35-42 days (described in Methods section above). The empirical results of this study and the allometric predictions are shown in Figure 16.

The empirical findings for the metabolic systems show no significant change in the glycolytic potential, as indicated by PFK activity. The allometric equation for PFK and heart mass and the statistical comparisons of maximal activities among the different sized hearts indicated PFK activity is heart rate and heart mass independent. The allometric equation for PFK and heart rate (i.e., PFK = 19 HR$^{0.14}$, r = 0.65) predicted a 15% increase, which is within 1 standard deviation (SD) from the mean of the determined PFK activity. The experimental findings for Krebs cycle (CS activity) and fat oxidation (HADH activity) capacities showed a 20% and a 42% increase, respectively. The respective predicted changes were 39% and 57%. The allometric predictions for the CS activity in the paced hearts were within 2 SD of the empirical activity, and the predicted HADH activity was less than 1/2 of an SD from the actual mean activity.

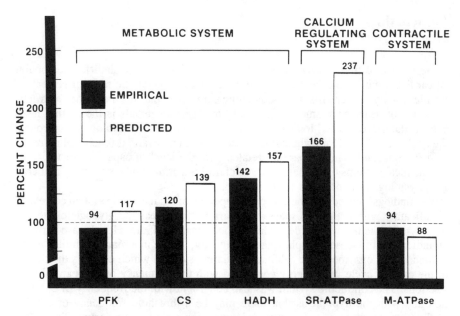

Figure 16. Comparison of the empirical findings from cardiac pacing to that of the allometric predictions. Empirical findings are illustrated as solid bars, predicted findings as open bars. These data represent the close association of myocardial chronotropism with the biochemical character of the muscle.

The sarcoplasmic reticulum Ca^{2+}-pumping capacity, as predicted from the comparative heart data, was expected to increase to accommodate chronic tachycardia. The allometric equation used in this prediction was $SR = 9.5 \times 10^{-4} HR^{1.26}$. This equation took into consideration that these were not adult pigs and were pigs with estimated heart rates of approximately 90 bpm. The predicted percentage of change in SR-Ca^{2+} ATPase was 137%; the actual observed change was 66% (Figure 16). Although the empirical findings were less than predicted, they are in agreement with the hypothesis that heart rate is a determinant of myocardial SR-Ca^{2+} ATPase activity.

The biochemical markers used for the contractile system remained unchanged following tachycardia. The myosin ATPase activity was similar in both the paced and the nonpaced hearts (Figure 16). The electrophoretogram of nondisassociated myosin exhibited only a single band that migrated at the same rate as that of the nonpaced heart (i.e., V_3). The predicted outcome from the comparative heart data was that myosin ATPase and the myosin phenotype would remain the same at a heart rate of 180 bpm. A change in myosin would not be expected to occur until a heart rate of approximately 300 bpm was reached. Thus, the empirical and predicted results are in agreement.

In summary, these experiments have tested the hypothesis that comparative myocardial chronotropism is the hemodynamic correlate, and possibly the determinant, of the capacities of the three major biochemical systems of cardiac muscle. Chronic experimental tachycardia was imposed on the hearts of pigs; the empirical findings are in agreement with the allometric predictions and therefore support the above hypothesis.

Conclusion

Hearts from different-sized mammals are required to accomplish different amounts of cardiac minute work because of the differences in metabolic rates of larger and smaller mammals. The main hemodynamic parameter that sets the higher energetic demands of heart from smaller compared to larger mammals is the resting heart rate. It therefore seemed logical that by using a comparative biological approach, we could gain insight into whether the differences in myocardial functional demands of different-sized mammals are correlated with the level of capacities of the three biochemical systems (i.e., metabolic, calcium-regulating, and contractile) that confer physiological expression to muscle.

The findings showed that the aerobic component of the metabolic system correlated significantly with both heart mass and heart rate, whereas the glycogenolytic and glycolytic capacities were independent of heart mass and rate. Hexokinase activity, an indicator of glucose phosphorylating capacity, scaled in a manner similar to the mitochondrial enzymes. The calcium-regulating system, which controls the timing of the cardiac cycle, was highly correlated with the frequency of myocardial contractions. The contractile system was also congruent with the frequency of contraction and with the hypothesis that there may be a threshold frequency of cardiac contractions at which a switch in myosin phenotypic expression occurs. To further test whether inherent myocardial chronotropism is the physiological parameter that sets the level of biochemical capacities of cardiac muscle, experimental tachycardia was imposed on hearts of swine. The empirical findings agreed with the allometric predictions from the comparative findings and therefore support the hypothesis. The general conclusion from these findings is that resting heart rate is the hemodynamic correlate of the capacities of the three biochemical systems that bestow physiological expression to cardiac muscle.

Acknowledgments

The authors wish to thank Mary Lou Ashton for her excellent technical assistance in accomplishing the electron microscopy and Valerie Baddon for her excellent secretarial support in preparing this manuscript. The studies summarized in this paper were supported by grants from the Ontario Heart and Stroke Foundation and the Natural Sciences and Engineering Research Council of Canada.

References

1. Alpert, N.; Mulieri, L. Heat, mechanics, and myosin ATPase in normal and hypertrophied heart muscle. Fed. Proc. 41:192-198; 1982.
2. Baldwin, K.M., Cooke, D.A.; Cheadle, W.G. Time course adaptations in cardiac and skeletal muscle to different running programs. J. Appl. Physiol. 42:267-272; 1977.

3. Baldwin, K.M.; Hooker, A.M.; Herrick, R.E. Schrader, L.F. Respiratory capacity and glycogen depletion in thyroid-deficient muscle. J. Appl. Physiol. 49:102-106; 1980.

4. Barany, M. ATPase activity of myosin correlated with speed of muscle shortening. J. Gen. Physiol. 40:197-216; 1967.

5. Bass, A.; Brdiczka, D.; Eyer, P.; Hofer, S.; Pette, D. Metabolic differentiation of distinct muscle types at the level of enzymatic organization. Eur. J. Biochem. 10:198-206; 1969.

6. Beatty, C.H.; Peterson, R.D.; Basinger, G.M.; Bocek, R.M. Major metabolic pathways for carbohydrate metabolism of voluntary skeletal muscle. Am. J. Physiol. 210:404-410; 1966.

7. Beatty, C.H.; Young, M.K.; Bocek, R.M. Respiration and metabolism by homogenates of various types of muscle. Am. J. Physiol. 223:1232-1236; 1972.

8. Biology data book. 2d ed. Altman, P.L.; Dittmer, D.S., eds. Bethesda, MD: Fed. Soc. Exp. Biol.; 1979:1688-1692. (Vol. 3).

9. Blank, S.; Chen, V.; Hamilton, N.; Salerno, T.; Ianuzzo, C.D. Metabolic characteristics of mammalian myocardia. (Unpublished manuscript).

10. Blank, S., Chen, V.; Ianuzzo, C.D. Biochemical characteristics of mammalian diaphragms. Respir. Physiol. 74:115-126; 1988.

11. Canadian Council on Animal Care. Guide to the care and use of experimental animals. Ottawa: Author; 1980:83. (Vol. 1).

12. Carafoli, E. The homeostasis of calcium in heart cells. J. Mol. Cell. Cardiol. 17:203-212; 1985.

13. Cooney, G.; Taegtmeyer, H.; Newsholme, E.A. Tricarboxylic acid cycle flux and enzyme activities in the isolated working rat heart. Biochem. J. 200:701-703; 1981.

14. Coulson, R.; Hernandez, T.; Herbert, J. Metabolic rate, enzyme kinetics *in vivo*. Comp. Biochem. Physiol. 56A:251-262; 1977.

15. Delcayre, C.; Swynghedauw, B. A comparative study of heart myosin. Pflügers Arch. 355:39-47; 1975.

16. Emmett, B.; Hochachka, P. Scaling of oxidative and glycolytic enzymes in mammals. Respir. Physiol. 45:261-272; 1981.

17. Forbes, M., Hawkey, L.; Jirge, S.; Sperelakis, N. The sarcoplasmic reticulum of mouse heart: its divisions, configurations and distribution. J. Ultrastr. Res. 93:1-16; 1985.

18. Hamrell, B.; Low, R. The relationship of mechanical V_{max} to myosin ATPase activity in rabbit and marmot ventricular muscle. Pflügers Arch. 377:119-124; 1978.

19. Harigya, S.; Schwartz, A. Rate of calcium binding and uptake in normal animal and failing human cardiac muscle. Circ. Res. 25:781-794; 1969.

20. Henderson, A.; Craig, R.; Sonnenblick, E.; Urschel, C. Species differences in intrinsic myocardial contractility. Proc. Soc. Exp. Biol. Med. 134:930-932; 1970.

21. Henriksson, J.; Chi, M.; Hintz, C.; Young, D.; Kaiser, K.; Salmons, S.; Lowry, O.H. Chronic stimulation of mammalian muscle: changes in enzymes of six metabolic pathways. Am. J. Physiol. 251:C614-C632; 1986.

22. Hoh, J.F.Y.; McGrath, P.A.; Hale, P.T. Electrophoretic analysis of multiple forms of rat cardiac myosin: effects of hypophysectomy and thyroxine replacement. J. Mol. Cell. Cardiol. 10:1053-1076; 1978.

23. Holloszy, J.; Booth, F. Biochemical adaptations to endurance exercise in muscle. Annu. Rev. Physiol. 38:273-291; 1976.

24. Holt, J., Rhode, E.; Kines, H. Ventricular volumes and body weights in mammals. Am. J. Physiol. 215:704-715; 1968.

25. Hoppeler, H.; Lindstedt, S.; Classen, H.; Taylor, R.; Mathieu, O.; Weibel, E. Scaling mitochondrial volumes in heart to body mass. Respir. Physiol. 55:131-137; 1984.

26. Larsson, M.; Pettersson, T.; Carlstrom, A. Thyroid hormone binding in serum of 15 vertebrate species: isolation of thyroxine binding globulin and prealbumin analog. Gen. Comp. Endocrinol. 58:360-375; 1985.

27. Lee, R.M.; McKeenzie, R.; Kobayashi, K.; Garfield, R.E.; Forrest, J.B.; Daniel, E.E. Effects of glutaraldehyde fixation osmolarities on smooth muscle cell volume and osmotic reactivity of cells after fixation. J. Microsc. 125:77-88; 1982.

28. Lompre, A.M.; Mercadier, J.; Wesnewsky, C.; Bouveret, P.; Pantaloni, C.; D'Albio, A.; Schwartz, K. Species- and age-dependent changes in the relative amounts of cardiac myosin isoenzymes in mammals. Dev. Biol. 84:286-290; 1981.

29. Lowry, O.H.; Rosebrough, N.J.; Farr, A.L.; Randall, R.J. Protein measurement with the Folin phenol reagent. J. Biol. Chem. 193:265-275; 1951.

30. Morkin, E.; Flink, I.; Goldman, S. Biochemical and physiologic effects of thyroid hormone on cardiac performance. Prog. Cardiovasc. Dis. 25:435-464; 1983.

31. Nakanishi, T.; Nagae, M.; Takao, A. Developmental changes in contractile protein adenosine 5'-triphosphatase in rabbit heart. Circ. Res. 58:890-895; 1986.

32. Noble, E.G.; Ianuzzo, C.D. Influence of training on skeletal muscle enzymatic adaptations in normal and diabetic rats. Am. J. Physiol. 249:E360-E365; 1985.

33. O'Brien, P.; Ling, E.; Williams, H.; Brotherton, S.; Salerno, T.A.; Lumsden, J.H.; Ianuzzo, C.D. Compensatory adaptation of the heart to chronic rate overload: increase in Ca^{2+} transport ATPase activity of myocardial sarcoplasmic reticulum. Can. J. Cardiol. 4:243-250; 1988.

34. O'Brien, P.J. Porcine malignant hyperthermia susceptibility: increased calcium sequestering activity of skeletal muscle sarcoplasmic reticulum. Can. J. Vet. Res. 50:329-337; 1986.

35. Pagani, E.D.; Solaro, R.J. Swimming exercise, thyroid state, and the distribution of myosin isoenzymes in rat heart. Am. J. Physiol. 245:H713-H720; 1983.

36. Rall, J. Energetic aspects of skeletal muscle contraction: implications of fiber types. Exerc. Sport Sci. Rev. 13:33-74; 1985.

37. Reap, M.; Cass, C.; Hightower, D. Thyroxine and triiodothyronine levels in ten species of animals. Southwestern Vet. 31:31-34; 1978.

38. Rodgers, R.; Black, S.; Katz, S.; McNeill, J. Thyroidectomy of SHR: effects on ventricular relaxation and on SR calcium uptake activity. Am. J. Physiol. 250:H861-H865; 1986.

39. Rupp, H. Polymorphic myosin as the common determinant of myofibrillar ATPase in different haemodynamic and thyroid states. Basic Res. Cardiol. 77:34-46; 1982.

40. Shonk, C.E.; Boxer, G.E. Enzyme patterns in human tissue: I. Method for determination of glycolytic enzymes. Cancer Res. 24:709-721; 1964.

41. Solaro, R.J.; Pang, D.C.; Briggs, F.N. Purification of cardiac myofibrils with Triton X-100. Biochim. Biophys. Acta 245:259-262; 1971.

42. Srere, P.A. Citrate synthase. Methods Enzymol. 13:3-8; 1969.

43. Stahl, W. Organ weights in primates and in other mammals. Science 150:1039-1042; 1965.

44. Steel, R.G.D.; Torrie, J.H. Principles and procedures of statistics: a biometrical approach. 2d ed. New York: McGraw-Hill Book Co.; 1980.

45. Swynghedauw, B. Developmental and functional adaptation of contractile proteins in cardiac and skeletal muscle. Physiol. Rev. 66(3):710-771; 1986.

46. Taylor, R. Structural and functional limits to oxidative metabolism: Insights from scaling. Annu. Rev. Physiol. 49:135-146; 1987.

47. Williams, H.; Ianuzzo, C.D. The effects of triiodothyronine on cultured neonatal rat cardiac myocytes. J. Mol. Cell. Cardiol. 20:689-699; 1988.

48. Wilson, D.; Nishiki, K.; Erecinska, M. Energy metabolism in muscle and its regulation during individual contraction-relaxation cycles. TIBS 6:16-19; 1981.

PART IV

Muscle Bioenergetics

The Role of the Phosphocreatine Energy Shuttle in Exercise and Muscle Hypertrophy

Samuel P. Bessman and Fatemeh Savabi

University of Southern California, Los Angeles, California, U.S.A.

The conventional view of the energy transfer leading to muscle contraction is depicted in Figure 1, which shows that ATP is formed in mitochondria and diffuses to myofibrils. ADP, formed on muscle contraction, diffuses back to the mitochondria, stimulating respiratory activity in the process called respiratory control. The first evidence for the important role of phosphocreatine (PCr) in muscle metabolism was demonstrated by Belitzer (1). He observed that creatine added to muscle minces stimulated oxygen uptake. The creatine (Cr) was converted to PCr, believed to be the energy compound for muscle contraction. In 1966 Bessman and Fonyo (4) presented quantitative data for the respiratory control of pigeon breast muscle mitochondria by Cr, which led to the suggestion of the feedback regulation of respiration in response to muscle contraction, accomplished through a reciprocal diffusion of Cr and PCr between mitochondria and myofibrils (Figure 2), called the phosphocreatine energy shuttle (5). For the past decade, data have accumulated supporting the existence of this shuttle in muscle. We will attempt here to clarify this shuttle and its connection to the growth response of muscle to emphasize the similarity that exists between the action of insulin and exercise.

Phosphocreatine Energy Shuttle

Phosphocreatine was until recently considered to act as a buffer for the resynthesis of ATP (Figure 1). This explanation, however, was inadequate to explain the outcome of many biochemical, physiological, and isotopic studies. The phosphocreatine energy shuttle (Figure 2) was first postulated by Bessman in 1954 (2). It was based on the metabolic similarity between muscle work and the administration of insulin to the diabetic (Figure 3). The following facts are the basis for the phosphocreatine energy shuttle: (a) the ability of Cr to stimulate mitochondrial respiration (4); (b) cessation of ischemic heart and skeletal muscle contraction while a large fraction of ATP still remained (18, 41); (c) evidence of compartmentation of adenine nucleotides (18, 35); (d) existence of localized specific isoenzymes of CPK at the mitochondria and myofibrils (34).

The phosphocreatine energy shuttle (Figure 2) includes three parts. First, there is the peripheral terminus of the shuttle, where the transport form of energy (PCr) is utilized by the bound CPK to rephosphorylate the ADP produced by the myofibrillar

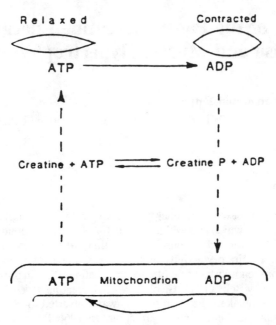

Figure 1. The energy transport–respiratory control system of muscle based on ATP-ADP shuttle and a buffer system of creatine and phosphocreatine (creatine P).

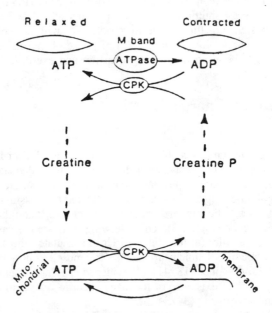

Figure 2. The phosphocreatine energy shuttle, showing the traffic of energy between two isoenzymes of creatine phosphokinase, one bound to the mitochondrion and one to the myofibril.

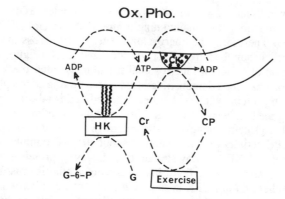

Figure 3. The acceptor role of insulin action, through hexokinase, and of exercise in the electron transport system of the mitochondrion.

ATPase. PCr is thus transduced to ATP, the utilizable form of energy, in situ as need arises (e.g., in muscle contraction). The chemical signal that muscle has contracted is the liberation of free Cr at or in the immediate vicinity of the contractile site. This signal then enters the intervening space (the second part of the shuttle), in which Cr and PCr diffuse in opposite directions. Cr arrives at the mitochondrial site, the energy-generating terminus (the third part) of the shuttle, where it interacts with the mitochondrial isoenzyme of CPK, which is bound closely to the translocase site, where the conditions are faborable for PCr production by transphosphorylation to Cr from the gamma phosphate of nascent ATP. These three processes, structurally immobilized as clusters of enzymes at mitochondrion and myofibril, permit immediate respiratory control, with the formation of ATP as needed for contraction. There is much experimental evidence for the presence of close functional interaction between CPK isoenzymes and the sites of ATP utilization and production, evidence in which the product of one is used as a substrate for the other. For example, at the mitochondrial site, the nascent ATP produced by mitochondrial oxidative phosphorylation has more favorable access to mitochondrial bound CPK for production of PCr than does extra mitochondrial ATP (12, 13). At the myofibrillar site, the ATP made via rephosphorylation of ADP by bound CPK using PCr, has better access to myofibrillar ATPase than does the general pool of ATP (7, 37, 38).

It has recently been shown that CPK is attached to many sites of ATP utilization, such as sarcoplasmic reticulum (24), sarcolemmal membrane (42), and ribosomes (25). Both skeletal and heart muscle sarcoplasmic reticulum contain significant CPK activity. The close spatial proximity between CPK and Ca^{2+}-dependent ATPase in the skeletal muscle sarcoplasmic reticulum already has been demonstrated by Khan et al. (24). It has been shown that CPK bound to the membrane maintains a much higher rate of Ca^{2+} uptake in the presence of PCr than with an added ATP regenerating system at the same adenine nucleotide concentration (27). It is evident that CPK bound to the sarcoplasmic reticulum represents an effective transphosphorylation system, maintaining the concentration of ATP available for the Ca^{2+} pump above the critical level necessary for rapid calcium sequestration during active relaxation in both cardiac and skeletal muscle. It has also been shown that in the presence of

PCr, plasma membrane CPK immediately rephosphorylates ADP produced in the Na⁺-K⁺ATPase reaction, thus maintaining a high and constant ATP:ADP ratio in the system (42). Therefore, the energy for ion transport across the surface membrane of the cell is supplied from PCr via localized CPK (Figure 4).

The association of CPK with microsomal fractions isolated from brain, skeletal muscle, and heart has been demonstrated (25, 32). The role of the phosphocreatine energy shuttle in protein synthesis has been studied in our laboratory by Carpenter et al. (9). Using the highly specific CPK inhibitor 2,4 dinitrofluorobenzene (DNFB), they showed that protein synthesis in diaphragm was inhibited in parallel with the inhibition of CPK activity to a maximum of about 70%. The inhibition was not due to a direct effect of DNFB on any step in the pathway of protein synthesis, for the same concentrations of DNFB didn't inhibit protein synthesis in isolated liver cells that contain neither PCr nor CPK in significant amounts. Further work has revealed that microsomal protein synthesis was supported more efficiently by phosphocreatine than by the regenerating system for ATP (36). The microsome is another example of a terminus for the PCr energy shuttle (Figure 4).

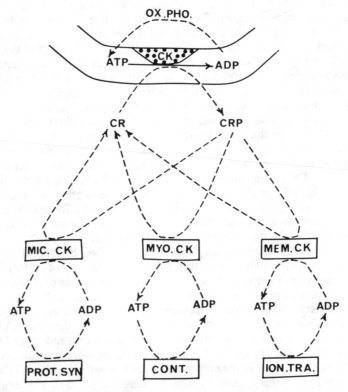

Figure 4. Schematic representation of the role of the phosphocreatine energy shuttle in various endergonic processes, such as protein synthesis, contraction, and ion transport. MYO, myofibril; MIC, microsome; MEM, membrane.

The Phosphocreatine Energy Shuttle in Muscle

The question of the necessity of the phosphocreatine energy shuttle for optimal muscle function has been debated for the last few years. When animals were fed beta-guanidinopropionic acid (β-GPA), an analog of Cr, their muscle Cr and PCr were replaced by β-GPA and phosphorylated β-guanidinopropionate (β-GPAP) (16). The total Cr concentration fell from 39 to 9.6 μmol/g, and the PCr concentration dropped from more than 20 to less than 2 μmol/g. Concomitantly, the ATP concentration fell from 6.8 to 3.2 μmol/g. In association with these biochemical changes, there were functional and structural changes as well (26, 33, 43). The functional changes, however, have been found to be considerable by some and less marked by others (28, 33, 43). Some investigators have therefore postulated that Cr and PCr are not critical for muscle function (28, 29), even though diseased and atrophied muscle are low in Cr and patients with muscle disease usually have abnormal Cr metabolism (14).

Careful analysis of the data from the laboratories of Fitch and others on this subject demonstrates a consistent relationship between the use of high-energy phosphate and tension development, which suggests the ability of β-GPAP to substitute for PCr (15). Although β-GPAP is a very poor substrate for CPK in vitro (10), it might be a rather good substrate in vivo due to compartmentation of enzymes and substrate, as its in vivo utilization suggests. The other factor that might be responsible for the discrepancy noted is that only a small portion of the intracellular Cr and PCr is involved in the energy transport process. We have recently shown that only about 8% of the total intracellular Cr is actually free to participate in the process of energy transport in heart (Savabi, submitted for publication). More than 55% of total intracellular Cr is present as PCr; the rest is somehow bound and not easily available for phosphorylation. We have also shown that the PCr pool is not a homogeneous pool, for ^{14}C-Cr labeling studies show that the most recently formed PCr breaks down most slowly during anoxia. Therefore, if only 8% of the normal amount of intracellular Cr remains after a few weeks of β-GPA feeding (as has been reported) or if β-GPA and β-GPAP can act as free Cr and PCr, then little, if any, functional disability would be apparent in this model of Cr-depleted muscle. If, on the other hand, as in the conventional view, there are homogenous pools of ATP and PCr, we should be able to see a much greater decrease in ATP in the Cr-depleted muscle than in the control after finite periods of muscular contraction. In fact, a smaller than expected drop in available ATP has been reported (15). This is apparently due to the fact that muscle performance is reduced somewhat in Cr-depleted muscles; the remaining Cr and PCr and their accumulated analogs are sufficient to maintain the energy shuttle.

The structural changes and atrophy seen in Cr-depleted muscles (26, 43) might be due either to the loss of bound Cr from intracellular protein (14), the cofactor effect of Cr on myosin synthesis, and/or the inability of the PCr energy shuttle to provide sufficient energy for protein synthesis. This is explained in the next section.

Creatine has been shown to stimulate the biosynthesis of myofibrillar protein in differentiating skeletal muscle cells both in vivo and in vitro (20-22). The response is concentration-dependent over the range of 10-100 μM and maximal over the range of 100 μM to 250 μM Cr. Note that the normal plasma concentration of Cr is 100 μM. The stimulation is specific because the rates of total protein and DNA synthesis are increased and the rate of degradation is not changed significantly.

Creatine also stimulates the uptake of amino acids into the contractile proteins. This finding is of considerable biological interest because if applicable to adult tissue, it suggests that the amount of load-bearing protein could hypertrophy in proportion to the rate of PCr hydrolysis, whereas an unused muscle that does not hydrolyze PCr and liberate free Cr rapidly would atrophy.

The importance of the intracellular Cr concentrations per se in the regulation of contractile proteins in mature muscle in vivo is not so clear. Studies by Hofmann et al. (19) have shown that the hydrolysis of PCr was the same after heavily and lightly loaded contractions, suggesting that the hypertrophy of isometric exercise may not be mediated by the intracellular Cr concentration. Although in this type of study the measured concentration of Cr or PCr might not change significantly, the rate of turnover might increase dramatically during heavily loaded contraction. On the other hand, according to our and others' studies, it seems that during the process of PCr synthesis or breakdown, there is a significant change only in free (unbound) Cr concentration (31, 40). Because most of the intracellular free Cr is bound and not available for phosphorylation (Savabi, submitted for publication), it is probably not available for participation in any other process such as energy transport for protein synthesis. The concentration of Cr per se might not be responsible for the stimulation of protein synthesis seen in physiologically active muscle; it might well be the increased transport of PCr in the intervening space during contraction that makes more energy available to the ribosomes (Figure 4). In other words, increased energy transport by the phosphocreatine energy shuttle during muscle contraction could be responsible for muscle growth.

Phosphocreatine Energy Shuttle and Hypertrophy of Exercised Muscle

It is well known that muscle size is influenced by its pattern of activity. Increased work demands lead to growth, and disuse induces tissue atrophy (8, 44). Growth of muscle correlates with the change in rates of protein synthesis and breakdown, with the return of full activity stimulating synthesis and inhibiting breakdown (17). The above changes are accompanied by changes in energy metabolism in the cell. An increased PCr content in skeletal muscle of dogs after training, but not in myocardium, has been reported by Keul et al. (23). This appears to be a physiologically valid difference in behavior, compatible with our proposal that exercise acts to stimulate protein synthesis by the increased contractile activity that causes more transport of PCr.

Apart from neuronal and hormonal effects on the structure and function of muscle (23, 45) that might cause changes in the rate of protein synthesis, the PCr energy shuttle can also increase the rate of protein synthesis by the contracting muscle. Figure 4 shows the way that the PCr energy shuttle can affect the rate of protein synthesis. As described in the previous section, there is close connection between CPK isoenzymes and many of the sites of ATP utilization (ATPases) and production (mitochondrial oxidative phosphorylation and adenine nucleotide translocase). During contraction Cr is liberated at utilization sites and returns to the mitochondria (in red muscles) to be rephosphorylated to PCr, at the same time stimulating oxidative phosphorylation (respiratory control). It can also diffuse to ATP-producing sites of glycolysis to stimulate this pathway, thus stimulating anaerobic energy production (ATP). The PCr generated in these pathways can be utilized for all endergonic functions such as contraction, protein synthesis, ion transport (Figure 4), and perhaps other transport such as amino acids, depending upon whether there is an isoenzyme of CPK available at that site to transduce the PCr to ultimately used ATP. The increase in muscle protein synthesis, for example, would result in increased myosin ATPase (21, 22, 46), which constitutes a major part of muscular adaptation to physical exercise.

The heart behaves differently from skeletal muscle, and this appears to be clearly related to the shuttle. The resistance of the heart to severe loss of substance in prolonged bed rest, paralysis, or starvation, compared to the wastage of skeletal muscle under the same conditions, is apparently due to the fact that heart is continually contracting, thereby maintaining its own respiratory control and energy economy. On the other hand, cardiac hypertrophy seen in hypertension might occur through an oversupply of PCr. Early in hypertension there seems to be a proportional increase in mitochondria and myofibrils and an increase in cardiac mass, which can maintain the heart's function as a pump. Whenever loading is prolonged, there is a change in organization and properties of myocardial cells, which results in diminished contractile function and eventually heart failure (48). If, during this prolonged hypertension, myofibrils are being synthesized at a higher rate than mitochondria, it would result in a thicker and wider myofibrillar section, so that the distance between mitochondria and the center of myofibrils is increased (48). This would result in a diminished energy delivery (as PCr) from mitochondria to the myofibrillar ATPase sites, causing reduced contractile efficiency and, finally, failure.

Functional Similarity of Exercise and Insulin

The PCr energy shuttle was predicted from the mitochondrial-hexokinase theory of insulin action (2). It has been postulated that insulin acts by connecting hexokinase to mitochondria, where it phosphorylates glucose with nascent ATP and resupplies ADP efficiently for respiratory control (Figure 3). This would explain the generally anabolic effects of insulin, for the acceptor process increases energy delivery to all the anabolic processes, such as membrane transport and protein, fat, and carbohydrate synthesis. The insulin-like action of exercise in diabetic comes from the same type of "acceptor" mechanism, which is generated by muscle contraction. Exercise liberates Cr, which returns to mitochondria, where it accelerates respiratory control by its phosphorylation to PCr in a close interaction between mitochondrial translocase and CPK (12, 13, 35, 39, 47).

Recently, it has been shown that insulin stimulates mitochondrial oxidation (47), confirming the hexokinase theory. We have observed that insulin does not increase mitochondrial oxidation by spontaneously beating isolated atria (6). However, if the

CPK is inhibited, there is clear insulin stimulation of residual mitochondrial oxidation (unpublished data). These preliminary experiments also reveal a small difference between skeletal and cardiac muscle. In skeletal muscle the PCr energy shuttle appears to have a much greater role in protein synthesis than in cardiac muscle. CPK inhibition results in about 70% decrease in protein synthesis in diaphragm muscle (9). The remaining 30% is that portion of protein synthesis that depends on carbohydrate metabolism and is stimulated by insulin (3, 30). Experiments by DeSchepper et al. (11) showed that insulin acts on only 30% of the protein synthesis of diaphragm. That is equal to the portion that remains after PCr energy shuttle inhibition by DNFB. With the above findings in mind, one would expect that at rest the diabetic heart should lose much less weight than skeletal muscle.

We have recently found that the hearts of diabetic rats are smaller than the control hearts almost to the same extent as the loss of their total body weight (submitted for publication). Only about 40% of the total body weight consists of muscle, and this is the tissue that suffers the significant weight loss. Therefore, the weight loss in the heart of diabetic rats is at about half the rate of loss of skeletal muscle. If exercise were the only factor in weight maintenance, the loss would seem to be larger than expected.

We have found that there is also a loss of up to 50% in total heart protein, which suggests that not only the insulin-dependent portion of protein synthesis is diminished, but the phosphocreatine energy shuttle might also be affected to some extent. In fact, we have observed about 30% reduction in mitochondrial CPK activity in diabetic rat heart. These mitochondria also had lower oxidative phosphorylation capacity and diminished response to the stimulatory effects of creatine. The lower mitochondrial oxidative phosphorylation ability and the lower CPK activity could both be the result of a diminished insulin-related portion of protein synthesis, perhaps the synthesis of the isoenzymes of CPK. Therefore, inadequate mitochondrial energy production in the form of PCr could contribute further to the weight loss of diabetic heart. The same defect could also be responsible for the diabetic cardiomyopathy unrelated to atherosclerotic disease and hypertension.

Conclusion

A factor that has not been considered in the growth response of muscle to exercise until recently (8, 44) is the effect of exercise on energy metabolism and, through this process, its effects on muscle protein synthesis. We propose that a mechanism for these changes is to be found in overactivity or deterioration of the phosphocreatine energy shuttle.

The ultimate source of oxidative energy for all endergonic processes is ATP. PCr is synthesized by mitochondrial CPK, using preferentially the mitochondrial-produced ATP through close functional interaction with translocase or through the cytoplasmic CPK using glycolytic ATP, depending on the type of muscle. PCr then moves toward the myofibrils or those other energy-utilizing sites to which some isozyme of CPK is attached, where it can rephosphorylate the locally produced ADP through close functional interaction among the locally attached enzymes. The released Cr (i.e., the product of muscle contraction) then returns to the mitochondrial or gly-colytic sites, where it stimulates more ATP production (Figure 4). This system of energy transport in heart and skeletal muscle is called the phosphocreatine energy shuttle. During muscle contraction the increased rate of turnover of PCr can be responsible for muscle hypertrophy, for the stimulated phosphocreatine energy shuttle enhances mitochondrial energy production, which then provides more energy for protein synthesis (Figure 4).

It has been shown that 70% of the protein synthesis is dependent on the source of energy from the phosphocreatine energy shuttle; the rest (30%) depends on the source of energy that is stimulated by insulin. The above finding explains why heart does not atrophy in prolonged bed rest. It explains why there is cardiac hypertrophy in chronic hypertension, for the increased work of the myocardium stimulates Cr turnover and production of PCr. It would also clarify the insulin-like action of exercise in diabetics, for both insulin and exercise act as respiratory control stimulants of ATP production for all the endergonic processes.

This review emphasizes the important fact that the molecular form in which energy is distributed in an organ depends upon the enzymes that are closely attached to the sites of energy formation and utilization. It explains why one process of energy utilization (e.g., muscle contraction) can affect the availability of energy for other endergonic processes.

References

1. Belitzer, V.A. La regulation de la respiration musculaire par le transformation du phosphagene. Enzymalogia 6:1-5; 1939.

2. Bessman, S.P. A contribution to the mechanism of diabetes mellitus. In: Najjar, V., ed. Fat metabolism. Baltimore: Johns Hopkins Press; 1954:133-137.

3. Bessman, S.P. Insulin and the energetics of protein synthesis. In: Ebashi, S., ed. Cellular regulation and malignant growth. Tokyo: Japan Sci. Soc. Press; and Berlin: Springer-Verlag; 1985:276-282.

4. Bessman, S.P.; Fonyo, A. The possible role of mitochondrial bound creatine kinase in regulation of mitochondrial respiration. Biochem. Biophys. Res. Commun. 22:597-602; 1966.

5. Bessman, S.P.; Geiger, P.J. Transport of energy in muscle. Science 211:448-452; 1981.

6. Bessman, S.P.; Mohan, C.; Zaidise, I. The intracellular site of insulin action— the mitochondrial Krebs cycle. Proc. Natl. Acad. Sci. USA 83:5067-5070; 1986.

7. Bessman, S.P.; Yang, W.C.T.; Geiger, P.J.; Erickson-Viitanen, S. Intimate coupling of creatine phosphokinase and myofibrilar adenosinetriphosphatase. Biochem. Biophys. Res. Commun. 96:1414-1420; 1980.

8. Booth, F.W.; Gollnick, P.D.; Effect of disuse on the structure and function of skeletal muscle. Med. Sci. Sports Exerc. 15:415-420; 1983.

9. Carpenter, C.L.; Mohan, C.; Bessman, S.P. Inhibition of protein synthesis in muscle by 2,4 dinitrofluorobenzene, an inhibitor of creatine phosphokinase. Biochem. Biophys. Res. Commun. 111:884-889; 1983.

10. Chevli, R.; Fitch, D.C. Beta-guanidinopropionate and phosphorylated beta-guanidinopropionate as substrates for creatine kinase. Biochem. Med. 21:162-167; 1979.

11. DeSchepper, P.J.; Toyoda, M.; Bessman, S.P. A requirement for carbohydrate metabolism for the stimulation of amino acid incorporation into protein by insulin. J. Biol. Chem. 240:1670-1674; 1965.

12. Erickson-Viitanen, S.; Geiger, P.J.; Viitanen, P.; Bessman, S.P. Compartmentation of mitochondrial creatine phosphokinase: II. The importance of the outer mitochondrial membrane for mitochondrial compartmentation. J. Biol. Chem. 257:14405-14411; 1982.

13. Erickson-Viitanen, S.; Viitanen, P.; Geiger, P.J.; Yang, W.C.T.; Bessman, S.P. Compartmentation of mitochondrial creatine phosphokinase: I. Direct demonstration of compartmentation with the use of labeled precursors. J. Biol. Chem. 257:14395-14404; 1982.

14. Fitch, C.D. Significance of abnormalities of creatine metabolism. In: Rowland, L.P., ed. Pathogenesis of human muscular dystrophies. Amersterdam: Excerpta Medica; 1927:328-340.

15. Fitch, C.D.; Jellinek, M.; Fitts, R.H.; Baldwain, K.M.; and Holloszy, J.O. Phosphorylated beta-guanidinopropionate as a substitute for phosphocreatine in rat muscle. Am. J. Physiol. 228:1123-1125; 1975.

16. Fitch, C.D.; Mueller, E.J. Experimental depletion of creatine and phosphocreatine from skeletal muscle. J. Biol. Chem. 249:1060-1063; 1974.

17. Goldspink, D.F. The influence of immobilization and stretch on protein turnover of rat skeletal muscle. J. Physiol. (Lond.) 264:267-282; 1977.

18. Gudbjarnason, S.; Mathes, P.; Ravens, K.A. Functional compartmentation of ATP and creatine phosphate in heart muscle. J. Mol. Cell. Cardiol. 1:325-339; 1970.

19. Hofmann, W.W.; Butte, J.; Leon, H.A. Relationship of intracellular creatine concentration and uptake to muscle mass in vivo. Am. J. Physiol. 235:C199-C203; 1978.

20. Ingwall, J.S. Creatine and the control of muscle-specific protein synthesis in cardiac and skeletal muscle. Circ. Res. 38(Suppl. I):I-115–I-123; 1976.

21. Ingwall, J.S.; Morales, M.F.; Stockdale, F.E. Creatine and control of myosin synthesis in differentiating skeletal muscle. Proc. Natl. Acad. Sci. USA, 69:2250-2253; 1972.

22. Ingwall, J.S.; Weiner, C.D.; Morales, M.F.; Davis, E.; Stockdale, F.G. Specificity of creatine in the control of muscle protein synthesis. J. Cell Biol. 62:145-151; 1974.

23. Keul, J.; Doll, E.; Keppler, D. The adaptation of the energy supply in muscle to physical activity. In: Jokl, E., ed. Energy of metabolism in human muscle. Baltimore: Univ. Park Press; 1972:244-260.

24. Khan, M.A.; Holt, P.G.; Papadimitriou, J.M.; Knight, J.O.; Kakulas, B.A. Histochemical localization of creatine kinase in skeletal muscle by the tetrazolium and the incubation film-lead precipitation techniques. In: Basic research in myology. Amsterdam: Excerpta Medica; 1971:96-101. (International Congress Series).

25. Klein, T.O. Localization of creatine kinase in microsomes and mitochondria of human heart and skeletal muscle and cerebral cortex. Nature 207:1393-1394; 1965.

26. Laskowski, M.B.; Chevli, R.; Fitch, C.D. Biochemical and ultrastructural changes in skeletal muscle induced by a creatine antagonist. Metabolism 30:1080-1085; 1981.

27. Levitsky, D.O.; Levchenko, T.S.; Saks, V.A.; Sharov, V.G.; Smirnov, V.N. The functional coupling between Ca^{2+}-ATPase and creatine phosphokinase in heart muscle sarcoplasmic reticulum. Biokhimiia 42:1766-1773; 1977.

28. Meyer, R.A.; Brown, T.R.; Kushmerick, M.J. CK kinetics in phosphocreatine depleted rat hearts. Biophys. J. 45:91a; 1984.

29. Meyer, R.A. Sweeney, H.L.; Kushmerick, M.J. A simple analysis of the "phosphocreatine shuttle." Am. J. Physiol. 246:C365-C377; 1984.

30. Mohan, C.; Bessman, S.P. Effect of insulin on the metabolic distribution of carbons 1, 2, and 3 of pyruvate. Arch. Biochem. Biophys. 248:190-199; 1986.

31. O'Brien, S.A.; Nutbeam, A.R. Creatine release from the isolated perfused rat heart. In: Harris, P.; Biong, A.J.; Fleckentein, A., eds. Recent advances in studies on cardiac structure and metabolism. Baltimore: Univ. Park Press; 1973:177-181.

32. Oganro, E.A.; Peters, T.J.; Hearse, D.J. Subcellular compartmentation of creatine kinase isoenzymes in guinea pig heart. Cardiovasc. Res. 11:250-259; 1977.

33. Petrofsky, J.S.; Fitch, C.D. Contractile characteristics of skeletal muscle depleted of phosphocreatine. Pflügers Arch. 384:123-129; 1980.

34. Saks, V.A.; Rosenshtraukh, L.V.; Smirnov, V.N.; Chazov, E.I. Role of CK in cellular function and metabolism. Can. J. Physiol. Pharmacol. 56:691-706; 1978.

35. Savabi, F.; Bessman, S.P. Recovery of isolated rat atrial function related to ATP under different anoxic conditions. Arch. Biochem. Biophys. 248:151-157; 1986.

36. Savabi, F.; Carpenter, C.L.; Bessman, S.P. The polysome as a terminal for the creatine phosphate energy shuttle. Biochem. Med. Metab. Biol. 40:29-298; 1988.

37. Savabi, F.; Geiger, P.J.; Bessman, S.P. Kinetic properties and functional role of creatine phosphokinase in glycerinated muscle fibers—further evidence for compartmentation. Biochem. Biophys. Res. Commun. 114:785-790; 1983.

38. Savabi, F.; Geiger, P.J.; Bessman, S.P. Myofibrillar end of the creatine phosphate energy shuttle. Am. J. Physiol. 247:C424-C432; 1984.

39. Savabi, F.; Geiger, P.J.; Bessman, S.P. Three-step preparation and purification of phosphorus-33-labeled creatine phosphate of high specific activity. Anal. Biochem. 138:384-389; 1984.

40. Savabi, F.; Geiger, P.J.; Bessman, S.P. Post-anoxic recovery of spontaneously beating isolated atria: pH-related role of adenylate kinase. Biochem. Med. Metab. Biol. 35:345-355; 1986.

41. Seraydarian, M.; Mommaerts, W.F.H.M.; Wallner, A. The amount and compartmentalization of adenosine diphosphate in muscle. Biochim. Biophys. Acta 65:443-460; 1962.

42. Sharov, V.G.; Saks, V.A.; Smirnov, V.N.; Shazov, E.I. An electron microscopic histochemical investigation of the localization of creatine phosphokinase in heart cells. Biochim. Biophys. Acta 468:495-501; 1977.

43. Shields, R.P.; Whitehair, C.K.; Carrow, R.E.; Heusner, W.W.; Van Huss, W.D. Skeletal muscle function and structure after depletion of creatine. Lab. Invest. 33:151-158; 1975.

44. Van Der Meulen, J.P.; Peckham, P.H.; Mortimer, J.T. Use and disuse of muscle. Ann. N.Y. Acad. Sci. 228:177-189; 1974.

45. Wildenthal, K.; Griffin, E.E.; Ingwall, J.S. Hormonal control of cardiac protein and amino acid balance. Circ. Res. 38(Suppl. I):I-138–I-144; 1976.

46. Wilkerson, J.; Evonuk, E. Changes in cardiac and skeletal muscle myosin ATPase activities after exercise. J. Appl. Physiol. 30:328-330; 1970.

47. Yang, W.C.T.; Geiger, P.J.; Bessman, S.P.; Borrebaek, B. Formation of creatine phosphate from creatine and ^{32}P-labeled ATP by isolated rabbit heart mitochondria. Biochem. Biophys. Res. Commun. 76:882-887; 1977.

48. Zak, R. Cardiac hypertrophy. Biochemical Hospital Practice. 18:85-97; 1983.

The Role of Subcellular Organization of Kinases in Energy Metabolism

Dieter Brdiczka, Volker Adams, Matthias Kottke, Gabriella Sandri, and Enrico Panfili

University of Constance, Konstanz, F.R.G. and University of Triest, Triest, Italy

The metabolic pathways that produce cellular ATP provide a high phosphorylation potential in the extramitochondrial compartment, whereas the intramitochondrial ATP/ADP energy potential is significantly lower (37). The high cytosolic phosphorylation potential, which is only slightly altered during biological work (19), on the one hand agrees with the physiologically low flux through the glycolytic ATP production relative to the high rate of oxidative phosphorylation, and on the other hand excludes a direct equilibration of the mitochondrial phosphorylation potential with that in the cytosol. The data thus underline the importance of the ATP/ADP translocation process in the adaptation of the rate of oxidative phosphorylation according to the requirements of the cell. The asymmetric ATP export performed by the translocator is driven electrogenically by the mitochondrial membrane potential (25). Thus, the intramitochondrial ATP gains phosphorylation energy during export when it is exchanged against external ADP. When the export of ATP was studied in competitive in vitro experiments, the membrane potential was able to generate a concentration of ATP 13 times higher than ADP (25).

If we consider the existence of an ATP/ADP quotient in the cytosol of 10 in the liver (37) and of approximately 40 in muscle (19), it goes without saying that the translocation process would be at equilibrium and therefore would have low rates (Table 1). However, it cannot be easily dismissed that under physiological conditions the flux rate in the mitochondrial ATP/ADP exchange is high in spite of a high phosphorylation potential in the cytosol. A satisfying answer to this problem has to be given in terms of a mechanism that keeps the translocator away from equilibrium. At this point the functional coupling of kinases to the translocator comes into effect. The existence of this interaction has been described for hexokinase in mitochondria from liver (6, 16), muscle (39), and brain (20), and also for creatine kinase in muscle mitochondria by several authors (4, 15, 22, 35, 40). Provided that we agree to the functional coupling between translocator and kinases, it would be a promising mechanism to dislocate the translocator from equilibrium because the direct interaction with kinases would cause an immediate transfer of the phosphorylation energy from the exported ATP to metabolites that are not substrates for the translocator.

Table 1   Intra- and Extramitochondrial ATP/ADP Quotients

Source	ATP/ADP
Perfused liver	
Cytosol	10.3
Mitochondria	0.18
Mm. gastrocnemius	
Cytosol	40.0
Mitochondria	1.6
Energized	
liver mitochondria	
Efflux, competitive	12.5

Note. The data physiologically observed in liver (37) and muscle (19), are compared to the asymmetric ATP/ADP export in energized liver mitochondria. The latter values were determined by Klingengberg and Heldt (25) in competitive in vitro experiments.

Apart from hexokinase and creatine kinase, there are quite a number of different kinases situated outside the inner membrane at the mitochondrial periphery (Figure 1) that may be involved in this postulated mechanism. Of these kinases, two groups can be defined with respect to location and to function: (a) those that bind to the outer membrane pore protein at the surface of the membrane (for example hexokinase, glycerolkinase [14]); and (b) others located between the two boundary membranes, for example, adenylate kinase (7), nucleoside diphosphate kinase (23), and creatine kinase (21). The enzymes of the former group will be called "energy-consuming kinases," the products of which are phosphorylated metabolites not directly equilibrating with the extramitochondrial phosphorylation potential. The function of the latter kinases, called "energy-transmitting kinases," is to exchange mitochondrial phosphorylation energy between different high-energy compounds.

Studies of the subcellular organization of these kinases have revealed that the peripheral energy-consuming kinases, depending on the metabolic situation, exist in a free as well as in a mitochondrial-bound state (1, 32). In contrast to the latter kinases, of the energy-transmitting kinases in the intermembrane space, a second corresponding isozyme is present in the cytosol. Such an intracellular organization allows the free, energy-consuming kinases or the cytosolic isozymes of energy-transmitting kinases to equilibrate with the extramitochondrial ATP/ADP. In accordance to the above-mentioned arguments, we postulate, however, that the mitochondrial-bound as well as the intermembrane kinases have access to a different ATP/ADP pool between the two boundary membranes. An important assumption of this view is a disequilibrium of high-energetic compounds across the outer membrane pore, which may be dynamically controlled by the formation of contacts between the two boundary membranes. We shall explain in this article how the inner membrane potential may affect the outer membrane pore and limit its conductivity. Furthermore, the importance of the contact sites in this type of regulation

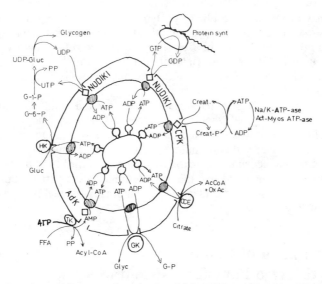

Figure 1.   Location of kinases at the mitochondrial periphery. Energy-consuming kinases: hexokinase (HK); glycerol kinase (GK) bound to the outer membrane pore (14); this may be assumed also for fatty acid activating enzyme (TK [33]) and ATP-citrate lyase (CCE [24]). Energy-transmitting kinases: mitochondrial isozymes located between the two boundary membranes, adenylate kinase (AdK [7]), nucleoside diphosphate kinase (NUDIKI [23]), creatine kinase (CPK [21]).

will be emphasized by the description of the preferential organization of several peripheral kinases in these sites as observed by electron-microscopic and biochemical investigations. We want to discuss, as the final topic, the relevance of this dynamic compartmentation of kinases in the regulation of fluxes in the glycolysis or oxidative phosphorylation by demonstrating its absence in tumor cells.

Energy-Consuming Kinases

It has been observed that hexokinase and glycerolkinase bind to the pore protein in the mitochondrial outer membrane and can compete for the same binding site (14). However, in the livers of starved rats, the activity of mitochondrial-bound glycerolkinase increases while that of hexokinase decreases (32). The desorption upon starvation of hexokinase II, which is predominant in liver, has been explained by the increase of repulsive forces between the negatively charged enzyme and the mitochondrial membrane surface (13, 26). As has recently been demonstrated, the latter can result from increased levels of free fatty acids in starved rats (43).

The regulatory consequence of the hexokinase desorption is 3-fold: First, the free enzyme becomes accessible to inhibition by glucose-6-phosphate (42); second, the activity of isozyme II, especially, is significantly reduced (1, 41) by debinding; and third, the enzyme utilizes cytosolic (glycolytic) ATP. This brings us to the important topic we want to discuss later, namely, that the energy-consuming kinases would increase the glycolytic flux in the free state and, conversely, would reduce it by becoming bound. The latter implies a functional coupling to the inner mitochondrial compartment, which has been demonstrated for hexokinase in brain, (20), liver (6, 16), and muscle (39).

The location of hexokinase at the surface of rat liver and brain mitochondria was analyzed using immuno-gold labeling techniques (28, 41). By analyzing the distribution of gold grains, it was observed that the enzyme was predominantly located in areas where the inner and outer mitochondrial boundary membranes were close together. Taking into account that hexokinase binds specifically to the pore protein (14, 29), this result suggested that the enzyme might preferentially bind to outer membrane pore proteins in the contact sites or, alternatively, that pores are concentrated only in these sites.

Characterization of Contact Sites
Between the Two Boundary Membranes

The existence of contact sites between the two boundary membranes has been demonstrated by three different methods: electron microscopy, isolation and biochemical characterization, and treatment with digitonin. Contact sites between the two mitochondrial boundary membranes were first described by Hackenbrock (17) in thin sections of rat liver mitochondria. These contacts have been assumed to be responsible for the atypical behavior of the fracture plane in freeze-fractured mitochondria, which is characterized by frequent jumping of the fracture plane between the two membranes (38). Supposing that fracture plane deflections would occur only in the contact sites, we suggested that the frequency of these deflections would directly correlate to the frequency of contacts. Based on these considerations, we determined the frequency of fracture plane deflections in freeze-fractured samples of mitochondria in different metabolic states. We observed a significantly larger frequency of contacts (fracture plane deflections) in phosphorylating mitochondria compared to mitochondria in States 4 and 1 (26, 27). Uncoupling of the mitochondria by dinitrophenole or glycerination caused a further reduction of the contacts. In view of these findings, we concluded that the contacts might be regulated by the activity of the oxidative phosphorylation.

From the results described above, we decided to judge hexokinase as a good marker enzyme for the contact fraction when we attempted to isolate the contact fraction from osmotically disrupted liver mitochondria by density gradient centrifugation (31). We were able to separate a fraction in the density gradient, which was distinct from the main outer and inner membrane fractions and was characterized by a high hexokinase activity (Figure 2). Furthermore, it contained inner and outer membrane components. Consistent with the results in liver, we obtained this fraction also from brain (28) and kidney mitochondria. The presumptive contact fraction was further characterized by recentrifugation on a second discontinuous density gradient after decoration of hexokinase by specific antibodies and protein-A-gold.

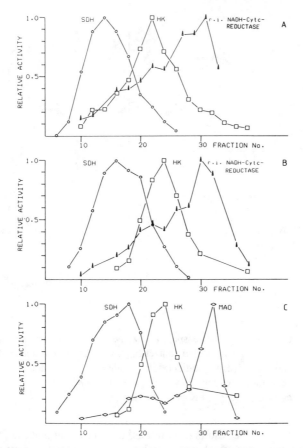

Figure 2. Subfractionation of osmotically lysed mitochondria by sucrose density gradient centrifugation. Isolated mitochondria from brain (A), kidney (B), and liver (C) were disrupted by swelling (20 mM phosphate buffer), shrinking (30% sucrose), and sonification. The enzyme activities are expressed relative to the maximum activity in the peak fraction of the respective enzyme and are mean values of four experiments. SDH, succinate dehydrogenase, HK, hexokinase, MAO, monoamine oxidase, r.i. NADH-Cytc-REDUCTASE, rotenone insensitive –.

Although this procedure exclusively increased the density of hexokinase, we observed a comigration of the inner and outer membrane components with the hexokinase activity (Figure 3), suggesting the existence of a complex between the enzyme and the two boundary membranes. Considering that hexokinase specifically binds to the pore protein in the outer membrane, and taking into account the preferential binding of the enzyme in the contacts, we turned our curiosity on the distribution of the pore protein at the mitochondrial surface and observed a random distribution all over the outer membrane (31). These results brought up the idea of a specific structure of the pore protein in the contacts, which will be discussed later. The structure of the isolated contact fraction was further analyzed by surface proteolysis and

184   Brdiczka, Adams, Kottke, Sandri, and Panfili

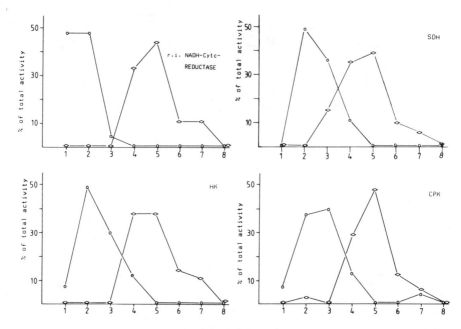

Figure 3. Distribution of contact-site–specific enzymes in a density gradient after immuno-gold labeling of hexokinase. The labeled contact fraction from brain mitochondria was centrifuged on a discontinuous density gradient: left to right 40%, 45%, and 50% sucrose w/v. Open circles show enzyme activity profiles in the gradient loaded with unlabeled contact fraction. Abbreviations as in Fig. 2, CPK=creatine kinase.

freeze-fracturing (31). The results of both methods agreed in that the fraction contained right-side-out outer membrane vesicles that enwrapped an inner membrane vesicle.

From the nonrandom distribution of hexokinase and the fracture plane deflections between the two boundary membranes at specific points of contact, a heterogeneous composition of the outer membrane inside and beyond the contact sites was to be expected. The dissimilar effect of digitonin on the outer membrane may result from this heterogeneity because it is characterized by a relatively specific detachment of those parts of the outer membrane that are outside the contacts (8, 18). In accordance with this, the activity of enzymes residing in the contact zones, like hexokinase, could not be removed by digitonin treatment, whereas the activity of adenylate kinase was liberated parallel to the desorption of the outer membrane and marker enzymes like monoamine oxidase (28, 31). When we studied the digitonin effect on mitochondria in different functional states, we observed that more pore protein remained bound to the mitoplast fraction of phosphorylating mitochondria, whereas a significantly higher amount of pore protein was removed by digitonin from uncoupled (DNP) or glycerol-treated mitochondria (2, 31). This result was directly comparable with the observations in electron microscopy, where uncoupling and incubation with glycerol reduced the frequency of contacts, whereas they were increasing in phosphorylating mitochondria (27). The amount of hexokinase activity that remained bound to the mitoplast fraction correlated with the concentration of porin, meaning that the frequency of contacts, in addition to changes in surface charge (43), regulates the formation of the hexokinase-porin complex (2). Thus, digitonin treatment proved to be quite a good method to indicate the presence of contact sites and to characterize the mitochondrial surface inside the contacts.

Energy-Transmitting Kinases

Having previously accepted the fact that hexokinase, representing peripheral energy-consuming kinases, resided almost specifically inside the contacts, we now turned our interest to the distribution of energy-transmitting kinases. The mitochondrial isozymes of creatine kinase (21), nucleoside diphosphate kinase (23), and adenylate kinase (7) are located in the intermembrane space, a location that allows direct interaction with the adenine nucleotide translocator. To localize the energy-transmitting kinases, we applied the same methods as described for hexokinase.

When freshly isolated mitochondria were treated with increasing concentrations of digitonin, nucleoside diphosphate kinase and creatine kinase, in contrast to adenylate kinase, became incompletely extracted from the mitoplast fraction of brain (Figure 4A) and liver (Figure 4B). This pointed to a different location of the three kinases in the intermembrane space, in that adenylate kinase appeared to be outside the contact zones.

The conclusion drawn from digitonin treatment completely agreed with the distribution of the energy-transmitting kinases in the mitochondrial subfractions. We isolated the contact fraction analogous to the experiment shown in Figure 2 from osmotically disrupted brain, kidney, and liver mitochondria. The activity profiles in the density gradient derived from the three different types of mitochondria (Figure 5) resulted in a concentration of nucleoside diphosphate kinase and creatine kinase activity (not present in liver mitochondria) in the contact site fraction. The activity of adenylate kinase, however, remained on top of the gradients and thus appeared to reside outside these structures.

Regulation of the Outer Membrane Pore by the Membrane Potential

Provided that we are allowed to take for granted this difference in location of adenylate kinase and the other kinases, a satisfying explanation for this may be the possibility to regulate the outer membrane pore permeability specifically in the contact sites. In agreement with this, several authors (9, 12) have observed a regulatory effect of the outer membrane on creatine kinase activity that persisted even after digitonin treatment (5). To explain the regulation of the outer membrane pore, it seems plausible to think of a property distinct from bacterial porins, namely, the voltage dependence. When reconstituted in planar bilayers, the pore can switch to a lower conducting state, depending on the applied voltage (34, 36). Taking into account the high ion conductivity of the pore, the existence of an electrochemical potential across the outer membrane can be excluded. However, in the contact sites,

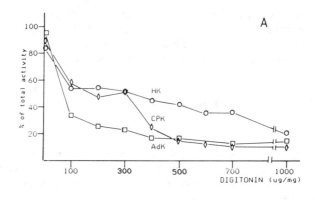

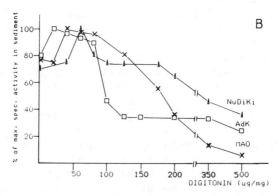

Figure 4. Effect of digitonin on the desorption of peripheral mitochondrial enzymes. Mitochondria of brain (A) and liver (L) were incubated for 1 min in mannitol/sucrose medium with increasing concentrations of digitonin and subsequently centrifuged. The data are means of three experiments. Abbreviations as in Fig. 2 and 3; AdK, adenylate kinase, NuDiKi, nucleoside diphosphate kinase.

a transduction of the inner membrane potential across the outer membrane appears possible and would lead to a dynamic compartmentation at the mitochondrial surface, regulated by the formation of the contact sites and the fluctuations of the inner membrane potential.

At a voltage between 30 and 60 mV, the pore switches to a lower conductivity (10, 34) and becomes cationically selective (30). We have recently observed that the pore in the low-conducting state was impermeable for ADP and ATP (3), suggesting that the inner membrane potential might exert control on the adenine nucleotide transport in the contacts by forcing the pore to the low-conducting state, thereby preventing equilibration of anionic metabolites with the cytosol (5). Supposing that low-conducting pores are present in the contact sites, we were then at liberty to expect the pores in the open state beyond the contacts to be characterized by high conductivity and low anion selectivity (10).

Our experience with the specific binding of hexokinase activity to the pores prepared us to study whether the low- and high-conducting states of the pore could exist in the outer membrane at the same time. We found that isolated pure outer membrane had a lower affinity for hexokinase compared to the outer membrane in

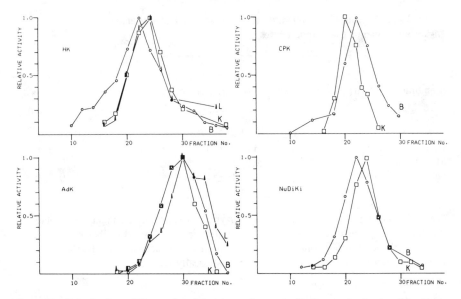

Figure 5. Distribution of kinases in subfractions of osmotically disrupted mitochondria. Fragments of mitochondria from brain (B), kidney (K), and liver (L) were subfractionated by density gradient centrifugation as in Fig. 2. The four panels depict relative activity profiles of the respective kinases in gradients which separate the membrane fragments of the different types of mitochondria.

the contact fraction. Furthermore, the half-saturation constant of the contacts for hexokinase resembled that determined in phosphorylating mitochondria (Table 2), which led us to conclude that, physiologically, hexokinase may bind to the low-conducting form of the pore in the contacts. To explain how in this case the enzyme can get access to intramitochondrial ATP, we have to consider that the membrane potential across the inner membrane is not constant. Thus, the voltage-dependent regulation of the pore, which may come into existence in the contacts, could result in a frequent change between anion and cation selectivity, according to the fluctuations of the inner membrane potential.

On the whole it emerged, from the different affinities of hexokinase to the outer membrane inside and outside the contacts, that the pore may exist in the outer membrane in two distinct states at the same time. This suggests that the equilibration of energy-transmitting kinases located in the contacts, like creatine kinase, may be controlled by the membrane potential, in contrast to kinases beyond the contact sites, like adenylate kinase (Figure 6).

Regulation of Energy Metabolism

With respect to the restricted transport properties of the pore protein in the contacts and the location of several kinases in these sites, there are two ways of considering the regulatory role of this organization in energy metabolism. One way

Table 2   Half-Saturation Constants for Hexokinase I of Outer Membrane Inside and Beyond the Contact Sites

Membrane fraction	KS (nM HK I)	Binding capacity (mU/μg Porin)
Contact sites	43.9 $\pm$ 7.2	0.44 $\pm$ 0.1
Outer membrane	131.0 $\pm$ 82.5	1.60 $\pm$ 0.3
Mitochondria phosphorylating	46.1 $\pm$ 17.1	1.10 $\pm$ 0.4

Note. The binding of isolated hexokinase isozyme I was performed in sucrose isolation medium in the presence of 5 mM $MgCl_2$ and glucose. The assay for phosphorylating mitochondria additionally contained 5 mM phosphate and succinate and 1 mM ADP. The probability that the different groups are statistically identical: $p = 1\%$.

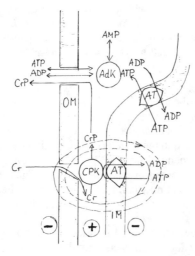

Figure 6.   Scheme showing how regulated and unregulated outer membrane pores may affect mitochondrial peripheral kinases. The model assumes a capacitative coupling between inner (IM) and outer (OM) membrane in the contact sites. The resulting membrane potential across the outer membrane changes the pore structure in the contacts to the low conductance, cationic-selective state. Consequently these pores would become impermeable for phosphocreatine (CrP) ATP and ADP. AT, adenylate translocator.

concerns the possibility of directing the load of energy production either to the glycolysis or to the oxidative phosphorylation by binding or debinding the energy-consuming kinases. The other regulatory role concerns the effect of all contact-specific kinases on the mitochondrial ATP/ADP exchange. The latter regulatory function refers to the asymmetric ability of the adenylate translocator for active export of ATP without active uptake of ADP, although the ADP gradient across the inner membrane is directed out of the mitochondria (Table 1). To meet these specifications, two aspects come into existence inside the contact sites: the restriction of the transport through the outer membrane pore, governed by the inner membrane potential, which excludes equilibration with the phosphorylation potential in the cytosol; and second, the direct communication of kinases with the translocator. Both effects would serve to dislocate the ATP translocation process from equilibrium and thus maintain high flux rates.

To base this view on some evidence, we started to investigate the organization of kinases in tumor cells. The energy metabolism of many tumor cells is characterized by an imbalance between the two ATP-supplying metabolic pathways: glycolysis and oxidative phosphorylation. Consequently, when we analyzed the contribution of these two metabolic systems to cellular ATP in highly glycolytic HT 29 cells, we observed that the oxidative phosphorylation produced only 50% of the total ATP (11). In contrast to this, in a low glycolytic subpopulation of these cells (obtained by adaptation to glucose-free medium), oxidative phosphorylation contributed more than 80% to the cellular ATP (Table 3). Both subpopulations of the HT 29 cells contained the same amount of well-coupled mitochondria, so the only satisfying explanation for the difference in energy metabolism appeared to be in terms of an insufficient mitochondrial ADP supply in the highly glycolytic cells.

Table 3   Relative Contribution of Glycolysis and Oxidative Phosphorylation to Cell ATP Production in Different Subpopulations of Human Adenocarcinoma (HT 29) Cells

	HT 29 Cells	
Source of ATP	Undifferentiated	Differentiated
Glycolysis		
nmol/min/mg	18.9 ± 3.4	7.0 ± 2.1
% of total ATP	45.4	17.2
Oxidative phosphorylation		
nmol/min/mg	21.9 ± 1.1	33.7 ± 3.0
% of total ATP	54.7	82.8
Total ATP		
nmol/min/mg	40.1	40.8

Note. The rate of glycolytic ATP synthesis was calculated from the lactate production (1 mol ATP per mol lactate). The production of ATP by the oxidative phosphorylation was calculated from the respiratory rates of the tumor cells in the presence of glucose (2.5 mol ATP per mol of oxygen). The data are taken from ref. 11.

Because of the assumption that the contact sites may provide an important structural basis in the ATP/ADP exchange, we looked for these structures at the mitochondrial periphery in freeze-fractured samples of the different HT 29 subpopulations. The answer we arrived at was the almost complete absence of contact sites in the highly glycolytic cells, whereas the sites' frequency was normal in the low glycolytic population (11, Table 4).

Table 4   Frequency of contact sites in Mitochondria of Freeze-Fractured Differentiated and Undifferentiated Human Adenocarcinoma (HT 29) Cells

Cells	$L(\mu m/\mu m^2)$	%
Hepatocytes	15.0 + 7.0	100
HT 29 cells		
differentiated	23.0 + 10.3	150
undifferentiated	4.8 + 1.7	32

Note. HT 29 adenocarcinoma cells grown in the presence of glucose (undifferentiated) and cells of the same cell line adapted to glucose-free medium (differentiated) were fixed by rapid freezing techniques and freeze-fractured. The length of the edge (L), where the fracture plane deflects, was examined as described by Knoll and Brdiczka (27). The determination was made 2 days after readdition of glucose to the differentiated cells. The probability that the different experimental groups are statistically identical: $p = .2\%$. The data of HT 29 cells are taken from ref. 11.

In view of these findings, the disregulation of tumor energy metabolism appeared to be a good example to make the point about the importance of the dynamic organization of kinases at the mitochondrial periphery in which contact site formation is involved. Irrespective of the amount of kinase activity (which is typically very high in tumor cells) bound to the mitochondrial surface, the ADP supply of the oxidative phosphorylation seemed to depend on the organization of kinases in the contact sites. Considering the specific location of hexokinase in the contact sites, a plausible reason for this could be to provide a direct coupling of the enzyme via the pore protein to the ATP/ADP translocator. Consequently, glucose would be phosphorylated at the expense of mitochondrial ATP, thus saving 25% of the glycolytic ATP production. It goes without saying that this would exert a great influence on the glycolytic flux. In view of these considerations, we finally arrived at the assumption that the rate of glycolysis may be basically regulated by the formation of contacts, which itself depends on the activity of the oxidative phosphorylation.

References

1. Adams, V.; Bosch, W.; Hämmerle, T.; Brdiczka, D. Activation of low Km hexokinases in purified hepatocytes by binding to mitochondria. Biochim. Biophys. Acta 932:195-205; 1988.

2. Adams, V.; Brdiczka, D.; Bosch, W. Functional coupling of kinases to the oxidative phosphorylation is important for the regulation of glycolytic flux. 5th EBEC Short Reports. (1988). p. 281.

3. Benz, R.; Wojtczak, L.; Bosch, W.; Brdiczka, D. Inhibition of adenine nucleotide transport through the mitochondrial porin by a synthetic polyanion. FEBS Lett. 210:75-80; 1988.

4. Bessman, S.P.; Carpenter, C.L. The creatine-phosphate energy shuttle. Annu. Rev. Biochem. 54:831-865; 1985.

5. Brdiczka, D.; Adams, V.; Kottke, M.; Benz, R. Topology of peripheral kinases: its importance in transmission of mitochondrial energy. In: Azzi, A.; Nalecz, K.A.; Nalecz, M.J.; Wojtczak, L., eds. Anion carriers of mitochondrial membranes. Berlin: Springer (in press).

6. Brdiczka, D.; Knoll, G.; Riesinger, I.; Weiler, U.; Klug, G.; Benz, R.; Krause, J. Microcompartmentation at the mitochondrial surface: its function in metabolic regulation. In: Brautbar, N., ed. Myocardial and skeletal muscle bioenergetics. New York: Plenum Press; 1986:55-69.

7. Brdiczka, D.; Pette, D.; Brunner, G.; Miller, F. Kompartimentierte Verteilung von Enzymen in Rattenlebermitochondrien. Eur. J. Biochem. 294-304; 1968.

8. Brdiczka, D.; Schumacher, D. Iodination of peripheral mitochondrial membrane proteins in correlation to the functional states of the ADP/ATP carrier. Biochem. Biophys. Res. Commun. 73:823-832; 1976.

9. Brooks, S.P.J.; Suelter, C.H. Compartmented coupling of chicken heart creatine kinase to the nucleotide translocase requires the outer membrane. Arch. Biochem. Biophys. 257:144-153; 1987.

10. Colombini, M. A candidate for the permeability pathway of the outer mitochondrial membrane. Nature 279:643-645; 1979.

11. Denis-Pouxviel, C.; Riesinger, I.; Bühler, C.; Brdiczka, D.; Murat, J.-C. Regulation of mitochondrial hexokinase in cultured HT 29 human cancer cells. Biochim. Biophys. Acta 902:335-348; 1987.

12. Erickson-Viitanen, S.; Viitanen, P.; Geiger, P.J.; Yang, W.C.; Bessman, S.P. Compartmentation of mitochondrial creatine phosphokinase. J. Biol. Chem. 257:14395-14404; 1982.

13. Felgner, P.L.; Wilson, J.E. Effect of neutral salts on the interaction of rat brain hexokinase with the outer mitochondrial membrane. Arch. Biochem. Biophys. 182:282-294; 1977.

14. Fiek, C.; Benz, R.; Roos, N.; Brdiczka, D. Evidence for identity between the hexokinase-binding protein and the mitochondrial porin in the outer membrane of rat liver mitochondria. Biochim. Biophys. Acta 688:429-440; 1982.

15. Gellerich, F.N.; Schlame, M.; Bohnensack, R.; Kunz, W. Dynamic compartmentation of adenine nucleotides in the mitochondrial intermembrane space of rat-heart mitochondria. Biochim. Biophys. Acta 890:117-126; 1987.

16. Gots, R.E.; Bessman, S.P. The functional compartmentation of mitochondrial hexokinase. Arch. Biochem. Biophys. 163:7-14; 1974.

17. Hackenbrock, C.R. Chemical and physical fixation of isolated mitochondria in low-energy and high-energy states. Proc. Natl. Acad. Sci. USA 61:598-605; 1968.

18. Hackenbrock, C.R.; Miller, K.J. The distribution of anionic sites on the surface of mitochondrial membranes. J. Cell Biol. 65:615-630; 1975.

19. Hebisch, S.; Sies, H.; Soboll, S. Function dependent changes in the subcellular distribution of high energy phosphates in fast and slow rat skeletal muscles. Pflügers Arch. 406:20-24; 1986.

20. Inui, M.; Ishibashi, S. Functioning of mitochondria-bound hexokinase in rat brain in accordance with generation of ATP inside the organelle. J. Biochem. 85:1151-1156; 1979.

21. Jacobs, H.; Held, H.W.; Klingenberg, M. High activity of creatine kinase in mitochondria from muscle and brain. Evidence for a separate mitochondrial isozyme of creatine kinase. Biochem. Biophys. Res. Commun. 16:516-521; 1964.

22. Jacobus, W.E. Respiratory control and the integration of heart high-energy phosphate metabolism by mitochondrial creatine kinase. Annu. Rev. Physiol. 47:707-725; 1985.

23. Jacobus, W.E.; Evans, J.J. Nucleoside diphosphokinase of rat heart mitochondria. Dual localization in matrix intermembrane space. J. Biol. Chem. 252:4232-4241; 1977.

24. Janski, A.M.; Cornell, N.W. Association of ATP citrate lyase with mitochondria. Biochem. Biophys. Res. Commun. 92:305-312; 1980.

25. Klingenberg, M.; Heldt, H.W. The ADP/ATP translocation in mitochondria and its role in intracellular compartmentation. In: Sies, H., ed. Metabolic compartmentation. New York: Acad. Press, 1982:101-122.24.

26. Klug, G.; Krause, J.; Östlund, A.K.; Knoll, G.; Brdiczka, D. Alteration in liver mitochondrial function as a result of fasting and exhaustive exercise. Biochim. Biophys. Acta 764:272-282; 1984.

27. Knoll, G.; Brdiczka, D. Changes in freeze-fracture mitochondrial membranes correlated to their energetic state. Biochim. Biophys. Acta 733:102-110; 1983.

28. Kottke, M.; Adams, V.; Riesinger, I.; Bremm, G.; Bosch, W.; Brdiczka, D.; Sandri, G.; Panfili, E. Mitochondrial boundary membrane contact sites in brain: points of hexokinase and creatine kinase location and control of Ca^{2+} transport. Biochim. Biophys. Acta 395:807-832; 1988.

29. Lindén, M.; Gellerfors, P.; Nelson, B.D. Pore protein and the hexokinase-binding protein from the outer membrane of rat liver mitochondria are identical. FEBS Lett. 141:189-192; 1982.

30. Ludwig, O.; Benz, R.; Schultz, I.E. Porin of paramecium mitochondria: isolation, characterization and ion selectivity of the closed state. Biochim. Biophys. Acta 978:319-327; 1989.

31. Ohlendieck, K.; Riesinger, I.; Adams, V.; Krause, J.; Brdiczka, D. Enrichment and biochemical characterization of boundary membrane contact sites in rat-liver mitochondria. Biochim. Biophys. Acta 860:672-689; 1986.

32. Östlund, A.K.; Göhring, U.; Krause, J.; Brdiczka, D. The binding of glycerol kinase to the outer membrane of rat liver mitochondria: its importance in metabolic regulation. Biochem. Med. 30:231-245; 1983.

33. Pande, S.V.; Blanchear, M.C. Preferential loss of ATP-dependent long-chain fatty acid activating enzyme in mitochondria prepared using Nargase. Biochim. Biophys. Acta 202:43-48; 1970.

34. Roos, N.; Benz, R.; Brdiczka, D. Identification and characterization of the pore-forming protein in the outer membrane of rat liver mitochondria. Biochim Biophys. Acta 686:204-214; 1982.

35. Saks, V.A.; Rosenshtraukh, L.V.; Smirnov, N.; Chazov, E.I. Role of creatine phosphokinase in cellular function and metabolism. Can. J. Physiol. Pharmacol. 56:691-706; 1987.

36. Schein, S.J.; Colombini, M.; Finkelstein, A. Reconstitution in planar bilayers of a voltage-dependent anion-selective channel obtained from paramecium mitochondria. J. Membr. Biol. 30:99-120; 1976.

37. Soboll, S.; Scholz, R.; Heldt, H.W. Subcellular metabolite concentrations. Dependence of mitochondrial and cytosolic ATP systems on the metabolic state of perfused liver. Eur. J. Biochem. 87:377-390; 1978.

38. Van Venetie, R.; Verkleij, A.J. Possible role of non-bilayer lipids in the structure of mitochondria. Biochim. Biophys. Acta 692:397-405; 1982.

39. Viitanen, P.V.; Geiger, P.J.; Erickson-Viitanen, S.; Bessman, S.P. Evidence for functional hexokinase compartmentation in rat skeletal muscle mitochondria. J. Biol. Chem. 259:9679-9684; 1984.

40. Wallimann, T.; Eppenberger, H.M. Localization and function of M-line bound creatine kinase. M-Band model and creatine phosphate shuttle. In: Shay, I.W., ed. Cell and muscle motility. New York: Plenum; 1985:239-285. (Vol. 6).

41. Weiler, U.; Riesinger, I.; Knoll, G.; Brdiczka, D. The regulation of mitochondrial-bound hexokinases in the liver. Biochem. Med. 33:223-235; 1985.

42. Wilson, J.E. Regulation of mammalian hexokinase activity. In: Beitner, R., ed. Regulation of carbohydrate metabolism. CRC Press; 1986:45-85. (Vol. 1).

43. Wojtczak, L.; Adams, V.; Brdiczka, D. Effect of oleate on the apparent Km of monoamine oxidase and the amount of membrane-bound hexokinase in isolated rat hepatocytes: further evidence for the controlling role of the surface charge in hexokinase binding. Mol. Cell. Biochem. 79:25-30; 1988.

Myosin Light Chain Phosphorylation in Striated and Smooth Muscles

James T. Stull, H. Lee Sweeney, and Kristine E. Kamm
University of Texas, Dallas and University of Texas at Austin, Austin, Texas, U.S.A.

Myosin, the primary protein found in thick filaments of skeletal and smooth muscle cells, plays a central role in the contraction process. Thick filaments are composed of polymerized myosin monomers, and each myosin monomer consists of two heavy chain subunits (200 kDa) and two pairs of light chain subunits. The 20 kDa and 18.5 kDa myosin light chains of smooth and skeletal muscles, respectively, are also referred to as regulatory or phosphorylatable light chains. These light chains are phosphorylated by Ca^{2+}/calmodulin-dependent myosin light chain kinases (13, 41). Myosin light chain kinases are unique protein kinases that catalyze specifically the phosphorylation of myosin light chains with no other physiologically significant protein substrates. We have identified two classes of myosin light chain kinases that are represented by enzymes from skeletal and smooth muscles, respectively (20, 25-27).

In smooth muscle a cascade of cellular reactions leads to myosin light chain phosphorylation, which is necessary for contraction. In fast-twitch skeletal muscle, cytosolic Ca^{2+} levels are dynamically linked to myosin light chain phosphorylation, which appears to enhance muscle performance rather than being an integral component of the contractile mechanism. In this article we will briefly discuss the biochemical basis for two classes of myosin light chain kinases. In addition, the kinetic properties and physiological consequences of myosin light chain phosphorylation in smooth and striated muscles will be reviewed.

Myosin Light Chain Kinases

The relative masses of myosin light chain kinases from skeletal muscles have been examined by Western blotting procedures (26, 27). These myosin light chain kinases vary considerably in relative masses determined by SDS-PAGE and range from 68 kDa to 150 kDa (Table 1). The relative mass of myosin light chain kinase is constant within an animal species, regardless of the skeletal muscle fiber type (slow-twitch, red fibers versus fast-twitch, white). Western blot analyses have demonstrated that the masses of kinases in rabbit (87 kDa) and chicken (150 kDa) skeletal muscles in situ were identical to the purified enzymes. Thus, there are marked differences in sizes of myosin light chain kinases in skeletal muscle.

Considering the unique physiological properties of different smooth muscle tissues, it was of interest to determine whether there were also significant differences in the biochemical properties of smooth muscle myosin light chain kinases. The relative masses of three purified smooth muscle myosin light chain kinases were determined by SDS-PAGE (12). The masses of the three kinases were chicken gizzard, 130 kDa; bovine trachealis, 150 kDa; and porcine carotid artery, 140 kDa.

Monoclonal antibodies were raised against myosin light chain kinase from bovine trachealis (12). Western blot analyses indicated that two of the four monoclonal antibodies cross-reacted with all three purified smooth muscle myosin light chain kinases, whereas two of the antibodies reacted only with the mammalian myosin light chain kinases. Polyclonal and monoclonal antibodies were used for analyses of myosin light chain kinase masses in different smooth muscle tissues. The results indicate that the relative mass of smooth muscle myosin light chain kinase was the same in different tissues within a given animal species. For example, the mass of myosin light chain kinase was 150 kDa in bladder, aorta, trachea, and carotid artery from rabbit. Similar observations were made with other animal species. There were small but significant differences that ranged from 130 kDa to 150 kDa among different animal species (Table 1).

Monoclonal antibodies raised to rabbit skeletal muscle myosin light chain kinase did not cross-react with smooth muscle myosin light chain kinases, including enzyme in rabbit smooth muscles (25). Some of these monoclonal antibodies, however, inhibited enzyme activity, indicating that they bound to the catalytic domain. Likewise, antibodies raised to the smooth muscle myosin light chain kinases did not cross-react with enzyme from skeletal muscle tissues. Nunnally et al. (28) raised a monoclonal antibody to the calmodulin binding domain of the rabbit skeletal muscle myosin light chain kinase that did not bind to smooth muscle myosin light chain kinases. Thus, there appear to be major structural differences between myosin light chain kinases from smooth and those from skeletal muscles.

Table 1   Relative Masses of Myosin Light Chain Kinases

Animal species	Skeletal muscle[a]	Smooth muscle[a]
Chicken	150,000	130,000
Steer	108,000	150,000
Dog	100,000	140,000
Rabbit	87,000	150,000
Guinea pig	83,000	
Rat	82,000	
Mouse	75,000	
Human	68,000	

[a]The relative masses in daltons were determined by SDS-PAGE.

A unique feature of the phosphotransferase reaction catalyzed by myosin light chain kinases is the specificity for myosin light chains (41). It should be noted, however, that the catalytic properties of smooth versus skeletal muscle myosin light chain kinases are significantly different, with unique amino acid determinants for catalysts. The importance of primary structure around the phosphorylatable serine has been examined with synthetic peptide substrates homologous with the primary structure of chicken smooth and skeletal muscle myosin light chains:

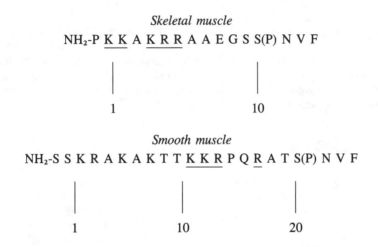

Skeletal muscle

NH$_2$-P $\underline{K}$ $\underline{K}$ A $\underline{K}$ $\underline{R}$ $\underline{R}$ A A E G S S(P) N V F

1   10

Smooth muscle

NH$_2$-S S K R A K A K T T $\underline{K}$ $\underline{K}$ $\underline{R}$ P Q $\underline{R}$ A T S(P) N V F

1   10   20

Synthetic peptide substrates with specific deletions or replacement of residues have been used with myosin light chain kinases from rabbit (87 kDa) and chicken (150 kDa) skeletal muscles (20). The conclusion has been reached that the 6-8 basic residues toward the amino terminus from the phosphorylatable serine are primary determinants for catalysis by skeletal muscle myosin light chain kinases. In addition, two basic amino acids located 10-11 residues toward the amino terminus from the phosphorylatable serine are important determinants. Thus, even though there are marked differences in the sizes of these two skeletal muscle kinases, their catalytic properties are essentially identical. The respective catalytic domains are probably highly conserved, although not identical in structure.

The basic residues that are in a homologous position in the smooth muscle myosin light chain (6-8 residues from the phosphorylatable serine) are also important determinants for gizzard smooth muscle myosin light chain kinase (29). The arginine residue at position 16 in smooth muscle myosin light chain is also an important determinant, whereas the homologous residue is a glutamic acid in the skeletal muscle light chain. Therefore, apparently, a basic residue at this position is not a determinant for catalysis by skeletal myosin light chain kinase. The catalytic properties of avian and mammalian smooth muscle myosin light chain kinases are very similar, if not identical (12). These results are analogous to results obtained from studies on the catalytic properties of avian and mammalian myosin light chain kinases from skeletal muscle.

These biochemical and immunological studies indicate that there are two classes of myosin light chain kinases. The marked differences in structural and catalytic properties suggest that the smooth and skeletal muscle enzymes are derived from two different genes.

Myosin Phosphorylation in Smooth Muscle

Initiation of smooth muscle contraction is thought to proceed primarily by a calmodulin-dependent pathway (14). A stimulus elicits an increase in the cytoplasmic Ca^{2+} concentration (Figure 1). There is an increase in Ca^{2+}/calmodulin, leading to activation of myosin light chain kinase and phosphorylation of the 20 kDa light chain subunit of myosin. Phosphorylated myosin then interacts with filamentous actin to produce contraction.

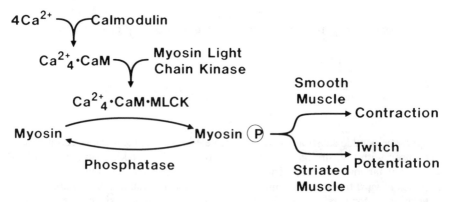

Figure 1.   Scheme for regulation of myosin light chain phosphorylation in smooth and skeletal muscles.

In response to excitation by receptor occupancy, Ca^{2+} is released into the cytoplasm from intracellular storage sites (e.g., sarcoplasmic reticulum). This is believed to occur in response to inositol 1,4,5-trisphosphate ($InsP_3$) (2, 40) generated from hydrolysis of phosphoinositides (9). If this is so, then an increase in intracellular $InsP_3$ should precede an increase in cytoplasmic Ca^{2+} and activation of myosin light chain kinase.

We have directed our attention to the first few seconds of contraction in neurally stimulated bovine tracheal smooth muscle (13, 15, 21). Previously, we observed a latency period of 500 ms between the onset of stimulation and significant changes in either active force or myosin light chain phosphorylation (15). We have determined some of the biochemical events during this period that may be associated with smooth muscle activation. In addition to assessing phosphoinositide metabolism, we measured calmodulin stimulation of cyclic nucleotide phosphodiesterase (37) to determine the apparent activation state of myosin light chain kinase both during the latency period and throughout the period of light chain phosphorylation. We were not able to directly assess myosin light chain kinase activation, due to technical difficulties (46). A key feature of the experimental approach is that activation begins with neurotransmitter (acetylcholine) release from electrically stimulated intrinsic nerves, producing synchronous activation of smooth muscle cells (13, 15).

Measurements of inositol phosphate formation in response to neural stimulation showed that $InsP_1$, $InsP_2$, and $InsP_3$ increased rapidly to values significantly different from control values by 500 ms of neural stimulation (21). $InsP_3$ levels doubled by 500 ms, but they were not significantly different from control values by 1 s. Duncan et al. (7) also observed a transient increase in $InsP_3$ when tracheal smooth muscle was stimulated with a high concentration of acetylcholine (10 μM). They found a 5-fold increase in $InsP_3$ at 1 s, which subsequently decreased to control values by 5 s. Our more rapid responses are probably smaller in magnitude due to the neural stimulation. However, it is clear that a physiological stimulus does increase $InsP_3$ levels before the development of force.

Ca^{2+}/calmodulin stimulation of cyclic GMP phosphodiesterase activity increased to a maximal extent by 500 ms after neural stimulation and remained elevated up to at least 4 s (Figure 2). If activation of phosphodiesterase and myosin light chain kinase follow the same time course, then myosin light chain kinase may be maximally activated by 500 ms. No significant change in the amount of monophosphorylated light chain (less than 10%) was observed during the first 500 ms. The apparent delay between onset of calmodulin-dependent enzyme activity and light chain phosphorylation may be attributed to the time required for conversion of the kinase from an inactive to an active form following binding of Ca^{2+}/calmodulin (11).

After 500 ms, monophosphorylation of light chain increased rapidly and transiently, reaching a maximum value of about 65% at 2 s (Figure 2). The earliest force generation occurred during the period of rapid light chain monophosphorylation. Contraction then proceeded at a lower rate, and active force continued to increase after monophosphorylation values had begun to decline. Diphosphorylation of myosin light chain occurred at a low rate, increasing to 5% of total light chain in the first 4 s and subsequently declining.

The transient myosin light chain phosphorylation observed during the early phase of smooth muscle contraction may result from the transient increase in cytoplasmic Ca^{2+} concentration (6, 36). We observed transients not only in amount of monophosphorylated and diphosphorylated light chain but also in calmodulin-stimulated cyclic nucleotide phosphodiesterase activity; the values for all three were reduced at 10 min compared to values at 4 s. At 10 min, however, maximal force was maintained. These responses are consistent with the notion that with continuous neural stimulation, the cytosolic Ca^{2+} concentration may increase only transiently in spite of force maintenance. The maintenance of force with reduced levels of cytosolic Ca^{2+} and myosin light chain phosphorylation, described as the latch state, is unique to smooth muscles (8).

Kamm and Stull (14) showed that neural stimulation of bovine tracheal smooth muscle resulted in a latency of 500 ms before there was any significant change in myosin light chain phosphorylation, force, or muscle stiffness. Once myosin light chain kinase was activated, myosin light chain was phosphorylated from 0.04 to 0.80 mol phosphate per mol light chain, with a pseudo–first-order rate of 1.1 per s. This rate of phosphorylation is similar to the maximal rate of phosphorylation observed in skeletal muscles (Table 2). There was no evidence of an ordered or

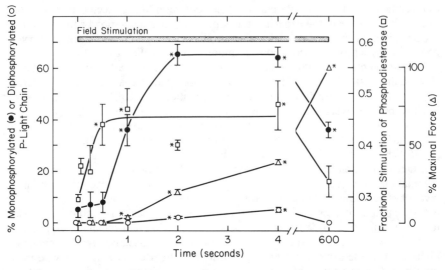

Figure 2.   Neural stimulation of calmodulin-sensitive phosphodiesterase, myosin light chain phosphorylation, and contraction in tracheal smooth muscle. *Values (mean ± S.E.M.) that are significantly different from control values at 0 s. *Note.* From "Biochemical Events Associated With Activation of Smooth Muscle Contraction" by W.C. Miller-Hance, J.R. Miller, J.N. Wells, J.T. Stull, and K.E. Kamm, 1988. Journal of Biological Chemistry, 263, p. 13979-13982. Copyright 1988 by Journal of Biological Chemistry. Adapted by permission.

Table 2   Properties of the Myosin Phosphorylation System in Smooth and Striated Muscles

Muscle	Maximal rate of phosphorylation[a]	Rate of dephosphorylation
Tracheal smooth[b]	31	0.25 s^{-1}
Fast-twitch, white[c]	50	0.007 s^{-1}
Slow-twitch, red[c]	17	0.027 s^{-1}
Heart[d]	0.30	0.023 min^{-1}

[a]μmol light chain phosphorylated per s per L intracellular H_2O. [b]From Kamm and Stull, 1985 (14). [c]From Moore and Stull, 1984 (23). [d]From Silver, Buja, and Stull, 1986 (38).

negatively cooperative process, as suggested from biochemical studies (14). The pseudo–first-order rate could be predicted from product inhibition of the phosphorylation reaction at high substrate concentrations (39) and is consistent with a random phosphorylation process in tracheal smooth muscle cells.

We developed a method for measuring nonphosphorylated, monophosphorylated, and diphosphorylated forms of myosin in tissue extracts to determine the distribution of myosin phosphate in relation to the extent of light chain phosphorylation (32). This analysis allowed us to determine directly whether the phosphorylation reaction in tracheal smooth muscle cells was random or negatively cooperative. In unstimulated bovine tracheal smooth muscle, the extent of light chain phosphorylation was 0.02 mol phosphate per mol light chain, with no measurable amount of phosphorylated myosin. Light chain phosphorylation rapidly increased to a maximal value of 0.78 mol phosphate per mol light chain. During the continuous neural stimulation, there was a proportionate increase in monophosphorylated and diphosphorylated forms of myosin. The relationship between the extent of light chain phosphorylation and the relative amount of diphosphorylated myosin was consistent with a random phosphorylation mechanism in bovine tracheal smooth muscle cells.

In summary, the 500 ms latency in myosin light chain phosphorylation and mechanical activation in neurally stimulated smooth muscle is associated with biochemical processes required for activation of myosin light chain kinase. InsP$_3$ formation is fast enough to serve as a second messenger; in addition, calmodulin activation of cyclic nucleotide phosphodiesterase (hence, probably myosin light chain kinase, also) precedes myosin light chain phosphorylation. Once myosin light chain kinase is activated, myosin light chain is rapidly and randomly phosphorylated. Mechanical activation is associated with myosin light chain phosphorylation.

Myosin Phosphorylation in Skeletal Muscles

Although phosphorylation of myosin light chain was first described for rabbit skeletal muscle myosin (31) and myosin light chain kinase was first purified from rabbit skeletal muscle (35), the role of myosin phosphorylation in striated muscle contraction has been more difficult to elucidate. It is clear that myosin phosphorylation does not play a dominant or obligatory role in contraction, as is suggested for myosin phosphorylation in smooth muscle. However, recent biochemical and physiological experiments indicate that myosin light chain phosphorylation may have a role in potentiating striated muscle contraction.

Pemrick (30) first demonstrated an effect of phosphorylation of light chain on the actin-activated MgATPase activity of rabbit skeletal muscle myosin. Phosphorylation increased MgATPase activity by decreasing the K_{app} of actin for myosin with no effect on the V_{max} value. These observations were made with both myosin and the proteolytic fragment of myosin, heavy meromyosin. Persechini and Stull (33) also demonstrated a decrease in the K_{app} of actin after phosphorylation, with no change in the V_{max} value. The phosphorylation response was labile, and conditions used by many investigators for the preparation and assay of myosin could result in the loss of the phosphorylation effect. Phosphorylated myosin dissociates from actin at higher pyrophosphate concentrations than does nonphosphorylated myosin (19). These data collectively indicate that phosphorylated skeletal muscle myosin has an apparent higher affinity for actin.

Muscle fibers can be made permeable by mechanical or chemical treatments that remove membrane structures, allowing for the control of the internal environment surrounding the myofilament lattice. The Ca^{2+} concentration can be controlled with divalent metal buffer systems, and MgATPase can be added for phosphorylation or contraction. This experimental approach has been used to study the effect of myosin light chain phosphorylation on isometric force in rabbit skeletal muscle fibers at 0.6 and 10 μM Ca^{2+} (34). The lower Ca^{2+} concentration produced 10-20% of the maximal isometric force obtained at 10 μM Ca^{2+}. Phosphorylation of myosin light chain from 0.10 to 0.80 mol of phosphate per mol of light chain resulted in a 100% increase in isometric force at the lower Ca^{2+} concentration (Figure 3). Addition of a protein phosphatase dephosphorylated light chain and reversed the isometric tension response. At the higher Ca^{2+} concentration, light chain phosphorylation was found to have little effect on isometric force. Permeable fibers were also isolated under conditions in which there was 0.80 mol of phosphate per mol of light chain. Addition of protein phosphatase to fibers incubated at 0.60 μM Ca^{2+} caused a decrease in isometric force associated with dephosphorylation of light chain. Thus, light chain phosphorylation increases force at Ca^{2+} concentrations less than those required for maximal activation of the thin filament regulatory proteins.

The effect of myosin light chain phosphorylation on force produced over a wide range of Ca^{2+} concentrations has also been examined in permeabilized rabbit skeletal muscle fibers. There was no effect at Ca^{2+} concentrations that produced 50% or greater activation of contraction (43). However, myosin phosphorylation increased force at less than 50% of maximal activation by Ca^{2+}, with a leftward shift of the

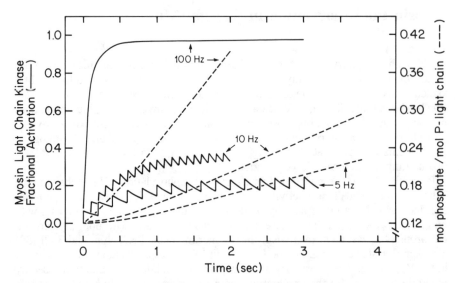

Figure 3. Myosin light chain kinase activation and light chain phosphorylation in response to stimulation of fast-twitch skeletal muscle. Curves were derived from computer simulation in which the activation-inactivation properties of myosin light chain kinase and the total activities of myosin light chain kinase and phosphatase were used. *Note.* From "Myosin Light Chain Phosphorylation in Fast and Slow Skeletal Muscles in Situ" by R.L. Moore and J.T. Stull, 1984, *American Journal of Physiology, 247,* p. C462-C471. Copyright 1984 by *American Journal of Physiology.* Adapted by permission.

pCa^{2+} concentration-force relationship (44). This shift was due to a decrease in the slope of the Ca^{2+}-force relationship. Similar results have also been obtained with cardiac fibers, another striated muscle with a thin filament troponin-tropomyosin, Ca^{2+} regulatory system (24, 44). Myosin light chain phosphorylation does not appear to alter the kinetics of the cross-bridge cycle, as assessed by the force-velocity relationship (34, 43). Therefore, myosin phosphorylation is probably not altering the time a myosin cross-bridge remains attached to actin, but it may increase the probability of myosin cross-bridge interaction with actin at submaximal levels of Ca^{2+} activation (44). Although the mechanism for this potentiation response has not been fully described, it appears that myosin phosphorylation affects the response to Ca^{2+} activation of thin filaments of skeletal muscle fibers and is not required for contraction per se.

In order to determine the function of myosin light chain phosphorylation in living muscle, it is important to understand how myosin light chain phosphorylation is regulated in vivo. In mammalian striated muscles, there are several key properties of the phosphorylation system: An increase in the phosphate content of myosin light chain is dependent upon the frequency of muscle stimulation; the maximal rate of light chain phosphorylation exceeds the maximal rate of light chain dephosphorylation by 10- to 60-fold; the maximal rates of phosphorylation and dephosphorylation are much slower than the rates of contraction and relaxation (17, 18, 23). Based upon these properties, a quantitative model has been proposed for explaining the contraction-frequency dependence of myosin light chain phosphorylation (23, 42). When previously quiescent muscle is stimulated in a very rapid and repetitive fashion to produce a tetanic contraction (200 Hz), myosin light chain kinase is fully activated due to a rapid and sustained increase in sarcoplasmic Ca^{2+} concentrations; the rate of light chain phosphorylation is dependent upon the amount of myosin light chain kinase in muscle. However, a single rise and fall in sarcoplasmic Ca^{2+} concentration, as a result of a single twitch stimulus, results in the rapid activation of a small portion of myosin light chain kinase. This activation is followed by a relatively slow rate of inactivation (1 s^{-1}) after the decrease in sarcoplasmic Ca^{2+} concentrations and relaxation. The critical feature of this hypothesis is related to the slow rate of inactivation of myosin light chain kinase (seconds) relative to the rapid rate of decrease in sarcoplasmic Ca^{2+} concentrations and relaxation (milliseconds). The fraction of myosin light chain kinase in the active form will thus be dependent upon the relative magnitudes of the activation and inactivation processes. An increase in the frequency of contraction at physiological rates (0.5 to 30 Hz) increases the extent of fractional activation because a greater number of Ca^{2+} transients results in a greater incremental increase in the active form of the enzyme for a given period of time (Figure 3). In addition, the time between Ca^{2+} transients, during which myosin light chain kinase inactivation occurs, is decreased. With a continuous repetitive stimulation, therefore, the fractional activation of myosin light chain kinase increases until an equilibrium is established between the activation and inactivation processes.

The model presented (23, 42) has used quantitative information regarding the intracellular content of calmodulin, myosin light chain kinase activity, myosin light chain phosphatase activity, and estimates of the rates of myosin light chain kinase activation and inactivation as a result of increases and decreases in sarcoplasmic Ca^{2+} concentrations. This model shows that transient increases and decreases in the amount of activated myosin light chain kinase resulting from the cyclic activation and inactivation of the enzyme are evident at lower, physiologically relevant contraction frequencies, that is, between 1 and 30 Hz. It is important to emphasize that myosin light chain kinase can be activated during repetitive stimulation at these low-frequency ranges that occur in vivo, despite the fact that the muscle is relaxed (sarcoplasmic Ca^{2+} concentrations are low) during most of the period between each stimulation (16). A plateau in fractional activation that results from an equilibrium being established between the activation and inactivation processes is apparent with prolonged periods of stimulation or at higher contraction frequencies. These predicted extents of light chain phosphorylation are in good agreement with experimentally determined values.

Because experimentally observed and simulated rates of myosin light chain phosphorylation are similar (23, 42), the primary regulation mechanisms proposed for the activation and inactivation of myosin light chain kinase, and the relative activities of myosin light chain kinase and myosin light chain phosphatase, appear to be sufficient to describe the effect of contraction frequency on light chain phosphorylation in white, fast-twitch skeletal fibers. However, there are differences in the responses to repetitive stimulation in different types of striated muscle fibers. In red, slow-twitch muscle, the myosin light chain kinase and myosin light chain phosphatase activities are 3 times lower and 4 times higher, respectively, than the same activities in white, fast-twitch skeletal muscle fibers (Table 2). There are even greater differences in comparing these values to cardiac muscle. Thus, there is approximately a 12-fold decrease in the potential for phosphorylation. Computer simulation with these biochemical properties for red, slow-twitch muscle indicate that much higher contraction frequencies are required for a small increase in phosphorylation. These predicted results are confirmed by direct experimental observations (23).

It is clear that myosin light chain phosphorylation is not required for actin-activation of myosin MgATPase activity or contraction of permeable striated muscle fibers. Therefore, myosin light chain phosphorylation in vivo would not be expected to be obligatory for contraction. Myosin light chain phosphorylation in intact skeletal muscle fibers has no significant effect on maximal force development (1, 5, 17, 18) or the maximal shortening velocity (3). At this time, the only correlation of myosin light chain phosphorylation to a physiological property of striated muscles is to the contraction-induced potentiation of isometric twitch tension in fast-twitch fibers (10, 16-18, 22, 23). Potentiation of isometric twitch tension is a response intrinsic to fast-twitch, but not slow-twitch, skeletal muscle fibers. Phosphate incorporation into myosin light chain resulting from contraction of slow-twitch skeletal muscles is rarely observed and occurs only in response to muscle stimulation at frequencies and durations that exceed those observed in vivo. Although there is one report claiming a high extent of myosin light chain phosphorylation in slow-twitch skeletal muscle (45), these results are contrary to numerous other studies (1, 5, 10, 18, 23) and can probably be explained by technical artifacts (22).

Potentiation of isometric twitch tension in fast-twitch fibers occurs either following a tetanus (post-tetanic) or upon repetitive stimulation of contractile twitches (staircase). There is a direct correlation between the extent of isometric twitch tension potentiation following the tetanus or during the staircase response under a variety of experimental conditions (10, 16-18, 22, 23). In relation to recent data obtained with permeable fibers, Ca^{2+} activation of thin filaments during a twitch would have to be less than maximal for myosin phosphorylation to be a mechanism for potentiation of isometric twitch tension. Recent modeling of Ca^{2+} movements in skeletal muscle upon activation suggest that the maximal amount of Ca^{2+} binding to troponin during an isometric twitch is probably not saturating the troponin Ca^{2+} binding sites (4). The Ca^{2+} binding-time integral during a twitch shows less than 50% saturation during the transient increase and decrease in sarcoplasmic Ca^{2+} concentrations. Thus, phosphorylation of myosin could result in potentiation of isometric tension during twitches because less than 50% saturation is achieved during much of the Ca^{2+} transient time. In the case of a tetanus, phosphorylation would not result in potentiation because Ca^{2+} binding sites on troponin are greater than 50% saturated.

In summary, myosin light chain is phosphorylated under physiological conditions of repetitive, low-frequency stimulation in fast-twitch skeletal muscle. Phosphorylation under these conditions can be accounted for by the activation-inactivation properties of myosin light chain kinase, in addition to the relative and total amounts of myosin light chain kinase and myosin light chain phosphatase activities. In fast-twitch skeletal muscle, myosin phosphorylation increases actin-activated myosin MgATPase activity, increases tension at levels of Ca^{2+} that produce partial activation in permeable fibers, and correlates with potentiation of isometric twitch tension following repetitive stimuli. This myosin phosphorylation plays a modulatory role in skeletal muscle contraction.

References

1. Barsotti, R.J.; Butler, T.M. Chemical energy usage and myosin light chain phosphorylation in mammalian skeletal muscle. J. Muscle Res. Cell Motil. 5:45-64; 1984.

2. Berridge, M.J.; Irvine, R.F. Inositol trisphosphate, a novel second messenger in cellular signal transduction. Nature 312:315-321; 1984.

3. Butler, T.M.; Siegman, M.J.; Mooers, S.U. Chemical energy usage during shortening and work production in mammalian smooth muscle. Am J. Physiol. 244:C234-C242; 1983.

4. Cannell, M.B.; Allen, D.G. Model of calcium movements during activation in the sarcomere of frog skeletal muscle. Biophys. J. 45:913-925; 1984.

5. Crow, M.T.; Kushmerick, M.J. Myosin light chain phosphorylation is associated with a decrease in the energy cost for contraction in fast twitch mouse muscles. J. Biol. Chem. 257:2121-2124; 1982.

6. DeFeo, T.T.; Morgan, K.G. Calcium-force relationships as detected with aequorin in two different vascular smooth muscles of the ferret. J. Physiol. (Lond.) 369:269-282; 1985.

7. Duncan, R.A.; Krzanowski, J.J.; Davis, J.S.; Polson, J.B.; Coffey, R.G.; Shimoda, T.; Szentivanyi, A. Rapid communications: polyphosphoinositide metabolism in canine tracheal smooth muscle (CTSM) in response to a cholinergic stimulus. Biochem. Pharmacol. 36:307-310; 1987.

8. Hai, C.M.; Murphy, R.A. Cross-bridge phosphorylation and regulation of latch state in smooth muscle. Am. J. Physiol. 254:C99-C106; 1988.

9. Hokin, L.E. Receptors and phosphoinositide-generated second messengers. Annu. Rev. Biochem. 54:205-235; 1985.

10. Houston, M.E.; Green, H.J.; Stull, J.T. Myosin light chain phosphorylation and isometric twitch potentiation in intact human muscle. Pflügers Arch. 403:348-352; 1985.

11. Johnson, J.D.; Holroyde, M.J.; Crouch, T.H.; Solaro, R.J.; Potter, J.D. Fluorescence studies of the interaction of calmodulin with myosin light chain kinase. J. Biol. Chem. 256:12194-12198; 1981.

12. Kamm, K.E.; Leachman, S.A.; Michnoff, C.H.; Nunnally, M.H.; Persechini, A.; Richardson, A.L.; Stull, J.T. Myosin light chain kinases and kinetics of myosin phosphorylation in smooth muscle cells. In: Siegman, M.J.; Somlyo, A.P.; Stephens, N.L., eds. Regulation and contraction of smooth muscle. New York: A. Liss, Inc.; 1987:183-193. (Vol. 245).

13. Kamm, K.E.; Stull, J.T. Myosin phosphorylation, force, and maximal shortening velocity in neurally stimulated tracheal smooth muscle. Am. J. Physiol. 249:C238-C247; 1985.

14. Kamm, K.E.; Stull, J.T. The function of myosin and myosin light chain phosphorylation in smooth muscle. Annu. Rev. Pharmacol. Toxicol. 25:593-620; 1985.

15. Kamm, K.E.; Stull, J.T. Activation of smooth muscle contraction: relation between myosin phosphorylation and stiffness. Science 232:80-82; 1986.

16. Klug, G.A.; Botterman, B.R.; Stull, J.T. The effect of low frequency stimulation on myosin light chain phosphorylation in skeletal muscle. J. Biol. Chem. 257:4688-4690; 1982.

17. Manning, D.R.; Stull, J.T. Myosin light chain phosphorylation and phosphorylase A activity in rat extensor digitorum longus muscle. Biochem. Biophys. Res. Commun. 90:164-170; 1979.

18. Manning, D.R.; Stull, J.T. Myosin light chain phosphorylation-dephosphorylation in mammalian skeletal muscle. Am. J. Physiol. 242:C234-C241; 1982.

19. Michnicka, M.; Kasman, K.; Kakol, I. The binding of actin to phosphorylated and dephosphorylated myosin. Biochim. Biophys. Acta 704:470-475; 1982.

20. Michnoff, C.H.; Kemp, B.E.; Stull, J.T. Phosphorylation of synthetic peptides by skeletal muscle myosin light chain kinases. J. Biol. Chem. 261:8320-8326; 1986.

21. Miller-Hance, W.C.; Miller, J.R.; Wells, J.N.; Stull, J.T.; Kamm, K.E. Biochemical events associated with activation of smooth muscle contraction. J. Biol. Chem. (in press).

22. Moore, R.L.; Houston, M.E.; Iwamoto, G.A.; Stull, J.T. Phosphorylation of rabbit skeletal muscle myosin in situ. J. Cell. Physiol. 125:301-310; 1985.

23. Moore, R.L.; Stull, J.T. Myosin light chain phosphorylation in fast and slow skeletal muscles in situ. Am. J. Physiol. 247:C462-C471; 1984.

24. Morano, I.F.; Hofmann, F.; Zimmer, M.; Ruegg, J.C. The influence of P-light chain phosphorylation by myosin light chain kinase on the calcium sensitivity of chemically skinned heart fibres. FEBS Lett. 189:221-224; 1985.

25. Nunnally, M.H.; Hsu, L.-C.; Mumby, M.C.; Stull, J.T. Structural studies of rabbit skeletal muscle myosin light chain kinase with monoclonal antibodies. J. Biol. Chem. 262:3833-3838; 1987.

26. Nunnally, M.H.; Rybicki, S.B.; Stull, J.T. Characterization of chicken skeletal muscle myosin light chain kinase: evidence for muscle-specific isozymes. J. Biol. Chem. 260:1020-1026; 1985.

27. Nunnally, M.H.; Stull, J.T. Mammalian skeletal muscle myosin light chain kinases. J. Biol. Chem. 259:1776-1780; 1984.

28. Nunnally, M.H.; Stull, J.T.; Blumenthal, D.K.; Krebs, E.G. Properties of a monoclonal antibody raised to the calmodulin-binding domain of myosin light chain kinase. Fed. Proc. 45:1551; 1986.

29. Pearson, R.B.; Jakes, R.; John, M.; Kendrick-Jones, J.; Kemp, B.E. Phosphorylation site sequence of smooth muscle myosin light chain (Mr = 20000). FEBS Lett. 168:108-112; 1984.

30. Pemrick, S.M. The phosphorylated L₂ light chain of skeletal myosin is a modifier of the actomyosin ATPase. J. Biol. Chem. 255:8836-8841; 1980.

31. Perrie, W.T.; Smillie, L.B.; Perry, S.V. A phosphorylated light-chain component of myosin from skeletal muscle. Biochem. J. 135:151-164; 1973.

32. Persechini, A.; Kamm, K.E.; Stull, J.T. Different phosphorylated forms of myosin in contracting tracheal smooth muscle. J. Biol. Chem. 261:6293-6299; 1986.

33. Persechini, A.; Stull, J.T. Phosphorylation kinetics of skeletal muscle myosin and the effect of phosphorylation on actomyosin adenosinetriphosphatase activity. Biochemistry 23:4144-4150; 1984.

34. Persechini, A.; Stull, J.T.; Cooke, R. The effect of myosin phosphorylation on the contractile properties of skinned rabbit skeletal muscle fibers. J. Biol. Chem. 260:7951-7954; 1985.

35. Pires, E.M.V.; Perry, S.V. Purification and properties of myosin light-chain kinase from fast skeletal muscle. Biochem. J. 167:137-146; 1977.

36. Rembold, C.M.; Murphy, R.A. Myoplasmic calcium, myosin phosphorylation, and regulation of the crossbridge cycle in swine arterial smooth muscle. Circ. Res. 58:803-815; 1986.

37. Saitoh, Y.; Hardman, J.G.; Wells, J.N. Differences in the association of calmodulin with cyclic nucleotide phosphodiesterase in relaxed and contracted arterial strips. Biochemistry 24:1613-1618; 1985.

38. Silver, P.J.; Buja, L.M.; Stull, J.T. Frequency-dependent myosin light chain phosphorylation in isolated myocardium. J. Mol. Cell. Cardiol. 18:31-37; 1986.

39. Sobieszek, A. Phosphorylation reaction of vertebrate smooth muscle myosin: an enzyme kinetic analysis. Biochemistry 24:1266-1274; 1985.

40. Somlyo, A.V.; Bond, M.; Somlyo, A.P.; Scarpa, A. Inositol trisphosphate-induced calcium release and contraction in vascular smooth muscle. Proc. Natl. Acad. Sci. USA 82:5231-5235; 1985.

41. Stull, J.T.; Nunnally, M.H.; Michnoff, C.H. Calmodulin-dependent protein kinases. In: Krebs, E.G.; Boyer, P.D., eds. The enzymes. Orlando, FL: Academic Press; 1986:113-166. (Vol. 17).

42. Stull, J.T.; Nunnally, M.H.; Moore, R.L.; Blumenthal, D.K. Myosin light chain kinases and myosin phosphorylation in skeletal muscle. In: Weber, G., ed. Advan. enzyme regul. Oxford and New York: Pergamon Press; 1985:123-140. (Vol. 23).

43. Sweeney, J.L.; Kushmerick, M.J. Myosin phosphorylation in permeabilized rabbit psoas fibers. Am. J. Physiol. 249:C362-C365; 1985.

44. Sweeney, J.L.; Stull, J.T. Phosphorylation of myosin in permeabilized mammalian cardiac and skeletal muscle cells. Am. J. Physiol. 250:C657-C660; 1986.

45. Westwood, S.A.; Hudlicka, O.; Perry, S.V. Phosphorylation in vivo of the P light chain of myosin in rabbit fast and slow skeletal muscles. Biochem. J. 218:841-847; 1984.

46. Zimmer, M.; Hofmann, F. Calmodulin antagonists inhibit activity of myosin light-chain kinase independent of calmodulin. Eur. J. Biochem. 142:393-397; 1984.

PART V

Muscle Metabolic Disorders: Exercise Implications

Disorders of Muscle Glycogenolysis/Glycolysis: The Consequences of Substrate-Limited Oxidative Metabolism in Humans

Steven F. Lewis and Ronald G. Haller

University of Texas Southwestern Medical Center and
Veterans Administration Medical Center, Dallas, Texas, U.S.A.

The importance of muscle glycogen as a substrate for human exercise performance was first demonstrated in a series of classical studies by Hultman, Bergstrom, Hermansen, Ahlborg, Saltin, and co-workers (1, 6, 29, 30, 64). At work loads above 50% of maximal oxygen uptake ($\dot{V}O_2$max), muscle glycogen was identified as the dominant fuel, and between 70-80% of $\dot{V}O_2$max, the duration of exercise performance was shown to be directly related to the initial glycogen content in active muscle, the point of fatigue corresponding closely to virtually complete glycogen depletion. The specific significance of glycogen as an oxidizable substrate during prolonged heavy exercise was evident from the relatively modest accumulation of muscle and blood lactate. To date, numerous studies on various aspects of human and animal glycogen metabolism have been reported (cf. 11, 16, 31, 56), but there is only limited information on the impact of a *lack* of available muscle glycogen on regulatory mechanisms during exercise in humans (cf. 37). Thus, the physiological significance of glycogen as the primary oxidizable fuel endogenous to skeletal muscle remains incompletely defined.

Unique models for studying this problem are provided by patients with disorders of muscle glycogenolysis/glycolysis. These are genetic defects consisting of an absent or, less frequently, a catalytically inactive enzyme protein in the metabolism of skeletal muscle glycogen. The known enzymatic defects are shown in Figure 1. Most of the data on exercise pathophysiology are available from patients with muscle glycogen phosphorylase deficiency (McArdle's disease), but an extensive series has recently been completed on human muscle phosphofructokinase (PFK) deficiency (7, 24, 34, 43, 47, 67). McArdle disease and PFK-deficient patients characteristically report a lifelong history of exercise intolerance, compatible with an inborn metabolic error, and demonstrate a lack of elevation in blood lactate levels during fatiguing ischemic exercise, the biochemical hallmark of absent glycolysis. The clinical hallmark of these disorders is the occurrence of an electrically silent muscle contracture resulting from intense or ischemic exercise. A rapid onset of fatigue related to a lack of glycogen availability observed in these patients after as little as 1-2 min of mild (by normal standards) nonischemic exercise is analogous to that experienced by healthy subjects with glycogen depleted muscles due to effort usually longer than 1 hour. The patients have a complete lack of access to glycogen, which cannot readily be duplicated by employing muscle glycogen depletion to create analogous models in healthy human or animal subjects. The problems (i.e., incomplete depletion, muscle glycogen restoration prior to testing, residual fatigue from exercise-induced depletion, unpleasant dietary restrictions) largely involve the achievement and maintenance of complete glycogen depletion in the muscles to be studied. These difficulties emphasize the uniqueness of studying patients with McArdle's disease and PFK deficiency. Animals with similar genetic errors of muscle glycogen metabolism are unavailable or not physiologically comparable (71, 73).

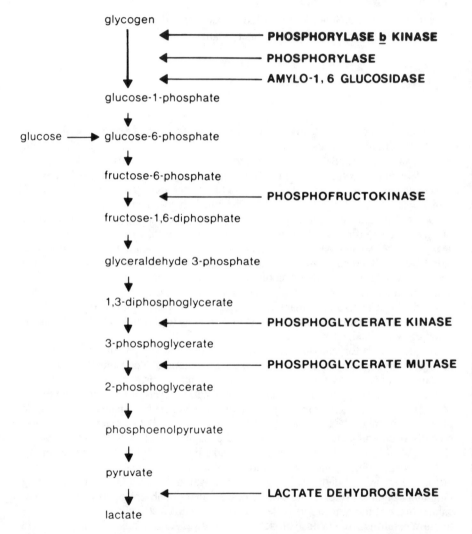

Figure 1.   Schematic of anaerobic glycogenolysis/glycolysis. Arrows indicating the reversibility of reactions have been omitted for simplicity. The sites of known human enzymatic defects are shown in bold type.

The Oxidative Defect in Glycogenolytic Disorders

Evaluation of the four modes of muscle ATP resynthesis/ADP removal—oxidative phosphorylation, anaerobic glycolysis, the creatine kinase reaction, and the adenylate kinase reaction (Table 1)—in patients with defects of glycogen metabolism, provides a framework for understanding the physiological implications of these defects. Oxidative metabolism is the major quantitative mode of ATP resynthesis and ADP removal in skeletal muscle, whereas glycolysis and the creatine kinase reaction play much more limited quantitative roles. The adenylate kinase reaction has a negligible capacity for ATP resynthesis and is coupled to that of AMP deaminase. The major function of the coupled adenylate kinase–AMP deaminase reactions appears to be to buffer increases in ADP when the rates of energy demand and ATP hydrolysis exceed the rates of ADP removal via oxidative phosphorylation, anaerobic glycolysis, and the creatine kinase reaction.

Table 1 ATP Resynthesis/ADP Utilization in Skeletal Muscle

1. Oxidative phosphorylation
   A. $glycogen_{(n)} + 6O_2 + 37P_i + 37ADP \rightarrow glycogen_{(n-1)} + 6CO_2 + 42H_2O + 37ATP$
   B. $glucose + 6O_2 + 36P_i + 36ADP \rightarrow 6CO_2 + 42H_2O + 36ATP$
   C. $palmitate + 23O_2 + 129P_i + 129ADP \rightarrow 16CO_2 + 145H_2O + 129ATP$

2. Anaerobic glycolysis
   A. $glycogen_{(n)} + 3P_i + 3ADP \rightarrow glycogen_{(n-1)} + 2\ lactate + 2H_2O + 3ATP$
   B. $glucose + 2P_i + 2ADP \rightarrow 2\ lactate + 2H_2O + 2ATP$

3. Creatine kinase reaction
   $ADP + PCr + H^+ \leftrightarrow ATP + Cr$

4. Adenylate kinase–AMP deaminase reactions
   $2ADP \leftrightarrow ATP + AMP/AMP + H_2O \rightarrow NH_3 + IMP + 2P_i$

Note. P_i, inorganic phosphate; ADP, adenosine diphosphate; ATP, adenosine triphosphate; PCr, phosphocreatine; Cr, creatine; AMP, adenosine monophosphate; IMP, inosine monophosphate. From ref. 38.

Overall assessment of oxidative metabolism consists of measuring $\dot{V}O_2max$ and its components, maximal arteriovenous oxygen difference and maximal cardiac output. In patients with McArdle's disease and PFK deficiency, $\dot{V}O_2max$ is 35-50% of normal (2, 23, 26, 37, 43). This is due to a markedly subnormal muscle oxygen extraction, which is reflected by a 25-50% rise in systemic arteriovenous oxygen difference from rest to maximal exercise, in contrast to the 3- to 4-fold elevation normally observed (Figure 2). Maximal cardiac output is within the normal range (Figure 2), indicative of a normal cardiac pump function, likely due to the presence of tissue-specific isozymes of phosphorylase (48) and phosphofructokinase (61). In direct contrast to McArdle and PFK-deficient patients, $\dot{V}O_2max$ and systemic arterio-venous oxygen difference are essentially normal in patients with a selective defect in muscle long chain fatty acid oxidation due to carnitine palmitoyltransferase deficiency (12, 25). These findings are consistent with evidence that the availability of muscle glycogen as an oxidizable substrate is critical for normal muscle O_2 extraction and the expression of maximal aerobic power (37). The depressed $\dot{V}O_2max$ in patients with McArdle's disease and PFK deficiency is associated with a virtual absence of muscle pyruvate (72), the preferred substrate for oxidative metabolism (22). It has been postulated (37) that in McArdle and PFK-deficient patients, a diminished supply of muscle pyruvate will limit the rate of production of acetyl CoA for incorporation into the citric acid cycle. This will in turn attenuate the maximal rates of formation of citrate and production of reducing potentials, chiefly NADH, resulting in a substrate-limited rate of oxygen uptake by the mitochondrial respiratory chain. The finding of subnormal levels of NADH in active muscle during maximal bicycle exercise in McArdle's disease (Sahlin, Haller, Henriksson, Areskog, Lewis, & Jorfeldt, unpublished observations) supports the concept of a substrate-limited oxidative metabolism in patients who lack the ability to oxidize muscle glycogen, the most abundant intramuscular oxidative fuel.

To What Extent Can Blood-Borne Substrates Compensate?

A substrate-limited oxidative metabolism in McArdle disease patients implies that the primary blood-borne oxidizable substrates, free fatty acids (FFA) and glucose, normally cannot provide sufficient energy to completely compensate for the unavailability of muscle glycogen during strenuous exercise. Utilization of FFA and glucose is dependent on the concerted action of several physiological systems, including (a) mobilization of these substrates from adipose tissue and liver, (b) their circulatory delivery to active muscle, (c) their transport into active muscle, and (d) their incorporation and oxidation by the appropriate intramuscular metabolic pathways. Available data are limited in McArdle disease and are largely lacking for patients with PFK deficiency, in whom glucose oxidation by muscle is blocked (Figure 1). Thus, the relative importance and limitations of each system cannot presently be discussed in detail. For McArdle disease, several pertinent issues can, however, be addressed. A compensatory increase in the availability of blood-borne substrate to active muscle could be accomplished merely by a larger than normal increase in blood flow to active muscle, which has been documented in patients with McArdle's disease (5, 41, 45); or it could be part of an integrated response including an enhanced adipose tissue lipolysis and hepatic glycogenolysis, possibly accompanied by increases in adipose tissue and splanchnic blood flow. A much steeper than normal increase in plasma norepinephrine in relation to systemic oxygen uptake occurs in McArdle patients (8), suggesting an increased signal for adipose tissue lipolysis and probably also for hepatic glycogenolysis. Measurements of adipose tissue and liver blood flow have not, to our knowledge, been reported during exercise in patients with glycogenolytic disorders, but there is evidence to suggest that flow to these organs is not abnormally large during exercise (45).

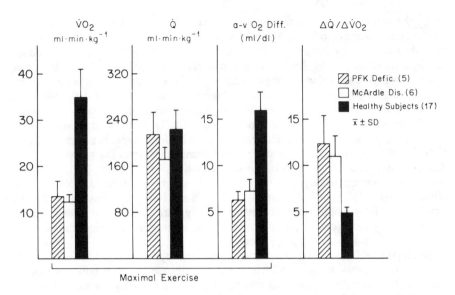

Figure 2. Oxygen uptake, cardiac output, and systemic arteriovenous oxygen difference ($\overline{X} \pm SD$) during maximal exercise performed 2-3 hours postprandially in patients with PFK deficiency (3 M, 2 F), McArdle's disease (4 M, 2 F), and healthy control subjects (9 M, 8 F). The mean regression slope ($\Delta\dot{Q}/\Delta\dot{V}O_2$; $\overline{X} \pm SD$) for each group is depicted in the rightmost panel. (Measurements as described by refs. 42, 69.)

The dynamics of glucose turnover in patients with McArdle's disease have not been studied in detail. There are, however, data indicating that the relative contribution of blood glucose to muscle ATP resynthesis during heavy exercise in McArdle patients can be considerably greater than in healthy subjects. Arterial or systemic venous blood glucose tends to fall during exercise in McArdle patients (9, 35, 53, 54, 66). Blood glucose concentration during exercise reflects the balance of the rates of hepatic glucose release and muscle glucose uptake (21). A decline in blood glucose would therefore imply that glucose uptake by active muscle is increasing more rapidly than hepatic glucose release. Measurements of leg blood flow and femoral arteriovenous glucose differences during maximal bicycle exercise in two patients with McArdle's disease studied under nonfasting conditions provide evidence for an increased muscle glucose utilization to support oxidative metabolism (Jorfeldt, Haller, Henriksson, Areskog, & Lewis, unpublished observations). Glucose uptake increased more than 4-fold and arterial glucose concentration fell between 7% and 21% from rest to maximal exercise in these patients. During maximal cycle exercise at a work load of 60-70 W, glucose uptake was similar in both patients, averaging 1.2 mmol/min (two-leg total). One mole of glucose yields 36 ATP when completely oxidized to CO_2 and H_2O. Leg O_2 uptake was similar in both patients, averaging 30 mmol/min (two-leg total).

Assuming that a mixture of fat and carbohydrate was oxidized, approximately 5.8 moles ATP can be produced per mole of O_2 consumed. Therefore, glucose taken up by the working legs, assuming complete oxidation from the virtual absence of lactate accumulation (Jorfeldt, Sahlin, Lewis, Henriksson, Areskog, & Haller, unpublished observations), can account for as much as 25% of the total ATP production by active muscle in McArdle patients. In contrast, arterial blood glucose increases during maximal exercise in healthy subjects (21, 33). Leg glucose uptake in healthy subjects, although much greater in absolute terms than that observed in the McArdle patients, can be calculated to account for only a few percent of the total ATP production during exercise at maximal oxygen uptake (33). This can be explained in part by the finding that free glucose accumulated in active leg muscle in normal subjects (33), suggesting that leg glucose utilization increased less than leg glucose uptake. The level of glucose-6-phosphate, a potent inhibitor of hexokinase (57), increases markedly in active muscle of healthy subjects at maximal exercise (33) but remains at very low levels in McArdle patients (67; Sahlin, Haller, Henriksson, Areskog, Lewis, & Jorfeldt, unpublished observations), suggesting that the glucose taken up can be readily incorporated into glycolysis in phosphorylase-deficient muscle, but not normal muscle, during heavy work.

Although blood glucose oxidation may normally support up to 1/4 of the maximal rate of oxidative resynthesis of ATP in McArdle's disease, its contribution is modest when contrasted with the fact that muscle glycogen is virtually the exclusive substrate fully oxidized by normal human skeletal muscle in maximal exercise (64). Elevation of blood glucose levels by approximately 70% during I.V. glucose infusion resulted in a 23% increase in $\dot{V}O_2$max in McArdle patients (26). However, blood glucose apparently cannot fully substitute for muscle glycogen as an oxidative substrate in short-term heavy exercise because $\dot{V}O_2$max and the proportion of carbohydrate oxidized (based on the respiratory exchange ratio) remained abnormally low in the McArdle patients after glucose infusion (26). The effect of larger elevations in blood glucose on $\dot{V}O_2$max in McArdle patients has not been systematically studied, but available data suggest that restoration of normal aerobic power is not likely to be achieved in this manner. *It is therefore apparent that a lack of availability of glycogen makes muscle heavily dependent on FFA as an oxidizable fuel.* This conclusion is particularly applicable to patients with PFK deficiency. PFK-deficient muscle is unable to oxidize glucose because its entry into glycolysis metabolically precedes the enzymatic defect.

Consequentially, it was postulated that in PFK deficiency $\dot{V}O_2$max is directly dependent on the availability of FFA. The hypothesis was confirmed in 4 PFK-deficient patients studied under three conditions in which mean plasma FFA varied nearly 6-fold: (a) intravenous glucose infusion, (b) fasting overnight, and (c) intravenous infusion of the triglyceride emulsion liposyn plus heparin injection (24). $\dot{V}O_2$max under conditions of increased FFA availability, that is, liposyn infusion and fasting, was 62% and 39% higher, respectively, than during glucose infusion, but it was far from fully normalized (Figure 3). Maximal cardiac output was similar under each condition, but maximal arteriovenous oxygen difference was larger the higher the level of plasma FFA, consistent with an increased O_2 extraction by working muscle when the substrate limitation to oxidative metabolism was partially removed by supplying increased FFA. In 4 PFK-deficient patients, $\dot{V}O_2$max was an average of 28% higher after fasting followed by 45 min of moderate exercise than under control conditions (2-hour postprandial) (Haller & Lewis, unpublished data). Also, when FFA availability was increased by fasting alone (13) or fasting followed by 45 min of moderate exercise (37) in McArdle patients, there was a 15-18% increase

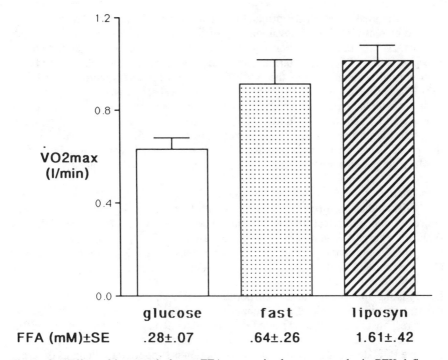

Figure 3. Effect of increased plasma FFA on maximal oxygen uptake in PFK deficiency ($n = 4$) (Haller & Lewis, unpublished data).

in $\dot{V}O_2$max over control levels. The similarity of $\dot{V}O_2$max in PFK deficiency and McArdle's disease under postprandial conditions (Figure 2) is consistent with the concept of a relatively limited overall contribution of blood glucose as a fuel for maximal exercise performance and with a strong dependency on FFA for oxidative metabolism in both of these glycogen storage diseases.

Compensatory Reactions in Active Muscle

In addition to the unavailability of muscle glycogen for ATP resynthesis via oxidative metabolism in McArdle's disease and PFK deficiency, there also is an obvious lack of anaerobic glycolysis, as demonstrated both by failure of muscle venous effluent lactate to rise (45) and by failure of muscle pH, as measured by ^{31}P-NMR, to fall (7, 18, 40, 58) as a result of ischemic or nonischemic exercise. A major consequence is the accumulation of ADP, which normally would be phosphorylated via glycolysis or carbohydrate-fueled oxidative phosphorylation. Muscle ADP accumulation has important implications for the creatine kinase reaction and adenylate kinase–AMP deaminase coupled reactions. The creatine kinase and adenylate kinase reactions are believed to be maintained near equilibrium (36). Over 50 years ago, Lohmann (44) showed that PCr breakdown was dependent on the presence of ADP. Also, ADP is a powerful activator of AMP deaminase (68, 74). Thus, ADP accumulation accelerates PCr breakdown, AMP production, and the deamination of AMP. An augmented increase in ADP removal via the creatine kinase and the coupled adenylate kinase–AMP deaminase reactions would be expected to lead to exaggerated muscle phosphocreatine (PCr) depletion and inorganic phosphate (P_i) accumulation and larger than normal accumulation of the AMP deamination products, ammonia and IMP (37). The postulated increase in creatine kinase flux has been proven correct in patients with McArdle's disease, in whom heavy exercise results in an exaggerated decline in muscle PCr and increase in muscle P_i for a given work load or force production (40, 59). Larger than normal elevations of ammonia (27, 62) and the IMP degradation products inosine and hypoxanthine (10, 47) in venous effluent from active muscle in McArdle patients are consistent with an increased flux through adenylate kinase and AMP deaminase.

In contrast to the accelerated depletion of PCr in McArdle's disease, recent ^{31}P-NMR studies performed on 5 patients with PFK deficiency have demonstrated a directly opposite effect, that is, attenuated depletion of PCr and accumulation of P_i during exercise in comparison to healthy subjects (7). Because PCr hydrolysis normally is the primary quantitative source of increase in free P_i in contracting muscle (15), the limited PCr depletion in active PFK-deficient muscle would partly explain the very modest accumulation of free P_i. Another reason for the subnormal rise in free P_i is the abnormally large incorporation of free P_i into phosphorylated glycolytic intermediates proximal to the enzymatic defect in PFK (14, 67). The mechanisms responsible for the unexpected finding of an attenuated PCr depletion in PFK deficiency are unknown but probably are not related to subnormal levels of ADP in active PFK-deficient muscle. This interpretation is supported by findings of larger than normal elevations of ammonia, inosine, and hypoxanthine in venous effluent from active muscle in PFK deficiency (34, 47) similar to those observed in McArdle's disease. In normal muscle, an increase in H^+ may be a major factor altering the equilibrium of the creatine kinase reaction toward PCr breakdown (63). However, a lack of increase in H^+ does not seem to interfere with PCr breakdown in phosphorylase-deficient muscle (40, 59). Therefore, the diminished decline in PCr in PFK-deficient muscle (7) does not appear to be due to an absent rise in H^+.

The capacities of the creatine kinase and adenylate kinase–AMP deaminase reactions to remove ADP are very minor relative to oxidative phosphorylation and glycolysis. The limited ADP utilization capacity of the adenylate kinase–AMP deaminase coupled reactions is illustrated by the very similar exercise capacity and fatigability in presumably rare cases of McArdle disease patients who lack AMP deaminase in addition to phosphorylase (28; Haller & Lewis, unpublished observations). Radda (55) has calculated, assuming a near equilibrium of the creatine kinase reaction (70), that free ADP can accumulate up to 240 μM in cramped phosphorylase-deficient muscle. This is approximately 6-fold the level in normal muscle at fatigue (55).

How Does the Circulatory System Compensate?

During dynamic exercise in humans, cardiac output ($\dot{Q}$) normally is closely coupled with VO_2 and increases by approximately 5-6 L for each L of increase in

$\dot{V}O_2$ (19, 42), that is, $\Delta\dot{Q}/\Delta\dot{V}O_2 \cong$ 5-6. Similarly, skeletal muscle blood flow increases approximately 6 L per L of increase in muscle O_2 uptake (3, 32). With a normal hemoglobin concentration and O_2 saturation, approximately 200 ml of O_2 are transported per L of arterial blood. Q and muscle blood flow must therefore increase approximately 5-6 L in order to transport each L of O_2 to working muscle. Thus, there normally is a tight, approximately 1:1 relation between the utilization and transport of O_2 both systemically and locally.

In contrast, in patients with PFK deficiency and McArdle's disease studied under nonfasted conditions, $\Delta\dot{Q}/\Delta\dot{V}O_2$ typically is 10 to 15 (39, 43) (Figure 2). Muscle blood flow data for PFK-deficient patients are lacking, but in McArdle's disease blood flow to active muscle is exaggerated (5, 45), increasing approximately 2-fold normally in relation to oxygen uptake (41). These data are basically consistent with a disruption of the normally tightly regulated delivery of O_2 to working muscle such that O_2 delivery increases at 2-3 times the normal rate with respect to O_2 utilization in these glycogenolytic defects.

This implies an increased substrate delivery, that is, an increased rate of perfusion of muscle with glucose and FFA, which may partially compensate for the substrate-limited oxidative metabolism. The signal for the exaggerated O_2 delivery may originate in working muscle and may be mediated by the effect of metabolites released from muscle causing both augmented local vasodilatation to increase muscle blood flow (65) and increased activation of metabolically sensitive types III and IV muscle afferents, which project to the central nervous cardiovascular control centers and result in a reflex autonomic outflow to the heart and blood vessels to increase cardiac output and muscle perfusion pressure (49). The common denominator responsible for the increased circulatory delivery of O_2 and substrate in PFK deficiency and McArdle disease is unknown but may relate to an exaggerated accumulation of muscle ADP resulting from the oxidative impairment and thus to an abnormally steep decline in the muscle phosphorylation potential, that is, [ATP]/[ADP] [P_i]. The results of Nuutinen, Wilson, Erecinska, and co-workers (51, 52) implicate an integral role for [ATP]/[ADP] [P_i] in the close coupling between myocardial O_2 delivery and demand.

Interventions to Increase or Reduce Substrate Availability

In McArdle and PFK-deficient patients, dietary modifications or intravenous infusions that increase the availability of oxidative substrates able to bypass the enzymatic defects in phosphorylase or phosphofructokinase result in enhanced muscle oxidative metabolism, reduced ADP accumulation, and more normal oxygen transport during exercise (Table 2). In contrast, interventions that reduce the availability of plasma FFA to working muscle, that is, oral nicotinic acid administration in McArdle's disease and glucose infusion in PFK deficiency, are associated with reduced $\dot{V}O_2$max and increased $\Delta\dot{Q}/\Delta\dot{V}O_2$ (24, 39). These findings link the subnormal $\dot{V}O_2$max and exaggerated $\Delta\dot{Q}/\Delta\dot{V}O_2$ during exercise in PFK deficiency and McArdle's disease with extramuscular fuel mobilization rate(s) insufficient to satisfy muscle oxidative demands.

**Table 2   Effects of Increased Substrate Availability
in PFK Deficiency and McArdle's Disease**

	$\dot{V}O_2max$	Muscle ADP[a]	$\Delta\dot{Q}/\Delta\dot{V}O_2$
PFK deficiency			
Lactate	↑	↓	↓
FFA	↑	?	↓
McArdle's disease			
Glucose	↑	↓	↓
FFA	↑	?	↓

Note. Increased lactate or glucose availability accomplished by I.V. infusion. Increased free fatty acid (FFA) availability accomplished by fasting overnight or I.V. liposyn plus heparin.

[a]Directional changes in muscle ADP estimated from changes in muscle phosphocreatine and inorganic phosphate (4, 40) and venous effluent ammonia (27, Haller & Lewis, unpublished observations), assuming creatine kinase and adenylate kinase reactions remain near equilibrium during muscle contraction (36, 70). ↓ = increased; ↑ = decreased; ? = unknown.

Muscle Fatigue in McArdle's Disease and PFK Deficiency

Increases in the delivery of blood-borne oxidizable substrates and in muscle ADP utilization in McArdle's disease and PFK deficiency are insufficient to compensate for the substrate-limited oxidative metabolism and to prevent premature muscle fatigue in these disorders. The metabolic factors normally correlated with human muscle fatigue are shown in Table 3. These factors include depletion of ATP and PCr and accumulation of H^+, P_i, diprotonated inorganic phosphate ($H_2PO_4^-$), and ADP. Because the clinically observed features of premature muscle fatigue are very similar in PFK deficiency and McArdle's disease, a metabolic common denominator is postulated. Gross muscle ATP depletion, long suspected as a cause of muscle contracture in McArdle disease and PFK deficiency, is an unlikely explanation because muscle ATP falls at most only modestly during fatigue or contracture (4, 7, 20, 40, 56, 60). This does not, however, rule out the possibility of fatigue due to depletion of a localized subcellular compartment of ATP in these defects. Depletion of PCr is not consistently related to fatigue in these defects. The decline in PCr is marked in McArdle's disease and attenuated in PFK deficiency. Muscle pH fails to decline with exercise in either defect, eliminating a role for H^+ accumulation. Findings to date imply that P_i accumulation could play an important role in fatigue in McArdle's disease but not in PFK deficiency. The increase of muscle P_i with respect to exercise intensity is exaggerated in McArdle's disease but is attenuated in PFK deficiency. Recent in vitro findings closely link diminished muscle force production with the accumulation of $H_2PO_4^-$ (50, 76). A relationship between increased muscle $H_2PO_4^-$ and fatigue has been corroborated in studies of voluntary muscle contractions performed by healthy human subjects (46, 77). Because H^+ accumulation does not occur in phosphorylase-deficient or PFK-deficient muscle, and because the elevation of

Table 3   Metabolic Correlates of Muscle Fatigue

	McArdle's disease	PFK deficiency
Depletion		
ATP	−	−
PCr	+	−
Accumulation		
H$^+$	−	−
P$_i$	+	−
H$_2$PO$_4^-$	−	−
ADP	+	+

Note. Minus = correlates with fatigue; plus = does not correlate with fatigue. Modified from reference 38.

muscle P$_i$ is exaggerated in McArdle's disease and subnormal in PFK deficiency, it is unlikely that muscle fatigue in these glycogenoses is attributable to H$_2$PO$_4^-$ accumulation.

In contrast to the metabolic factors discussed above, an obvious common denominator in PFK deficiency and McArdle's disease is ADP accumulation, which could result in fatigue due to product inhibition of the muscle ATPases. The extent of ADP accumulation in phosphorylase-deficient muscle calculated by Radda (55) is at or above a concentration equivalent to the K$_i$ for ADP of the myosin ATPase, that is, approximately 200 μM (17). The data of Cooke and co-workers (17), however, is inconsistent with an important role for ADP accumulation in the fall in muscle tension development due to product inhibition of myosin ATPase. Product inhibition by ADP of the Na$^+$-K$^+$ and/or Ca^{2+} ATPases is, however, an intriguing but as yet speculative explanation for the fatigue of glycogenolytic or glycolytic defects. Inhibition of the ATPases involved in ion pumping could cause a failure of electrical activation of the muscle or of muscle excitation-contraction coupling. The finding of a close temporal association between the decline in force production and the fall in the muscle action potential in phosphofructokinase- and phosphorylase-deficient muscle (75) is consistent with a role for impaired muscle excitation in fatigue in these disorders and identifies this as a potentially important future avenue of research.

Acknowledgments

Dr. Gunnar Blomqvist provided invaluable general support for the work related to this review. We appreciate the expert word processing assistance of Ms. Gladys Carter. Research funds for this work were provided by National Heart, Lung and Blood Institute Grant HL-06296, the Muscular Dystrophy Association, the Veterans Administration, and the Harry S. Moss Heart Center. S.F. Lewis is the recipient of Research Career Development Award HL-01581.

References

1. Ahlborg, B.; Bergstrom, J.; Ekelund, L.-G.; Hultman, E. Relationship between muscle glycogen concentration and exercise endurance time. Acta Physiol. Scand. 70:129-142; 1967.

2. Andersen, K.L.; Lund-Johansen, P.; Clausen G. Metabolic and circulatory responses to muscular exercise in a subject with glycogen storage disease (McArdle's disease). Scand. J. Clin. Lab. Invest. 24:105-113; 1969.

3. Andersen, P.; Saltin, B. Maximal perfusion of skeletal muscle in man. J. Physiol. (Lond.) 366:233-249; 1985.

4. Argov, Z.; Bank, W.J.; Maris, J.; Chance, B. Muscle energy metabolism in McArdle's syndrome by in vivo phosphorus magnetic resonance spectroscopy. Neurology 37:1720-1724; 1987.

5. Barcroft, H.; Greenwood, B.; McArdle, B.; McSwinney, R.R.; Semple, S.J.G.; Whelan, R.F.; Youlten, L.J.F. The effect of exercise on forearm blood flow and on venous blood flow in a subject with phosphorylase deficiency in skeletal muscle (McArdle's syndrome). J. Physiol. (Lond.) 184:44P-46P; 1966.

6. Bergstrom, J.; Hermansen, L.; Hultman, E.; Saltin, B. Diet, muscle glycogen and physical performance. Acta Physiol. Scand. 71:140-150; 1967.

7. Bertocci, L.A.; Nunnally, R.L.; Lewis, S.F.; Haller, R.G. Attenuated depletion of phosphocreatine in human muscle PFK deficiency during handgrip exercise. Soc. Mag. Res., Proc. 7th ann. meeting; 1988.

8. Blomqvist, C.G.; Lewis, S.F. Interaction between local and neurohumoral cardiovascular control mechanisms during dynamic and static exercise. In: Christensen, N.J.; Henriksen, O.; Lassen, N.A., eds. The sympathoadrenal system. Copenhagen: Munksgaard; 1986:188-202.

9. Braakhekke, J.P.; deBruin, M.I.; Stegeman, D.F.; Wevers, R.A.; Binkhorst, R.A.; Joosten, E.M.G. The second wind phenomenon in McArdle's disease. Brain 109:1087-1101; 1986.

10. Brooke, M.H.; Patterson, V.H.; Kaiser, K.K. Hypoxanthine and McArdle disease: a clue to metabolic stress in the working forearm. Muscle Nerve 6:204-206; 1983.

11. Brown, D.H. Glycogen metabolism and glycolysis in muscle. In: Engel, A.G.; Banker, B.Q., eds. Myology. New York: McGraw-Hill; 1986:673-695. (Vol. 1).

12. Carroll, J.E.; Brooke, M.H.; DeVivo, D.C.; Kaiser, K.K.; Hagberg, J.M. Biochemical and physiologic consequences of carnitine palmityltransferase deficiency. Muscle Nerve 1:103-110; 1978.

13. Carroll, J.E.; DeVivo, D.C.; Brooke, M.H.; Planer, G.J.; Hagberg, J.H. Fasting as a provocative test in neuromuscular diseases. Metabolism 28:683-687; 1979.

14. Chance, B.; Eleff, S.; Bank, W.; Leigh, J.S., Jr.; Warnell, R. ^{31}P NMR studies of control of mitochondrial function in phosphofructokinase-deficient human skeletal muscle. Proc. Natl. Acad. Sci. USA 79:7714-7718; 1982.

15. Chasiotis, D. The regulation of glycogen phosphorylase and glycogen breakdown in human skeletal muscle. Acta Physiol. Scand. (Suppl. 518):1-68; 1983.

16. Conlee, R.K. Muscle glycogen and exercise endurance: a twenty-year perspective. In: Pandolf, K.B., ed. Exercise and sport sciences reviews. New York: Macmillan; 1987:3-28. (Vol. 15).

17. Cooke, R. The inhibition of muscle contraction by the products of ATP hydrolysis (this volume). Champaign, IL: Human Kinetics Publishers; 1989.

18. Duboc, D.; Jehenson, P.; Tran Dinh, S.; Marsac, C.; Syrota, A.; Fardeau, M. Phosphorus NMR spectroscopy study of muscular enzyme deficiencies involving glycogenolysis and glycolysis. Neurology 37:663-671; 1987.

19. Durand, J.; Mensch-Dechene, J. Physiological meaning of the slope and intercept of the cardiac output–oxygen uptake relationship during exercise. Bull. Eur. Physiopathol. Respir. 15:977-998; 1979.

20. Edwards, R.H.T.; Dawson, M.J.; Wilkie, D.R.; Gordon, R.E.; Shaw, D. Clinical use of nuclear magnetic resonance in the investigation of myopathy. Lancet 725-731; 1982.

21. Galbo, H.; Sonne, B.; Vissing, J.; Kjaer, M.; Mikines, K.; Richter, E.A. Lack of accuracy of fuel mobilization in exercise. Proc. int. symp. prob. biochem. phys. exer. train., Amsterdam: Elsevier Science Publishers; 1986.

22. Gollnick, P.D. Metabolism of substrates: energy substrate metabolism during exercise and as modified by training. Fed. Proc. 44:353-357; 1985.

23. Hagberg, J.M.; Coyle, E.F.; Carroll, J.E.; Miller, J.M.; Martin, W.H.; Brooke, M.H. Exercise hyperventilation in patients with McArdle's disease. J. Appl. Physiol.: Respir. Environ. Exerc. Physiol. 52(4):991-994; 1982.

24. Haller, R.G.; DiMauro, S.; Vora, S.; Lewis, S.F. Glucose impairs exercise performance in muscle phosphofructokinase deficiency: the "out of wind" effect. Neurology 39(Suppl. 1):270; 1988.

25. Haller, R.G.; Lewis, S.F.; Cook, J.D.; Blomqvist, C.G. Hyperkinetic circulation during exercise in neuromuscular disease. Neurology 33:1283-1287; 1983.

26. Haller, R.G.; Lewis, S.F.; Cook, J.D.; Blomqvist, C.G. Myophosphorylase deficiency impairs muscle oxidative metabolism. Ann. Neurol. 17:196-199; 1985.

27. Haller, R.G.; Lewis, S.F.; Gunder, M.; Dennis, M. Ammonia production during exercise in McArdle's syndrome—an index of muscle energy supply and demand. Neurology 35:207; 1985.

28. Heller, S.L.; Kaiser, K.K.; Planer, G.J.; Hagberg, J.M.; Brooke, M.H. McArdle's disease with myoadenylate deaminase deficiency: observations in a combined enzyme deficiency. Neurology 37:1039-1042; 1987.

29. Hermansen, L.; Hultman, E.; Saltin, B. Muscle glycogen during prolonged severe exercise. Acta Physiol. Scand. 71:129-139; 1967.

30. Hultman, E. Studies on muscle metabolism of glycogen and active phosphate in man with special reference to exercise and diet. Scand. J. Clin. Lab. Invest. 19(Suppl. 94); 1967.

31. Hultman, E. Carbohydrate metabolism during hard exercise and in the recovery period after exercise. Acta Physiol. Scand. 128(Suppl. 556):75-82; 1986.

32. Jorfeldt, L.; Wahren, J. Leg blood flow during exercise in man. Clin. Sci. 41:459-473; 1971.

33. Katz, A.; Broberg, S.; Sahlin, K.; Wahren, J. Leg glucose uptake during maximal dynamic exercise in humans. Am. J. Physiol. (Endocrinol. Metab. 14) 251:E65-E70; 1986.

34. Kono, N.; Mineo, I.; Shimizu, T.; Hara, N.; Yamada, Y.; Nonaka, K.; Tarui, S. Increased plasma uric acid after exercise in muscle phosphofructokinase deficiency. Neurology 36:106-108; 1986.

35. Krzentowski, G.; Pallikarakis, N.; Pirnay, F. Metabolisme glucidique pendant l'exercice musculaire dans la maladie de McArdle. Acta Clin. Belg. 34:151-157; 1979.

36. Lawson, J.W.; Veech, R.L. Effects of pH and free Mg^+ on the Keq of the creatine kinase reaction and other phosphate transfer reactions. J. Biol. Chem. 254:6528-6537; 1979.

37. Lewis, S.F.; Haller, R.G. The pathophysiology of McArdle's disease: clues to regulation in exercise and fatigue. J. Appl. Physiol. 61:391-491; 1986.

38. Lewis, S.F.; Haller, R.G. Skeletal muscle disorders and associated factors that limit exercise performance. In: Pandolf, K.B., ed. Exercise and sport sciences reviews. Baltimore: Williams and Wilkins; (Vol. 17), 1989:67-113.

39. Lewis, S.F.; Haller, R.G.; Cook, J.D.; Blomqvist, C.G. Metabolic control of cardiac output response to exercise in McArdle's disease. J. Appl. Physiol. 57:1749-1753; 1984.

40. Lewis, S.F.; Haller, R.G.; Cook, J.D.; Nunnally, R.L. Muscle fatigue in McArdle's disease studied by ^{31}P-NMR: effect of glucose infusion. J. Appl. Physiol. 59:1991-1994; 1985.

41. Lewis, S.F.; Haller, R.G.; Henriksson, K.G.; Areskog, N.-H.; Jorfeldt, L. Availability of oxidative substrate and leg blood flow during exercise in McArdle's disease (abstract). Fed. Proc. 45:783; 1986.

42. Lewis, S.F.; Taylor, W.F.; Graham, R.M.; Pettinger, W.E.; Schutte, J.E.; Blomqvist, C.G. Cardiovascular responses to exercise as functions of absolute and relative workload. J. Appl. Physiol. 54:1314-1323; 1983.

43. Lewis, S.F.; Vora, S.; DiMauro, S.; Haller, R.G. Disordered oxidative metabolism in muscle phosphofructokinase deficiency. Neurology 38(Suppl. 1): 269; 1988.

44. Lohman, K. Uber die enzymatische aufspaltung de kreatinphosphorsaure; zugleich ein beitrag zum chemismus der muskelkontraktion. Biochem. Z. 271:264-277; 1934.

45. McArdle, B. Myopathy due to a defect in muscle glycogen breakdown. Clin. Sci. 10:13-33, 1951.

46. Miller, R.G.; Boska, M.D.; Moussavi, R.S.; Carlson, P.J.; Weiner, M.W. ^{31}P nuclear magnetic resonance studies of high energy phosphates and pH in human muscle fatigue. Comparison of aerobic and anaerobic exercise. J. Clin. Invest. 81:1190-1196; 1988.

47. Mineo, I.; Kono, N.; Hara, N.; Shimizu, T.; Yamada, Y.; Kawachi, M.; Kiyokawa, H.; Wang, Y.L.; Tarui, S. Myogenic hyperuricemia: a common pathophysiologic feature of glycogenosis types III, V, and VII. N. Engl. J. Med. 317(2):75-80; 1987.

48. Miranda, A.F.; Nette, E.G.; Hartlage, M.D.; DiMaruo, S. Phosphorylase isoenzymes in normal and myophosphorylase deficient human heart. Neurology 29:1538-1541; 1979.

49. Mitchell, J.H.; Schmidt, R.F. Cardiovascular reflex control by afferent fibers from skeletal muscle receptors. In: Handbook of physiology. The cardiovascular system. Bethesda, MD: Am. Physiol. Soc.; 1983:623-658. (Sect. 2, Vol. 3).

50. Nosek, T.M.; Fender, K.Y.; Godt, R.E. It is diprotonated inorganic phosphate that depresses force in skinned skeletal muscle fibers. Science 236:191-193; 1987.

51. Nuutinen, E.M.; Nelson, D.; Wilson, D.F.; Erecinska, M. Regulation of coronary blood flow: effects of 2,4-dinitrophenol and theophylline. Am. J. Physiol. 244 (Heart, Circ. Physiol. 13):H396-H405; 1983.

52. Nuutinen, E.M.; Nishiki, K.; Erecinska, M.; Wilson, D.F. Role of mitochondrial oxidative phosphorylation in regulation of coronary blood flow. Am. J. Physiol. 243 (Heart, Circ. Physiol. 12):H159-H169; 1982.

53. Pearson, C.M.; Rimer, D.G.; Mommaerts, W.H.F.M. A metabolic myopathy due to absence of muscle phosphorylase. Am. J. Med. 30:502-517; 1961.

54. Porte, D., Jr.; Crawford, D.W.; Jennings, D.B.; Aber, C.; McIlroy, M.B. Cardiovascular and metabolic responses to exercise in a patient with McArdle's syndrome. N. Engl. J. Med. 275:406-412; 1966.

55. Radda, G.K. Control of bioenergetics: from cells to man by phosphorus nuclear-magnetic-resonance spectroscopy. Biochem. Soc. Trans. 14:517-525; 1986.

56. Rennie, M.J.; Edwards, R.H.T. Carbohydrate metabolism of skeletal muscle and its disorders. In: Randle, P.J.; Steiner, D.; Whelan, W.J., eds. Carbohydrate metabolism and its disorders. New York: Academic Press; 1981:1-118. (Vol. 3).

57. Rose, J.A.; O'Connell, E.L. The role of glucose 6-phosphate in the regulation of glucose metabolism in human erythrocytes. J. Biol. Chem. 231:12-17; 1964.

58. Ross, B.D.; Radda, G.K. Application of ^{31}P n.m.r. to inborn errors of muscle metabolism. Biochem. Soc. Trans. 11(6):627-630; 1983.

59. Ross, B.D.; Radda, G.K.; Gadian, D.G.; Rocker, G.; Esiri, M.; Falconer-Smith, J. Examination of a case of suspected McArdle's syndrome by ^{31}P nuclear magnetic resonance. N. Engl. J. Med. 304:1338-1342; 1981.

60. Rowland, L.P.; Araki, S.; Carmel, P. Contracture in McArdle's disease. Arch. Neurol. 13:541-544; 1965.

61. Rowland, L.P.; DiMauro, S.; Layzer, R. Phosphofructokinase deficiency. In: Engel, A.G.; Banker, B.Q., eds. Myology. New York: McGraw-Hill; 1986: 1603-1617.

62. Rumpf, K.W.; Wagner, H.; Kaiser, K.; Meinck, H.M.; Gobel, H.H.; Scheler, F. Increased ammonia production during forearm ischemic exercise test in McArdle's disease. Klin. Wochenschr. 59:1319-1320; 1981.

226 Lewis and Haller

63. Sahlin, K.; Harris, R.C.; Hultman, E. Creatine kinase equilibrium and lactate content compared with muscle pH in tissue samples obtained after isometric exercise. Biochem. J. 152:173-180; 1975.

64. Saltin, B.; Karlsson, J. Muscle glycogen utilization during work of different intensities. In: Pernow, B.; Saltin, B., eds. Advances in experimental medicine and biology: muscle metabolism during exercise. New York-London: Plenum Press; 1971:289-299. (Vol. 11).

65. Shepherd, J.T. Circulation to skeletal muscle. In: Handbook of physiology. The cardiovascular system. Peripheral circulation and organ blood flow. Bethesda, MD: Am. Physiol. Soc.; 1983:319-370. (Vol. 3).

66. Slonim, A.E.; Goans, P.J. Myopathy in McArdle's syndrome. Improvement with a high protein diet. N. Engl. J. Med. 312:355-359; 1985.

67. Tarui, S.; Mineo, I.; Shimizu, T.; Sumi, S.; Kono, N. Muscle phosphofructo-kinase deficiency and related disorders. In: Serratrice, G.; Desnuell, C.; Pellissier, J.F.; Cros, D.; Gastraut, J.L.; Pouget, J.; Schiano, A., eds. Neuromuscular diseases. New York: Raven Press; 1984:71-77.

68. Terjung, R.L.; Dudley, G.A.; Meyer, R.A. Metabolic and circulatory limitations to muscular performance at the organ level. J. Exp. Biol. 115:307-318; 1985.

69. Triebwasser, J.H.; Johnson, R.L., Jr.; Burpo, R.P.; Campbell, J.C.; Reardon, W.C.; Blomqvist, C.G. Noninvasive determination of cardiac output by a modified acetylene rebreathing procedure utilizing mass spectrometer measurements. Aviat. Space Environ. Med. 48:203-209; 1977.

70. Veech, R.L.; Lawson, J.W.R.; Cornell, N.W.; Krebs, H.A. Cytosolic phosphorylation potential. J. Biol. Chem. 254:6538-6547; 1978.

71. Vora, S.; Giger, U.; Turchen, S.; Harvey, J.W. Characterization of the enzymatic lesion in inherited phosphofructokinase deficiency in the dog: an animal analogue of human glycogen storage disease type VII. Proc. Natl. Acad. Sci. USA 82:8109-8113; 1985.

72. Wahren, J.; Felig, P.; Havel, R.J.; Jorfeldt, L.; Pernow, B.; Saltin, B. Amino acid metabolism in McArdle's syndrome. N. Engl. J. Med. 288:774-777; 1973.

73. Walvoort, H.C. Glycogen storage disease in animals and their potential value as models of human disease. J. Inherited Metab. Dis. 6:3-16; 1983.

74. Wheeler, T.J.; Lowenstein, J.M. Adenylate deaminase from rat muscle. Regulation by purine nucleotides and orthophosphate in the presence of 150 mM KCl. J. Biol. Chem. 254:8994-8999; 1979.

75. Wiles, C.M.; Jones, D.A.; Edwards, R.H.T. Fatigue in human metabolic myopathy. In: Human Muscle Fatigue: Physiological mechanisms. Porter, R.; Whelan, J., eds. London: Pitman; 1981:264-277 (Ciba Found. Symp. 82).

76. Wilkie, D.R. Muscular fatigue: effects of hydrogen ions and inorganic phosphate. Fed. Proc. 45:2921-2923; 1986.

77. Wilson, J.R.; McCulley, K.K.; Mancini, D.M.; Boden, B.; Chance, B. Relationship of muscular fatigue to pH and diprotonated P_i in humans: a ^{31}P NMR study. J. Appl. Physiol. 64:2333-2339; 1988.

Disorders of Purine Nucleotide Metabolism in Muscle

Richard L. Sabina and Edward W. Holmes
Medical College of Wisconsin, Milwaukee, Wisconsin and
Duke University Medical Center, Durham, North Carolina, U.S.A.

Purine nucleotide synthesis is essential for maintaining steady state levels of high-energy phosphates in all cell types. This is accomplished in two ways: The first is *de novo* synthesis from the small precursor molecules ribose, glutamine, aspartate, glycine, formate, ATP, and CO_2 in a series of 11 reactions culminating in the formation of inosine monophosphate (IMP) (see Figure 1) (for review see ref. 66). Purine *de novo* synthetic activities are constitutively expressed in all cell types; *de novo* synthetic rates have been estimated in a number of tissues, including skeletal muscle, where it is relatively low (67). However, consideration of the proportion of body mass as skeletal muscle has led some authors to conclude that taken in total, this tissue is a major source of purine production in the body (12). The second route of purine nucleotide synthesis is salvage synthesis from preformed purine bases and nucleosides. This is accomplished either through the action of specific phosphoribosyl-transferases (for bases) or kinases (for nucleosides) present in all cell types. The rate-limiting factor in purine base salvage and *de novo* synthesis in all tissues appears to be the availability of $5'$ phosphoribosyl-1-pyrophosphate (PRPP).

PURINE BIOSYNTHESIS AND INTERCONVERSION

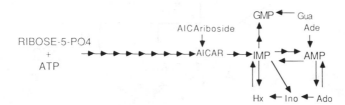

Figure 1. Purine *de novo* and salvage synthesis and interconversion in mammalian skeletal muscle. Ribose-5-PO_4, ribose-5-phosphate; ATP, adenosine triphosphate; AICA riboside, 5-amino-4-imidazolecarboxamide riboside; AICAR, 5-amino-4-imidazolecarboxamide ribotide; IMP, inosine monophosphate; GMP, guanosine monophosphate; AMP, adenosine monophosphate; Ado, adenosine; Ino, inosine; Hx, hypoxanthine; Ade, adenine; Gua, guanine.

Other purine enzymatic activities are involved in the catabolism and interconversion of nucleotides. One such activity, AMP deaminase, plays a specialized role in skeletal muscle, where its activity is almost two orders of magnitude higher than in any other nonmuscle tissue (39, 40). In skeletal muscle, AMP deaminase is the initial step in a series of three reactions termed the purine nucleotide cycle (see Figure 2). The anabolic arm of this cycle consists of two components, adenylosuccinate synthetase and adenylosuccinate lyase, the activities of which are higher in skeletal muscle than in other tissues (8, 35). The net effect of this cycle is to deaminate adenosine monophosphate (AMP) to IMP and then reaminate it back to AMP.

In the course of these events, the cycle consumes aspartate and guanosine triphosphate (GTP) and generates ammonia, guanosine diphosphate (GDP), fumarate, and inorganic phosphate. The anabolic arm of the cycle is rate-limiting, based on

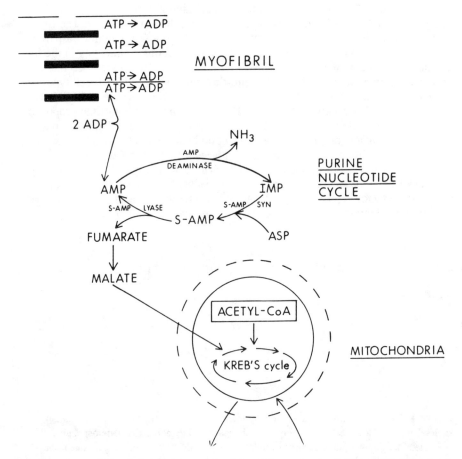

Figure 2. Schematic representation of the role of the purine nucleotide cycle in skeletal muscle energetics. Abbreviations as per Figure 1 except S-AMP Syn, adenylosuccinate synthetase; S-AMP lyase, adenylosuccinate lyase; NH_3, ammonia; Asp, aspartate.

the relative activity of AMP deaminase, which is 2 orders of magnitude higher than either adenylosuccinate synthetase or adenylosuccinate lyase (50). Finally, AMP deaminase activity is higher in glycolytic fibers than in oxidative fibers (43, 65), suggesting fiber-type–specific functions of the purine nucleotide cycle.

Role for the Purine Nucleotide Cycle in Skeletal Muscle Energetics

Several lines of evidence underscore the importance of a functional purine nucleotide cycle in skeletal muscle. These include the identification of muscle isozymes of purine nucleotide cycle components, proposed biochemical roles in skeletal muscle energy metabolism, physical association between purine nucleotide cycle components and contractile proteins, and animal and human models of myopathy associated with a disruption of the purine nucleotide cycle.

Isozymes of Purine Nucleotide Cycle Components

Isozymes for AMP deaminase have been described in a variety of organisms. Tissue surveys in the rat (39) and the human (40) have led to the identification of 3 and 4 isozymes, respectively. In both species 1 isozyme is found only in skeletal muscle, where it is named myoadenylate deaminase. Analysis of myogenesis in the chicken (49), the rat (31), and the human (23) has demonstrated a developmental program of isoform switching. In developing rat skeletal muscle, 3 peptides (embryonic, neonatal, and adult) have been identified. In addition, reports from rabbit (38, 42, 57), rat (42), and human (42) have presented evidence for 2 isoforms of AMP deaminase in adult skeletal muscle, although this has not been reproduced in the rat (36).

Two isoforms of adenylosuccinate synthetase have been described in the rat (for review, see 58), where they have been termed acidic and basic, depending on their absorption to ion-exchange columns. The basic isozyme is the only form detected in skeletal muscle and heart, whereas the spleen expresses the acidic form only. All other tissues examined contain both isozymes. Although isozymes for adenylosuccinate lyase have not been described, this activity has recently been purified from adult rat skeletal muscle (13). In addition, the discovery of a subset of autistic children exhibiting tissue-specific deficiencies of adenylosuccinate lyase provides evidence for the existence of several isozymes in the human (22, 64).

Biochemical Roles for the Purine Nucleotide Cycle in Skeletal Muscle

It is well established that energy generated in the mitochondrial oxidative and the glycolytic pathways is the main contributor to the maintenance of the high ATP:ADP ratio necessary for myofibrillar contraction. Energy produced in the mitochondrial reactions is transferred to the myofibril in the form of creatine phosphate, which is in turn converted to ATP by myofibrillar creatine kinase (11). In addition to providing more ATP for contractions, these reactions, also known as the creatine phosphate shuttle, consume ADP and H^+, thereby supplementing efforts to maintain a favorable ATP:ADP ratio. However, as the supply of substrates for energy generation are exhausted or when energy demand exceeds energy-generating capacities, creatine phosphate levels begin to decline, ultimately leading to a reduction in ATP. At this time, adenylate kinase, in concert with AMP deaminase, assumes the role of maintaining a favorable energy state by rapidly rephosphorylating half of the ADP produced at the expense of the other half and deaminating the resulting AMP (see Figure 2). In this fashion, the first proposed role for the purine nucleotide cycle in skeletal muscle energetics is the part that AMP deaminase plays in helping to maintain a high ATP:ADP ratio (29). In addition, it has been proposed that ammonia produced in the AMP deaminase reaction can serve to buffer the H^+ produced during contraction (21), although the in vivo significance of this proposal has been questioned (15, 25).

The products of the AMP deaminase reaction are reportedly in vitro effectors of key glycolytic enzymes. IMP activates glycogen phosphorylase b (3), and ammonia induces phosphofructokinase (59). The in vivo significance of these observations have also been questioned, however, due to the high levels of IMP required for activation and the lack of an ammonia effect at physiological potassium concentrations (25, 59). Furthermore, myoadenylate deaminase–deficient patients produce normal amounts of lactate despite a failure to produce ammonia during ischemic forearm exercise (17). Nevertheless, a 3- to 10-fold greater activity (43, 65) and transcript abundance (46) of AMP deaminase in glycolytic fibers, and elevated blood levels of ammonia (26, 44) and purine catabolites (10, 26), following ischemic exercise in patients with glycolytic defects, underscore an interdependence between the purine nucleotide cycle and anaerobic energy metabolism.

The reamination reactions of the purine nucleotide cycle are also proposed to play a role in skeletal muscle energy metabolism. The fumarate that is generated in the adenylosuccinate lyase reaction is subsequently converted to malate, in which form it can enter the mitochondria and contribute to the repletion, or the expansion, of tricarboxylic acid cycle intermediates (1, 2). The source of the fumarate produced in the adenylosuccinate lyase reaction is aspartate consumed in the adenylosuccinate synthetase reaction. However, through transamination reactions, a number of amino acids could ultimately serve as ammonia donors, which makes available the carbon skeletons of many amino acids for energy production (19).

At this point, it is worthwhile to mention that the term *cycle* may be a misnomer. Although some studies suggest both arms of the purine nucleotide cycle operate simultaneously during exercise (1, 2, 29, 30), other reports indicate that the catabolic and anabolic components of this cycle operate in series (33, 34). Specifically, deamination occurs during exercise and reamination occurs during the recovery phase. Regardless of whether the purine nucleotide cycle is turning during exercise, the much higher activity of AMP deaminase relative to the activity of the anabolic components of the cycle results in an accumulation of IMP during bouts of net ATP degradation in skeletal muscle.

Considered as a unit, the purine nucleotide cycle may also indirectly contribute to skeletal muscle energetics by preserving catabolized ATP as a nucleotide (i.e., IMP), thereby enabling rapid resynthesis of ATP following exercise (61). This can be appreciated by considering the consequences of myocardial ischemia, during which

bouts of net ATP degradation result in the loss of purine substrate as diffusible nucleosides and bases (62). This is primarily due to the fact that cardiac muscle contains
relatively low levels of AMP deaminase but a more active isoform of 5′ nucleo-
tidase (4, 39, 40). As a consequence, it may require days for normal ATP levels
to be restored following an ischemic insult (62). An analogous situation to the ischemic
myocardium is the myoadenylate deaminase–deficient patient who is capable of
performing enough work to result in net catabolism of ATP. In this case, there is
a significant loss of purine substrate during exercise (48).

In spite of the numerous proposed biochemical roles for the purine nucleotide cycle
in skeletal muscle energy metabolism, no one function fits all exercise situations.
None of these proposed functions are mutually exclusive, and it is quite likely that
different aspects of purine nucleotide cycle activity contribute to energy metabolism
in a fiber-type–specific manner.

Physical Association of Purine Nucleotide Cycle Components With Contractile Proteins

Reports of AMP deaminase binding to myosin and adenylosuccinate synthetase
to actin have provided physical evidence for a role of the purine nucleotide cycle
in skeletal muscle energetics. The majority of published data deals with the binding
of AMP deaminase to myosin. This phenomenon has been described in rabbit (5-7,
9, 27, 28) and rat (37, 51-53) skeletal muscle. In the rabbit, myoadenylate deaminase
has been found to bind to the subfragment-2 portion of myosin heavy chain in vitro
(5). This interaction is extremely tight, exhibiting a Kd of 14 × 10^{-8} M (5). The
maximal binding ratio, as determined by co-precipitation, has been observed to be
2 moles of myoadenylate deaminase bound per 1 mole of myosin heavy chain (5)
but only 1:2 in native thick filaments (27). The reason for the different observed
stoichiometries is not known but may be related to steric limitations in vivo (28).
This periodicity of binding in vivo may have a more physiological basis because
myoadenylate deaminase has been localized to the A band (7). Finally, the binding
of rabbit AMP deaminase to myosin heavy chain results in activation of the former
(6), and it is modulated by changes in pH over a physiological range (9).

Reports on the rat have shown that AMP deaminase binds to both heavy and light
meromyosin (52), indicating a different interaction in this species compared to the
rabbit. Nevertheless, the binding is also extremely tight, exhibiting a Kd of 6 ×
10^{-8} M (52). Similar to that observed in the rabbit, rat AMP deaminase is activated
by binding to myosin (53).

Although not investigated in the rabbit, controversy exists as to which isoforms
of AMP deaminase can bind to myosin in the rat. Shiraki et al. (52) report the binding to be specific for myoadenylate deaminase, whereas Ogasawara et al. (37) state
that all three AMP deaminase isozymes described in this rodent bind myosin to similar
degrees. Data have also been presented that suggest that the ratio of bound to unbound myoadenylate deaminase reversibly increases during electrical stimulation of
rat skeletal muscle (51). The identification of an unbound pool of myoadenylate
deaminase accessible to myosin during enhanced contractile activity further impli-
cates a role for this interaction in skeletal muscle energetics.

An association between adenylosuccinate synthetase and skeletal actin has also
been described in the rat (41). Evidence has been presented to show the specific

binding of the basic (i.e., muscle) isozyme to F-actin in vitro. The dissociation constant for this interaction in the rat was determined to be 72×10^{-8} M, and the stoichiometry of binding to be 1 mole of adenylosuccinate synthetase bound per 4 moles of F-actin.

No information is available regarding a potential interaction between adenylosuccinate lyase and the myofibrillar apparatus. However, the association of the other two components of the purine nucleotide cycle with contractile proteins presents physical evidence for compartmentalization of the purine nucleotide cycle in the myofibrillar network. What physiological significance these observations represent remains to be determined.

Myopathies Associated With Disruption of the Purine Nucleotide Cycle

Perhaps the most compelling evidence for a role of the purine nucleotide cycle in skeletal muscle energy metabolism are reports of myopathy associated with a disruption of this pathway. As such, these models may provide the most powerful tool to date for assessing the role of the purine nucleotide cycle in energy metabolism, myofibrillar structure, and skeletal muscle function.

The role of the purine nucleotide cycle in skeletal muscle function has been investigated utilizing rodent models of adenylosuccinate lyase inhibition (18, 60). The inhibition was achieved by bolus infusion of a ribosyl precursor to a purine de novo intermediate, 5-amino-4-imidazolecarboxamide riboside (AICA riboside). This compound is rapidly taken up and phosphorylated by mammalian cells (47), including skeletal muscle (45), where it enters the de novo pathway of purine nucleotide synthesis as 5-amino-4-imidazolecarboxamide ribotide (AICAR) (see Figure 1).

The efficient uptake and phosphorylation of AICA riboside relative to the limited capacity of the de novo pathway to rapidly metabolize AICAR to purine nucleotides results in the rapid intracellular accumulation of the latter (47). Adenylosuccinate lyase is a bifunctional enzyme in purine nucleotide biosynthesis, catalyzing the conversion of succinyl AICAR to AICAR as well as adenylosuccinate to AMP. The accumulation of the product of the former activity of the lyase (AICAR) effectively inhibits flux through the latter activity (adenylosuccinate AMP). Functional differences in resistance to fatigue between AICA riboside–treated and saline-control animals combined with biochemical evidence for inhibition of adenylosuccinate lyase (i.e., enhanced accumulation of adenylosuccinate during electrical stimulation) have been taken as evidence that a functional purine nucleotide cycle is necessary for normal skeletal muscle function.

Adenylosuccinate Lyase Deficiency in Humans

Recently, a subset of autistic children have been identified as exhibiting various tissue-specific deficiencies of adenylosuccinate lyase (22). These children were initially detected by the presence of succinylpurines in their bodily fluids (i.e., succinyl AICA riboside and succinyl adenosine). The description of tissue-specific deficiencies that vary among patients provides strong support for the existence of multiple isozymes of adenylosuccinate lyase in humans.

Since this initial report, additional patients have been identified (64). Relevant to this discussion, one of these children has been diagnosed as having a mild form of autism, myopathy, and a lack of adenylosuccinate lyase in muscle (as well as other tissues). Overall, this deficiency holds little promise as a human model of myopathy due to the associated symptoms of autism and other variable tissue-specific abnormalities. The consequences of the lack of purine *de novo* synthesis in these individuals outweigh any concerns regarding a disruption of the purine nucleotide cycle, although it is significant that the individual exhibiting a myopathy lacks adenylosuccinate lyase activity in muscle.

Similar to adenylosuccinate lyase deficiencies, adenylosuccinate synthetase deficiencies are also likely to be associated with other tissue-specific abnormalities. Complications associated with an inability to synthesize adenine nucleotides via the *de novo* pathway or through the salvage of inosine and hypoxanthine (the primary salvageable substrates in the blood) are likely to be life-threatening.

Myoadenylate Deaminase Deficiency in Humans

Unlike the reported deficiency of adenylosuccinate lyase and a suspected deficiency of adenylosuccinate synthetase, myoadenylate deaminase deficiency (MDD) presents as a suitable model of purine nucleotide cycle disruption for the following reasons: (a) Myoadenylate deaminase deficiency is confined to skeletal muscle; unlike the other components of the purine nucleotide cycle, myoadenylate deaminase is expressed only in skeletal muscle; and (b) AMP deaminase is a purine catabolic/interconverting enzymatic activity and as such does not normally play a vital role in cellular function. However, in skeletal muscle, where it is an essential component of an important energy-related pathway, a deficiency of myoadenylate deaminase may be associated with skeletal muscle abnormalities.

Myoadenylate deaminase deficiency is detected in approximately 2% of all people in whom biopsies are submitted for pathological evaluation (for review, see 61). Several highly sensitive laboratory procedures have been developed for detecting MDD. These include a standard blood test and histochemical and biochemical evaluation of muscle biopsy material.

The ischemic forearm exercise test, originally developed to screen for glycogenoses, has been applied to the detection of MDD. Diffusible muscle metabolites, such as lactate and ammonia, accumulate in blood after a brief period of intense anaerobic exercise. MDD is easily detected as a failure to produce a rise in blood ammonia following exercise. This test has been standardized by several laboratories (14, 56, 63), although it can still produce false positive results at a low frequency (i.e., 2-3%). Therefore, a positive test for MDD with ischemic forearm exercise is routinely followed up with biopsy for verification by histochemical stain or direct assay of AMP deaminase activity.

Biochemical and functional analysis of exercising MDD patients has provided evidence for myopathy associated with a disruption of the purine nucleotide cycle. Anaerobic exercise employing an ischemic forearm protocol (55) and a more aerobic one utilizing increasing work loads to fatigue on a bicycle ergometer (48) were performed with MDD and control individuals. Analysis of blood samples and muscle biopsies uncovered several metabolic abnormalities consistent with a deficiency of AMP deaminase (see Table 1). Significant differences in net energy consumption per unit work performed were observed between MDD and control individuals undergoing bicycle ergometry to fatigue, whereas no differences were apparent during anaerobic exercise.

Clinical features of MDD are presented in Table 2. Approximately 2/3 of all patients are males, with the onset of symptoms or age of diagnosis not confined to any particular age group. The most common symptom, reported in 88% of patients where information is available, is exercise-related easy fatigue, cramps, and myalgia. However, nearly half of all patients present with a variety of other associated neurological and rheumatological disorders. In addition, some deficient patients appear to be asymptomatic. This clinical heterogeneity has prompted some investigators to propose that MDD is simply a harmless genetic variant (20, 54).

Recently, Fishbein has reported evidence for multiple forms of MDD (16), which may serve as a basis for clarifying the confusing clinical picture associated with this metabolic myopathy. Based on a number of observations (see Table 3), Fishbein has proposed inherited and acquired forms of MDD. Inherited deficiency was proposed to be restricted to those individuals exhibiting exercise-related symptoms only and in whom it was also observed that residual activity was generally less than 2% of control and nonreactive with a muscle-specific antibody. Acquired deficiency includes those patients presenting with associated diseases. These individuals tend to have higher levels of residual activity, which also reacts with muscle-specific antibody. In addition, other muscle-specific enzymatic activities, such as creatine kinase and adenylate kinase, are reduced in acquired deficiency, although not as severely as AMP deaminase.

There is precedent for acquired MDD. In one study, biopsies from dystrophic patients and other individuals presenting with defined myopathies were assayed for endogenous AMP deaminase activity (24). Those individuals in whom the stage of disease was classified as severe exhibited markedly reduced or deficient levels of AMP deaminase activity relative to those who were in the early stages of disease.

**Table 1 Exercise-Induced Metabolic Alterations
Associated With Myoadenylate Deaminase Deficiency**

	Reference
Decreases	
Adenylate catabolism	48, 55
IMP accumulation	48, 55
.Plasma purine and ammonia levels	56
Increases	
Adenosine production	48
Energy substrate utilization per unit work	48

Table 2   Clinical Features of AMP Deaminase Deficiency

Sex: 87/128 male
Age at time of diagnosis
  Mean: 32 years
  Median: 30 years
  Range: < 1 to 70 years
Age at time of onset of symptoms
  Infancy (2 years): 1 out of 35 (3%)
  Childhood (2-12): 8 out of 35 (23%)
  Teenage (13-19): 9 out of 35 (26%)
  Young adult (20-40): 8 out of 35 (23%)
  Older adult (> 40): 9 out of 35 (26%)
Postexercise symptoms
  Easy fatigue, cramps: 49 out of 56 (88%)
  Myalgia
Other clinical diagnoses (presumably secondary deficiency)
  10 - Dystrophy
   9 - Neuropathy
   8 - Polymyositis
   7 - Atrophy
   3 - Collagen vascular disease
   2 - Amyotrophic lateral sclerosis
   2 - Progressive systemic sclerosis
   2 - Dermatomyositis
   2 - Hypotonia
   2 - Type I atrophy
   1 - Hypokalemic periodic paralysis
   1 - Kugelberg-Welander syndrome
   7 - Others
Laboratory abnormalities
  Failure to produce ammonia on ischemic testing
  Negative histochemical stain for AMP deaminase
  Diminished AMP deaminase activity on direct assay

Interestingly, creatine kinase activity, quantitated in the same biopsies, paralleled those of AMP deaminase, but reductions were not as severe. Utilizing a mouse model (C56BDyDy), other investigators provided evidence for a rapid and profound decrease in AMP deaminase activity upon denervation, approaching values found in a dystrophic counterpart (C56Bdydy) (32). The combined results of these two studies strongly suggest that AMP deaminase is extremely sensitive to pathological changes in skeletal muscle, a characteristic that would appear to play a significant role in the genesis of acquired myoadenylate deaminase deficiency.

**Table 3   Characteristics of Proposed Alternate Forms
of Myoadenylate Deaminase Deficiency**

	Clinical symptoms	Residual activity	Specificity
Primary	Exercise-related symptoms only	< 2%, not immunoreactive with muscle-specific antisera	Specific to AMP deaminase
Secondary	Other neuromuscular and rheumatological disorders	Up to 15%, immunoreactive with muscle-specific antisera	Reduction in other muscle-specific enzymatic activities

Molecular Biology as a Tool for Defining Myoadenylate Deaminase Deficiency

Clinical, biochemical, and immunological data derived from myoadenylate deaminase–deficient individuals have suggested multiple forms of this metabolic myopathy. Although there appears to be a distinct group of affected individuals in whom an inherited defect in AMP deaminase would be expected, it is also reasonable to assume at least one other cohort of patients who acquire a myoadenylate deaminase–deficient state secondary to pathological changes associated with the onset of a variety of primary neurological and rheumatological disorders. Moreover, there are likely to be multiple mechanisms responsible for myoadenylate deaminase deficiency. In order to identify these potential multiple mechanisms, it will be necessary to understand how AMP deaminase expression is regulated in the myocyte. In this light, efforts toward isolating the gene(s) for AMP deaminase and defining their regulation at the transcriptional and translational level now seem justified.

Recently, adult rat skeletal muscle myoadenylate deaminase cDNA has been isolated and sequenced (46). Utilizing this cDNA as a probe, a transcript has been identified in postnatal rat skeletal muscle whose abundance parallels that of AMP deaminase activity during development and in different adult skeletal muscle fibers. Analysis of DNA from a variety of organisms, again utilizing this rat cDNA as the probe, has demonstrated the myoadenylate deaminase gene to be highly conserved across mammalian species, including man. This should facilitate the cloning of the human myoadenylate deaminase gene for its use in delineating the molecular mechanisms associated with myoadenylate deaminase deficiency and, in a more general sense, in delineating the role of the purine nucleotide cycle in skeletal muscle energy metabolism.

Acknowledgments

The authors would like to acknowledge the expert secretarial assistance of Diane Dunlap in the preparation of this manuscript.

References

1. Aragon, J.J.; Lowenstein, J.M. The purine nucleotide cycle: comparison of the levels of citric acid cycle intermediates with the operation of the purine nucleotide cycle in rat skeletal muscle during exercise and recovery from exercise. Eur. J. Biochem. 110:371-377; 1980.

2. Aragon, J.J.; Tornheim, K.; Goodman, M.N.; Lowenstein, J.M. Replenishment of citric acid cycle intermediates by the purine nucleotide cycle in rat skeletal muscle. Curr. Top. Cell. Regul. 18:131-149; 1981.

3. Aragon, J.J., Tornheim, K.; Lowenstein, J.M. On a possible role of IMP in the regulation of phosphorylase activity in skeletal muscle. FEBS Lett. 117(Suppl.):K56-K64; 1980.

4. Arch, J.R.S.; Newsholme, E.A. Activities and some properties of 5-nucleotidase, adenosine kinase, and adenosine deaminase in tissues from vertebrates and invertebrates in relation to the control of the concentration and the physiological role of adenosine. Biochem. J. 174:965-977; 1978.

5. Ashby, B.; Frieden, C. Interaction of AMP aminohydrolase with myosin and its subfragments. J. Biol. Chem. 252:1869-1872; 1977.

6. Ashby, B.; Frieden, C. Adenylate deaminase: kinetic and binding studies on the rabbit muscle enzyme. J. Biol. Chem. 253:8728-8735; 1978.

7. Ashby, B.; Frieden, C.; Bischoff, R. Immunofluorescent and histochemical localization of AMP deaminase in skeletal muscle. J. Cell Biol. 81:361-373; 1979.

8. Barnes, L.B.; Bishop, S.H. Adenylosuccinate lyase from human erythrocytes. Int. J. Biochem. 6:497-503; 1975.

9. Barshop, B.A.; Frieden, C. Analysis of the interaction of rabbit skeletal muscle adenylate deaminase with myosin subfragments. J. Biol. Chem. 259:60-66; 1984.

10. Bertorini, T.E.; Shively, V.; Taylor, B.; Palmieri, G.M.A.; Fox, I.H. ATP degradation products after ischemic exercise: hereditary lack of phosphorylase or carnitine palmityltransferase. Neurology 35:1355-1357; 1985.

11. Bessman, S.P.; Geiger, P.J. Transport of energy in muscle: the phosphorylcreatine shuttle. Science 211:448-452; 1981.

12. Brosh, S.; Boer, P.; Zoref-Shani, E.; Sperling, O. De novo purine synthesis in skeletal muscle. Biochim. Biophys. Acta 714:181-183; 1982.

13. Casey, P.J.; Lowenstein, J.M. Purification of adenylosuccinate lyase from rat skeletal muscle by a novel affinity column. Biochem. J. 246:263-269; 1987.

14. Coleman, R.A.; Stajich, J.M.; Pact, V.W.; Pericak-Vance, M.A. The ischemic exercise test in normal adults and in patients with weakness and cramps. Muscle Nerve 9:216-221; 1986.

15. Dudley, G.A.; Terjung, R.L. Influence of aerobic metabolism on IMP accumulation in fast twitch muscle. Am. J. Physiol. 248:C37-42; 1985.

16. Fishbein, W.N. Myoadenylate deaminase deficiency: inherited and acquired forms. Biochem. Med. 33:158-169; 1985.

17. Fishbein, W.N.; Armbrustmacher, V.W.; Griffin, J.L. Myoadenylate deaminase deficiency: a new disease of muscle. Science: 545-548; 1978.

18. Flanagan, W.F.; Holmes, E.W.; Sabina, R.L.; Swain, J.L. Importance of purine nucleotide cycle to energy production in skeletal muscle. Am. J. Physiol. 251:C795-802; 1986.

19. Gorski, J.; Hood, D.A.; Brown, O.M.; Terjung, R.L. Incorporation of N-leucine amine into ATP of fast twitch muscle following stimulation. Biochem. Biophys. Res. Commun. 128:1254-1260; 1985.

20. Hayes, D.J.; Summers, B.A.; Morgan-Hughes, J.A. Myoadenylate deaminase deficiency or not? J. Neurol. Sci. 53:125-136; 1982.

21. Hochachka, P.W.; Mommsen, T.P. Protons and anaerobiosis. Science 219: 1391-1397; 1983.

22. Jaeken, J.; Van den Berghe, G. An infantile autistic syndrome characterized by the presence of succinylpurines in body fluids. Lancet ii: 1058-1061; 1984.

23. Kaletha, K.; Spychala, J.; Nowak, G. Developmental forms of human skeletal muscle AMP deaminase. Experientia 43:440-443; 1987.

24. Kar, N.C.; Pearson, C.M. Muscle adenylic deaminase activity: selective decrease in early-onset Duchenne muscular dystrophy. Neurology 23:478-482; 1973.

25. Katz, A.; Sahlin, K.; Henriksson, J. Muscle ammonia metabolism during isometric contraction in humans. Am. J. Physiol. 250:C834-840; 1986.

26. Kono, N.; Mineo, I.; Shimizu, T.; Hara, N.; Yamada, Y.; Nonaka, K.; Tarui, S. Increased plasma uric acid after exercise in muscle phosphofructokinase deficiency. Neurology 36:106-108; 1986.

27. Koretz, J.F. Structural studies of isolated native thick filaments from rabbit psoas muscle with AMP deaminase decoration. Proc. Natl. Acad. Sci. USA 79: 6205-6209; 1982.

28. Koretz, J.F.; Frieden, C. Adenylate deaminase binding to synthetic thick filaments of myosin. Proc. Natl. Acad. Sci. USA 77:7186-7188; 1980.

29. Lowenstein, J.; Tornheim, K. Ammonia production in muscle: the purine nucleotide cycle. Science 171:397-400; 1971.

30. Manfredi, J.P.; Holmes, E.W. Control of the purine nucleotide cycle in extracts of rat skeletal muscle: effects of energy state and concentrations of cycle intermediates. Arch. Biochem. Biophys. 233:515-529; 1984.

31. Marquetant, R.; Desai, N.M.; Sabina, R.L.; Holmes, E.W. Evidence for sequential expression of multiple AMP deaminase isoforms during skeletal muscle development. Proc. Natl. Acad. Sci. USA 84:2345-2349; 1987.

32. McCaman, M.W.; McCaman, R.E. Effects of denervation on normal and dystrophic muscle: DNA and nucleotide enzymes. Am. J. Physiol. 209:495-500; 1965.

33. Meyer, R.A.; Terjung, R.L. Differences in ammonia and adenylate metabolism in contracting fast and slow muscle. Am. J. Physiol. 237:C111-118; 1979.

34. Meyer, R.A.; Terjung, R.L. AMP deamination and IMP reamination in working skeletal muscle. Am. J. Physiol. 239:C32-38; 1980.

35. Muirhead, K.M.; Bishop, S.H. Purification of adenylosuccinate synthetase from rabbit skeletal muscle. J. Biol. Chem. 249:459-464; 1974.

36. Ogasawara, N.; Goto, H.; Watanabe, H.; Kawamura, T.Y.; Yoshino, M. Multiple forms of AMP deaminase in various rat tissues. FEBS Lett. 44:63-66; 1974.

37. Ogasawara, N.; Goto, H.; Yamada, Y. Effects of various ligands on interactions of AMP deaminase with myosin. Biochim. Biophys. Acta 524:442-446; 1978.

38. Ogasawara, N.; Goto, H.; Yamada, Y. AMP deaminase isozymes in rabbit red and white muscles and heart. Comp. Biochem. Physiol. 76:471-473; 1983.

39. Ogasawara, N.; Goto, H.; Yamada, Y.; Watanabe, T. Distribution of AMP deaminase isozymes in rat tissues. Eur. J. Biochem. 87:297-304; 1978.

40. Ogasawara, N.; Goto, H.; Yamada, Y.; Watanabe, T.; Asano, T. AMP deaminase isozymes in human tissues. Biochim. Biophys. Acta 714: 298-306; 1982.

41. Ogawa, H.; Shiraki, H.; Matsuda, Y.; Nakagawa, H. Interaction of adenylosuccinate synthetase with F-actin. Eur. J. Biochem. 85:331-337; 1978.

42. Raggi, A.; Bergamini, C.; Ronca, G. Isozymes of AMP deaminase in red and white skeletal muscles. FEBS Lett. 58:19-23; 1975.

43. Raggi, A.; Ronca-Testoni, S.; Ronca, G. Muscle AMP aminohydrolase. Biochim. Biophys. Acta 178:619-622; 1969.

44. Rumpf, R.W.; Wagner, H.; Kaiser, H.; Meinck, H.M.; Goebel, H.H.; Scheler, F. Increased ammonia production during forearm ischemic work test in McArdle's disease. Klin. Wochenschr. 59:1319-1320; 1981.

45. Sabina, R.L.; Kernstine, K.H.; Boyd, R.L.; Holmes, E.W.; Swain, J.L. Metabolism of 5-amino-4-imidazolecarboxamide riboside in cardiac and skeletal muscle. J. Biol. Chem. 257:10178-10183; 1982.

46. Sabina, R.L.; Marquetant, R.; Desai, N.M.; Kaletha, K.; Holmes, E.W. Cloning and sequence of rat myoadenylate deaminase cDNA. J. Biol. Chem. 262:12397-12400; 1987.

47. Sabina, R.L.; Patterson, D.; Holmes, E.W. 5-amino-4-imidazolecarboxamide riboside (Z-riboside) metabolism in eukaryotic cells. J. Biol. Chem. 260: 6107-6114; 1985.

48. Sabina, R.L.; Swain, J.L.; Olanow, C.W.; Bradley, C.W.; Fishbein, W.N.; DiMauro, S.; Holmes, E.W. Myoadenylate deaminase deficiency: functional and metabolic abnormalities associated with disruption of the purine nucleotide cycle. J. Clin. Invest. 73:720-730; 1984.

49. Sammons, D.W.; Chilson, O.P. AMP deaminase: stage-specific isozymes in differentiating chick muscle. Arch. Biochem. Biophys. 191: 561-570; 1978.

50. Schultz, V.; Lowenstein, J.M. Purine nucleotide cycle: evidence for the occurrence of the cycle in brain. J. Biol. Chem. 251:485-492; 1976.

51. Shiraki, H.; Miyamoto, S.; Matsuda, Y.; Momose, E.; Nakagawa, H. Possible correlation between binding of muscle type AMP deaminase to myofibrils and ammoniagenesis in rat skeletal muscle on electrical stimulation. Biochem. Biophys. Res. Commun. 100:1099-1103; 1981.

52. Shiraki, H.; Ogawa, H.; Matsuda, Y.; Nakagawa, H. Interaction of rat muscle AMP deaminase with myosin. I. Biochemical study of the interaction of AMP deaminase and myosin in rat muscle. Biochim. Biophys. Acta 566:335-344; 1979.

53. Shiraki, H.; Ogawa, H.; Matsuda, Y.; Nakagawa, H. Interaction of rat muscle AMP deaminase with myosin. II. Modification of the kinetic and regulatory properties of rat muscle AMP deaminase by myosin. Biochim. Biophys. Acta 566:345-352; 1979.

54. Shumate, J.B.; Katnik, R.; Ruiz, M.; Kaiser, K.; Frieden, C.; Brooke, M.H.; Carroll, J.E. Myoadenylate deaminase deficiency. Muscle Nerve 2:213-216; 1979.

55. Sinkeler, S.P.T.; Binkhorst, R.A.; Joosten, M.G.; Wevers, R.A.; Coerwinkel, M.M.; Oei, T.L. AMP deaminase deficiency: study of the human skeletal muscle purine metabolism during ischemic isometric exercise. Clin. Sci. 72:475-482; 1987.

56. Sinkeler, S.P.; Wevers, R.A.; Joosten, E.M.; Binkhorst, R.A.; Oei, L.T.; van'tHof, M.A.; deHaan, A.F. Improvement of screening in exertional myalgia with a standardized ischemic forearm test. Muscle Nerve 9:731-737; 1986.

57. Solano, C.; Coffee, C.J. Differential response of AMP deaminase isozymes to changes in the adenylate energy charge. Biochem. Biophys. Res. Commun. 85:564-571; 1978.

58. Stayton, M.M.; Rudolph, F.B.; Fromm, H.J. Regulation, genetics and properties of adenylosuccinate synthetase: a review. Curr. Top. Cell. Regul. 22:103-141; 1983.

59. Sugden, P.H.; Newsholme, E.A. The effects of ammonium, inorganic phosphate, and potassium ions on the activity of phosphofructokinase from muscle and nervous tissue of vertebrates and invertebrates. Biochem. J. 150:113-122; 1975.

60. Swain, J.L.; Hines, J.J.; Sabina, R.L.; Harbury, O.L.; Holmes, E.W. Disruption of the purine nucleotide cycle by inhibition of adenylosuccinate lyase produces skeletal muscle dysfunction. J. Clin. Invest. 74:1422-1427; 1984.

61. Swain, J.L.; Sabina, R.L.; Holmes, E.W. Myoadenylate deaminase deficiency. In: Stanbury, J.B.; Wyngaarden, J.B.; Fredrickson D.S.; Goldstein, J.C.; Brown, M.S., eds. The metabolic basis of inherited disease. 5th ed. New York: McGraw-Hill; 1983:1184-1191.

62. Swain, J.L.; Sabina, R.L.; McHale, P.A.; Greenfield, J.C., Jr.; Holmes, E.W. Prolonged myocardial nucleotide depletion after brief ischemia in the open-chested dog. Am. J. Physiol. 242:H818-826; 1982.

63. Valen, P.A.; Nakayama, D.A.; Veum, J.; Sulaiman, A.R.; Wortman, R.L. Myoadenylate deaminase deficiency and forearm ischemic exercise testing. Arthritis Rheum. 30:661-668; 1987.

64. Van den Berghe, G.; Jaeken, J. Adenylosuccinase deficiency. (Abstract). Pediatr. Res. 19:780; 1985.

65. Winder, W.W.; Terjung, R.L.; Baldwin, K.M.; Holloszy, J.O. Effect of exercise on AMP deaminase and adenylosuccinase in rat skeletal muscle. Am. J. Physiol. 227:1411-1414; 1974.

66. Wyngaarden, J.B.; Kelley, W.N. Gout. In: Stanbury, J.B.; Wyngaarden, J.B.; Fredrickson, D.S.; Goldstein, J.L.; Brown, M.S., eds. The metabolic basis of inherited disease. 5th ed. New York: McGraw-Hill; 1983:1043-1114.

67. Zimmer, H.G. Restitution of myocardial adenine nucleotides: acceleration by administration of ribose. J. Physiol. (Paris) 76:769-775; 1980.

Disorders of Lipid Metabolism in Muscle and Their Exercise Implications

Heinz Reichmann

University of Würzburg, Würzburg, West Germany

Fatty acids are preferentially used by muscle for energy production both at rest and during contraction. They are major substrates for energy production both in the absorptive and the postabsorptive state. There are several precursors of free fatty acids (FFA) that supply muscle. Very low density lipoproteins and chylomicrones are hydrolyzed to free fatty acids and glycerol by lipoproteinlipase, which is located on the surface of the endothelium. FFA enter muscle by diffusion. Intramuscular triglycerides are degraded by triglyceride lipase to FFA. Free fatty acids are activated by long-chain fatty acyl-CoA synthetase, which is located in the outer mitochondrial membrane. The long-chain acyl-CoA is converted to acylcarnitine by carnitine palmitoyltransferase (CPT 1), which is located in the outer surface of the inner mitochondrial membrane. Carnitine is required as an essential cofactor to allow transport across the inner mitochondrial membrane. Intramitochondrially, long-chain acyl-carnitine is converted by CPT 2 to acyl-CoA on the inner surface of the inner mitochondrial membrane. Acyl-CoA undergoes successively repeated cycles of beta-oxidation. Beta-oxidation of FA consists of four catalytic steps. The first step is catalyzation by various acyl-CoA dehydrogenases (DH) that are chain-length specific and dehydrogenate acyl-CoA to 2-trans-enoyl-CoA. Enoyl-CoA hydratase converts enoyl-CoA to hydroxyacyl-CoA, which is dehydrogenated to β-ketoacyl-CoA by hydroxyacyl-CoA DH. The last step is the cleavage of 3-ketoacyl-CoA, catalyzed by thiolase, resulting in acetyl-CoA and in acyl-CoA, two atoms shorter than the substrate, which successively enters the cycle again. Mitochondria contain ketoacyl-CoA thiolase for beta-oxidation and acetyl-CoA thiolase, which acts in ketone body metabolism. Acetyl-CoA either enters the tricarboxylic acid cycle or is used in ketone body metabolism. Thus, an impairment of one of these enzymatic steps should result in a lack of energy utilization of fatty acids.

In previous studies, we were able to show that increased muscle activity induced by electrical stimulation or strenuous training programs results in an increase in mitochondrial enzyme activities (4). For most intramitochondrial enzymes, there was a good correlation between their activities and the mitochondrial volume (8). In a new, more detailed study of all enzymes of the respiratory chain and of various enzymes of beta-oxidation of FA, we found increases in activities of up to 200% after 28d-stimulation (repeated cycles of 1-hour stimulation, 1-hour rest) of rabbit tibialis anterior (TA) muscle. All three enzymes measured (hydroxyacyl-CoA DH, crotonase [enoyl-CoA hydratase], thiolase) increased 1.5- to 3-fold in the stimulated muscle when compared to the contralateral control TA muscle (Figure 1). Similar results were obtained for carnitine palmityltransferase (CPT), which increased

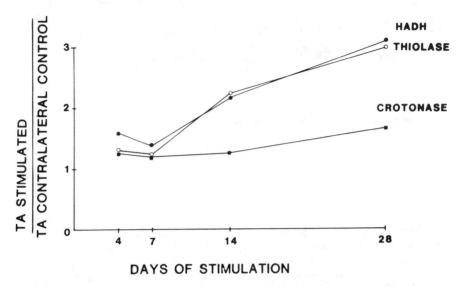

Figure 1. Beta-oxidation enzyme activity ratios from stimulated and contralateral control tibialis anterior muscle from rabbit. Animals were stimulated for up to 28 days by a frequency of 10 Hz, with 1 hour stimulation, 1 hour rest, and so on. HADH, hydroxyacyl-CoA dehydrogenase.

up to 3.3-fold (Figure 2). In contrast, free and total carnitine concentration showed only very slight increases (1.1- to 1.4-fold, respectively) (Figure 2). This discrepancy between mitochondrial enzymes and carnitine may be due to the fact that unlike the enzymes, carnitine is not produced inside the muscle fiber but has to be imported.

Rat treadmill training (15 weeks, 210 min training per day, 27 m/min at 15-degree grade) also resulted in increases in enzymes involved in the respiratory chain and beta-oxidation (Table 1). Thus, increased muscle activity is combined with increases in the enzymes of beta-oxidation, the enzyme CPT, and to a lesser degree the level of carnitine. That is why defects in beta-oxidation should cause an energy crisis when muscle is used for longer periods of time. Indeed, several diseases are connected to defects in beta-oxidation. At present, there are three major groups of lipid metabolism disorders that will be dealt with in this article: carnitine deficiency, CPT-disorder, and impairments of beta-oxidation enzymes (Table 2).

Carnitine is an essential cofactor permitting transport of long-chain FA across the inner mitochondrial membrane. Carnitine is acquired by diet (red meat, dairy products) or synthesized from lysine and methionine by the liver and to a lesser degree by the kidney. Carnitine is actively transported into muscle (6, 12). It is still not known what causes carnitine deficiency. In some patients a defect in the active transport of carnitine into muscle can be shown (7). During the last decade, up to 15 disorders that are associated with a secondary carnitine deficiency have been described. For example, acyl-CoA DH deficiencies are mostly associated with low free carnitine that is trapped as acylcarnitine in muscle and released in serum. For this reason it is debatable whether there exists a real primary carnitine deficiency. In spite of this consideration, clinicians differ between myopathic and systemic forms of carnitine deficiency.

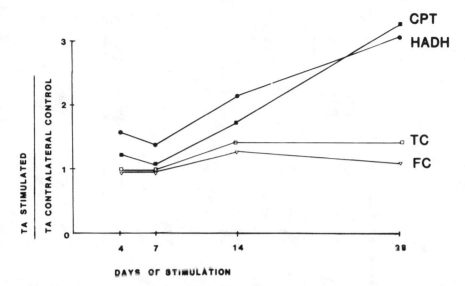

Figure 2. Enzyme activity ratio (carnitine palmitoyltransferase) and ratio of carnitine (free and total carnitine [FC and TC, respectively]) from stimulated and contralateral control tibialis anterior muscle from rabbit.

The myopathic form is characterized by progressive muscle weakness and high fat accumulation in muscle (3). Low carnitine concentrations (free and esterified) are found in muscle but not in liver and serum. The disease normally starts in childhood and involves proximal muscle weakness, myalgia, abnormal fatigability, rare myoglobinuria, creatinekinase increases, and sometimes hypertrophic cardiomyopathy. The disease seems to be autosomal-recessive (1). Morphological characteristics are fatty droplets, which are mostly found in type I and IIA muscle fibers. Mitochondria are normally structured. Low carnitine causes various problems in energy metabolism due to impaired lipid metabolism and ketone body production. The CoA:acyl-CoA ratio is decreased, and it is known that increased intramitochondrial acyl-CoA inhibits key enzymes of other pathways such as pyruvate dehydrogenase, CPT, or citrate synthetase (for review, see 2). Fasting periods are deleterious because of limited FA energy production and glycogen depletion, which results in hypoglycemia. Carnitine can be subdivided in muscle in free carnitine (74%), short- and medium-chain acylcarnitine (24%), and long-chain acylcarnitine (1.5%) (10).

Because myopathic carnitine deficiency is characterized by impairment of the transport of long-chain acyl-CoA through the inner mitochondrial membrane, we were interested in analyzing the subsequent enzymes of beta-oxidation (Table 3). Measurements of all the enzymes involved in beta-oxidation revealed no significant decrease in activity when compared to 10 normal controls. Thiolase was the only enzyme higher in the patients.

Systemic carnitine deficiency was first described by Karpati et al. in 1975 (5). In contrast to the myopathic form, systemic carnitine deficiency is a life-threatening disease. This form shows low (5-20% of normal) carnitine concentrations not only

Table 1 Enzyme Activities in Vastus Lateralis Muscle (Red and White Portion) From Control and Trained Rats

Enzyme	VL-W-Con	VL-W-Tr	Tr/Con	VL-R-Con	VL-R-Tr	Tr/Con
NADH dehydrogenase	40.7 ± 1.7	56.1 ± 11.7	1.38	74.1 ± 5.8	133 ± 42	1.79
NADH cytochrome c reductase	3.3 ± 0.7	5.4 ± 2.4	1.64	12.9 ± 4.9	15.5 ± 5.9	1.20
Succinate dehydrogenase	2.3 ± 0.6	3.3 ± 0.7	1.43	6.0 ± 2.1	7.8 ± 2.4	1.30
Succinate cytochrome c reductase	2.3 ± 0.6	3.1 ± 1.2	1.35	5.3 ± 1.2	8.0 ± 2.0	1.51
Cytochrome c oxidase	4.5 ± 0.8	6.6 ± 1.4	1.47	10.7 ± 4.6	11.3 ± 2.7	1.06
Palmitoyl-CoA dehydrogenase	0.77 ± 0.07	1.05 ± 0.2	1.36	1.14 ± 0.11	2.1 ± 0.9	1.84
Crotonase	6.9 ± 0.2	8.9 ± 1.8	1.29	3.3 ± 0.3	6.8 ± 0.8	2.06
Hydroxyacyl-CoA dehydrogenase	6.4 ± 1.1	8.7 ± 2.9	1.36	14.6 ± 1.7	19.7 ± 7.6	1.35
Thiolase	0.6 ± 0.1	0.8 ± 0.3	1.33			
Carnitine (free)	8.6 ± 1.6	7.85 ± .79	0.92	7.35 (2)	10.25 (2)	1.39
Carnitine (total)	10.2 ± 2.0	9.20 ± 1.2	0.9	8.75 (2)	12.9 (2)	1.47

Note. Enzyme activities are expressed as units/g muscle. In each group 4 animals were analyzed. The first 5 enzymes represent respiratory chain complexes; the next 4 enzymes belong to the beta-oxidation pathway. Carnitine is subdivided into free and total carnitine (nmoles/mg protein). For training protocol, see text.

Table 2   Disorders of Lipid Metabolism

Systemic carnitine deficiency
Myopathic carnitine deficiency
Long-chain acyl-CoA dehydrogenase deficiency
Medium-chain acyl-CoA dehydrogenase deficiency
Short-chain acyl-CoA dehydrogenase deficiency
Glutaric aciduria type I
Glutaric aciduria type II (multiple acyl-CoA DH deficiency)
β-ketothiolase deficiency

Table 3   Beta-Oxidation in Patients With a Myopathic Carnitine Deficiency and in Control Muscles

Enzyme	Controls (10)	Patients (5)
Butyryl-CoA dehydrogenase	8.0 ± 2.6	8.9 ± 4.8
Octanoyl-CoA dehydrogenase	7.5 ± 3.4	8.6 ± 3.8
Palmitoyl-CoA dehydrogenase	11.6 ± 7.7	10.7 ± 5.2
Crotonase	170 ± 69	232 ± 63
Hydroxyacyl-CoA dehydrogenase	30 ± 13	51 ± 16
Thiolase C10	18 ± 5.9	46 ± 19
Thiolase C4	51 ± 23	121 ± 50

Enzyme activities are expressed as units/mg protein.

in muscle but also in liver and serum. Serum carnitine is characterized by high proportions of short- and especially long-chain acylcarnitine (9). The disease starts in childhood with Reye-like symptoms due to hepatic encephalopathy. Characteristic findings are metabolic acidosis, hypoglycemia, hyperammonemia, elevated transaminase levels, and hypoprothrombinemia. Muscle weakness mostly follows liver impairment. Carnitine replacement therapy is beneficial in many instances, but not all patients improve. Carnitine can be administered intravenously and orally. Avoidance of fasting, frequent meals, and a high-carbohydrate, low-fat diet are usually suggested.

For CPT deficiency, on the contrary, there is no cure. Patients with a CPT deficiency have severe myoglobinuria associated with muscle "cramps" after severe exercise or high-intensity endurance training. Between attacks, patients show no symptoms and muscle morphology is normal. Attacks seem to be triggered by fasting, coldness, and endurance training, which should therefore be avoided by these patients. There is still controversy whether CPT 1 or 2 or both cause the problems. Short-time exercise is no problem for the patients because they use creatinephosphate and glycogen as energy supplies. The muscle weakness is preferentially found in proximal limb muscles but also in the respiratory muscles. Patients show no "second wind phenomenon"; because of the late onset of muscle tightness, they are not warned and continue with exercise, which is followed by myoglobinuria. Diagnosis is established between 15 and 30 years of age; for unknown reasons males are preferentially affected by the disease. An interesting new hypothesis suggests that in these patients there is a mutant enzyme that breaks down only when high palmitylcarnitine concentrations are present (as in fasting, coldness, or exercise) (13). Besides avoidance of the conditions likely to precipitate an attack, no real treatment of CPT deficiency is known. Diet should have high carbohydrate and low fat contents.

Disorders of beta-oxidation are normally due to a defect in one of the three acyl-CoA DH isozymes, which are chain-length specific and catalyze the first step of beta-oxidation. These enzyme defects have so far mostly been found in fibroblasts. The disease usually starts in childhood and shows Reye-like episodes. Muscles fatigue easily, and there is muscle hypotonia and hepatic encephalopathy. So far, no specific therapy is available. In 1984 Turnball et al. (11) reported on a defect of short-chain acyl-CoA DH in muscle. The patient was a 57-year-old female who suffered for 7 years from proximal muscle weakness. She also showed secondary carnitine deficiency. Muscle biopsy revealed lipid accumulation; endurance exercise resulted in lactic acidosis.

Taken together, impairment of lipid metabolism leads to problems in energy supply, especially when long-term muscle activity is required. Fasting is deleterious because of additional glycogen depletion. Liver involvement often causes hepatic encephalopathy. Muscle weakness is a common finding, and an increase in the lipid content of muscle is, with the exception of CPT deficiency, one of the hallmarks of the diseases. Treatment with carnitine is often effective in carnitine deficiency; however, there is no effective therapy for the other disorders of lipid metabolism.

Acknowledgment

This study was supported by the Deutsche Forschungsgemeinschaft (Re 265/5-3).

References

1. DiMauro, S.; Trevisan, C.; Hays, A.P. Disorders of lipid metabolism in muscle. Muscle Nerve 3:369-388; 1980.
2. Engel, A.G. Carnitine deficiency syndromes and lipid storage myopathies. In: Engel, A.G.; Banker, B.Q., eds. Myology. New York: McGraw-Hill; 1986: 1663-1696.
3. Engel, A.G.; Angelini, C. Carnitine deficiency of human skeletal muscle with associated lipid storage myopathy: a new syndrome. Science 179:899-902; 1973.
4. Green, H.J.; Reichmann, H.; Pette, D. Fibre type specific transformations in the enzyme activity pattern of rat vastus lateralis muscle by prolonged endurance training. Pflügers Arch. 399:216-222; 1983.
5. Karpati, G.; Carpenter, S.; Engel, A.G.; Walters, G.; Allen, J.; Rothman, S.; Klassen, G.; Mamer, O. The syndrome of systemic carnitine deficiency. Neurology 25:16-24; 1975.

6. Rebouche, C.J. Carnitine movement across muscle cell membrane—studies in isolated rat muscle. Biochim. Acta 471:145-155; 1977.

7. Rebouche, C.J.; Engel, A.G. Carnitine biosynthesis and metabolism in the primary deficiency syndromes. In: Serratrice, G., et al., eds. Neuromuscular diseases. New York: Raven Press; 1984:95-99.

8. Reichmann, H.; Hoppeler, H.; Mathieu-Costello, O.; van Bergen, F.; Pette, D. Biochemical and ultrastructural changes of skeletal muscle mitochondria after chronic electrical stimulation in rabbits. Pflügers Arch. 404:1-9; 1985.

9. Rimoldi, M.; DiDonato, S. Measurement of long-chain acylcarnitine. Neurology 32:916-917; 1982.

10. Trevisan, C.P.; Reichmann, H.; DeVivo, D.C.; DiMauro, S. Beta-oxidation enzymes in normal human muscle and in muscle from a patient with an unusual form of myopathic carnitine deficiency. Muscle Nerve 8:672-675; 1985.

11. Turnball, D.M.; Bartlett, K.; Stevens, D.L.; Albert, K.G.M.M.; Gibson, G.L.; Johnson, M.A.; McCulloch, A.J.; Sherratt, H.S.A. Short-chain acyl-CoA dehydrogenase deficiency associated with a lipid storage myopathy and secondary carnitine deficiency. N. Engl. J. Med. 311:1232-1236; 1984.

12. Willner, J.H.; Ginsburg, S.; DiMauro, S. Active transport of carnitine into skeletal muscle. Neurology 28:721-724; 1978.

13. Zierz, S.; Engel, A.G. Regulatory properties of a mutant carnitine palmitoyltransferase in human skeletal muscle. Eur. J. Biochem. 149:207-211; 1985.

Human Respiratory Chain Disorders: Implications for Muscle Oxidative Metabolism

Ronald G. Haller and Steven F. Lewis
Veterans Administration Medical Center and
University of Texas Southwestern Medical Center, Dallas, Texas, U.S.A.

Oxidative metabolism, the synthesis of ATP via oxidative phosphorylation, is the dominant source of energy for working muscle. Normal muscle oxidative metabolism depends upon the integrity of a metabolic network in which reducing equivalents (reduced nicotinamide adenine dinucleotide, NADH, and flavoproteins, e.g., $FADH_2$) produced in the course of substrate oxidation (i.e., glycolysis, β-oxidation, pyruvate dehydrogenase, Krebs cycle) are oxidized via the electron transport chain, where the reduction of molecular oxygen to water is coupled to the phosphorylation of ADP. Human muscle oxidative defects, correspondingly, can be considered to be of two major types (Figure 1). The first consists of disorders that impair substrate oxidation and thus modify the production of reducing equivalents. Examples include enzyme defects that selectively impair muscle carbohydrate or lipid oxidation. The second major class of oxidative defects impair the process by which NADH and $FADH_2$ are oxidized via electron transport. Rare biochemical defects that selectively disrupt the normal coupling of oxygen uptake to ADP phosphorylation (e.g., Luft's disease) or impair ATP synthase have been described (6). More common (though still rare) are defects in the mitochondrial respiratory chain that disrupt the flow of electrons from reduced cofactors (NADH, $FADH_2$) to oxygen.

The respiratory chain consists of four major enzyme complexes of the inner mitochondrial membrane, each comprised of multiple polypeptides that contain flavoproteins, iron-sulfur clusters, and/or heme proteins (cytochromes) that transfer electrons from substrate to oxygen (Figure 2). The energy generated in this process is conserved at three coupling sites (in complexes I, III, and IV) as a proton gradient between the inner (matrix) and outer surfaces of the inner mitochondrial membrane. The proton gradient is discharged in the presence of phosphate acceptor, ADP, with the synthesis of ATP, thus coupling phosphorylation to substrate oxidation. The formation of the respiratory chain complexes involves the interaction of proteins coded on the mitochondrial and nuclear genomes, thus requiring a complex process of synthesis, transport, and assembly of constituent proteins in the inner mitochondrial membrane. The enzyme complexes so formed comprise important structural as well as catalytic elements of the inner mitochondrial membrane. For example, cytochrome c oxidase (complex IV) alone constitutes roughly 15% of the inner membrane. It is not surprising, therefore, that respiratory chain defects are commonly associated with structural as well as functional mitochondrial changes.

252   Haller and Lewis

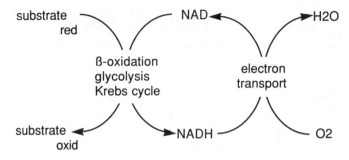

Figure 1. Schematic of the two major varieties of human muscle oxidative defects: (a) impairment of substrate oxidation and the production of reducing equivalents (e.g., NADH); (b) impairment of the oxidation of reducing equivalents via electron transport.

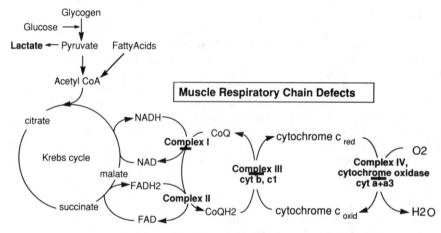

Figure 2. Diagram of the mitochondrial respiratory chain. The sites of well-defined human respiratory chain defects are indicated, and the relations between substrate oxidation and electron transport are shown.

Defects in the function and protein composition of the respiratory chain in human skeletal muscle involving complexes I, III, and IV have been characterized biochemically. Most commonly this has been accomplished through the isolation of mitochondria from biopsied skeletal muscle with subsequent assessment of substrate-specific oxygen uptake, quantitation of the content of mitochondrial cytochromes, and/or assay of specific mitochondrial enzymes. In some cases, immunologic, chromatographic, or electron paramagnetic resonance methods have been employed to characterize further the polypeptide or iron-sulfur components of the various respiratory chain complexes (7, 21, 28). The molecular mechanisms involved in the pathogenesis of these metabolic defects are incompletely understood, but genetic defects have been inferred from the presence of affected family members in approximately 30% of reported cases (6, 34). In some cases, the pattern of inheritance is compatible with an autosomal recessive trait, thus implying a nuclear genomic defect. In others, familial occurrence has been consistent with maternal inheritance (i.e., passed from affected females to their children). Because mitochondria are maternally inherited, this pattern suggests the presence of a defect in the mitochondrial genome. Holt and co-workers (18) demonstrated the presence of DNA deletions in muscle mitochondria in 9 of 25 patients with muscle respiratory defects, including many without evidently affected family members.

As a result of the usual requirement of very large muscle biopsies (typically 6-8 g) for the performance of oxygen electrode (polarographic) studies, and because of the need for substantial biochemical resources for these and related analyses, such mitochondrial studies have been undertaken at only a few medical centers. Furthermore, protocols employed for such mitochondrial studies are not strictly uniform, and in only a few cases is detailed information available regarding the molecular nature of these biochemical defects. Despite these limitations to precise comparisons of affected patients, common clinical, metabolic, and physiologic features of muscle respiratory chain disorders have emerged.

Clinical Manifestations of Respiratory Chain Defects

The clinical manifestations of human respiratory chain defects are diverse. This may relate to differing severity of the metabolic defect and to the fact that the distribution of the defect among tissues may vary. Thus, patients have been described in whom the biochemical defect and clinical symptoms are limited to skeletal muscle, whereas in others symptoms referable to the presence of the metabolic defect in the central nervous system, myocardium, or liver predominate (6). The most common clinical presentations of human respiratory chain defects are those of isolated or predominant skeletal muscle involvement, and of combined central nervous system and skeletal muscle involvement (mitochondrial "encephalomyopathies") in which muscle and central nervous system symptoms coexist. In the latter, seizures, stroke-like episodes, ataxia, or hearing or visual impairment may be present (6, 29, 34).

Symptoms attributable to respiratory chain defects in skeletal muscle consist predominantly of premature fatigability and, in many but not all cases, muscular weakness (inability to generate normal contractile force). The most severe respiratory chain defects are not compatible with life (7, 19, 28). In less severe oxidative defects, there typically is intolerance of physical activity, where trivial exercise induces a sense of heaviness and rapid loss of force-generating capacity of exercised muscles, shortness of breath, tachycardia, and high levels of blood lactate. This syndrome most commonly has been associated with respiratory chain defects involving complex I or III (8, 16, 21, 22, 30), though recently a patient with complex IV deficiency has been reported (15). When weakness is present in muscle respiratory chain defects, there is a propensity for the muscles involved in eye and lid movements to be affected, resulting in ophthalmoplegia. The variables responsible for persistent weakness in rested muscles in some patients are unknown but may relate to muscle fiber injury and atrophy as a consequence of the oxidative defect. The clinical and biochemical features of muscle respiratory chain defects have been the subject of excellent reviews (6, 7, 29, 34).

Mitochondrial Biogenesis
in Muscle Respiratory Chain Defects

The level of habitual physical activity of patients with muscle respiratory chain defects is markedly limited due to the fact that minor exertion induces rapid fatigue. Thus, such patients are remarkably sedentary. Skeletal muscle in these patients nevertheless reveals evidence of augmented mitochondrial biogenesis. This is manifest morphologically by increased mitochondrial numbers and biochemically by increases in the level of activity of certain oxidative enzymes. The presence of so-called ragged red fibers on histologic examination of muscle sections stained with Gomori trichrome is typical of these metabolic defects and represents the accumulation of increased numbers of mitochondria, especially in the subsarcolemmal area (32). Morphometric analysis has indicated that the proportion of cellular volume occupied by mitochondria may increase 2- to 3-fold or more in patients with such mitochondrial defects (11). Correspondingly, the yield of mitochondrial protein from muscle biopsy specimens is increased. In patients we recently have evaluated with mitochondrial defects, the protein yield was 1.5-2.5 times the level of controls; Hoppel and co-workers recently reported a child with fatal complex I deficiency in whom the mitochondrial yield was 4 times normal (19).

Mitochondrial composition also is typically abnormal. Ultrastructural analysis often reveals these mitochondria to be of bizarre shape and size and to contain anomalous arrays of cristae. Mitochondrial inclusions frequently are present. "Paracrystalline" inclusions representing the lattice-like deposition of apparent protein material are typical (6). Even when mitochondrial morphology appears normal, the distribution of respiratory proteins is disturbed, reflecting greatly diminished levels of defective portions of the respiratory chain and normal or increased levels of unaffected electron transport proteins and of other inner membrane and matrix oxidative enzymes. Patients with complex III or IV defects in whom levels of cytochromes b and/or aa_3 are deficient may have greater than normal levels of cytochrome $c + c_1$, resulting in highly deranged stoichiometry of these respiratory pigments (15, 25). Matrix (i.e., Krebs cycle) and inner membrane oxidative enzymes also may be dramatically increased to levels of 2- to 3-fold the mean of sedentary control subjects, whereas defective respiratory chain enzymes are reduced, often to 10-20% of normal levels (15). For example, the level of increase that we have found in the activity of muscle carnitine palmitoyl transferase and citrate synthase in whole muscle in such patients is roughly comparable to the increase in oxidative enzymes found in normal subjects with endurance training (Figures 3a and 3b) (12).

These findings indicate that skeletal muscle respiratory chain defects often markedly stimulate mitochondrial biogenesis and the synthesis of oxidative enzymes. This stimulus to increase oxidative metabolic machinery in muscle of patients with respiratory chain defects may in fact be comparable to or even surpass that associated with intense endurance training, though the level of habitual activity of these patients typically is profoundly limited due to premature fatigability. One may infer that metabolic factors that reflect the severe cellular oxidative deficit are responsible, rather than contractile activity per se. The biologic effect likely is adaptive to increase the level of the defective, rate-limiting enzyme. Nevertheless, the levels of defective respiratory chain components characteristically remain markedly subnormal, whereas other

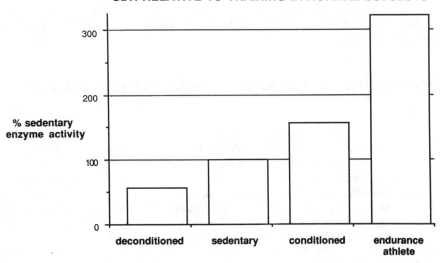

Figure 3a. Relative concentrations of a representative oxidative enzyme, succinate dehydrogenase (SDH), in normal subjects in relation to levels of habitual physical activity (data derived from reference 12).

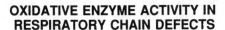

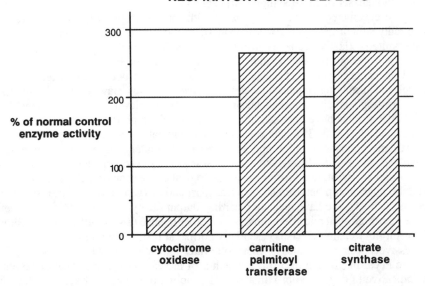

Figure 3b. Relative concentrations of citrate synthase (CS) and carnitine palmitoyl transferase (CPT) in 3 patients with muscle respiratory chain defects associated with low levels of muscle cytochrome c oxidase (COX) (physiological data for these patients are indicated in Table 1). Mean of sedentary control subjects = 100%.

oxidative enzymes may be greatly increased. Consequently, the usual close proportionality among oxidative enzymes of the electron transport chain, Krebs cycle, and lipid oxidation (33) is disrupted, and highly deranged stoichiometry of oxidative enzymes prevails.

Exercise Response in Muscle Respiratory Chain Defects

The pattern of exercise intolerance among muscle energy defects differs and reflects both the site of the metabolic block, which conditions energy availability under differing exercise conditions, and the local metabolic milieu that develops in exercise. In respiratory chain defects, anaerobic energy pathways are preserved, so isometric or ischemic exercise is relatively well tolerated, in contrast to muscle glycogenolytic defects. Also, the oxidative defect in muscle respiratory chain disorders cannot be modified by altering the availability of blood-borne oxidative substrates, as is the case in muscle glycolytic defects (23). The character of muscle fatigue in respiratory chain disorders also differs from that in glycolytic defects. Thus, exertional muscle cramping or myoglobinuria are not typical. Also, with fatiguing exercise, patients with electron transport defects develop a loss of muscle contractile force without the decrease in membrane excitability characteristic of severe glycolytic defects such as muscle phosphorylase deficiency (29). Intolerance of aerobic exercise in respiratory chain defects typically is associated with prominent systemic symptoms of shortness of breath and cardiac palpitations. Exercise testing has provided insight into the pathogenesis of these symptoms (Table 1).

Cycle ergometer VO_2max in patients with muscle respiratory chain defects is markedly subnormal, typically less than 1/2 that of healthy subjects (3, 8, 13, 15). The limited oxidative capacity in these patients is associated with an exaggerated increase in venous lactate and in the lactate:pyruvate ratio relative to work load and level of oxygen uptake (15). Also, the rate of fall of blood lactate after exercise is delayed, implying impaired lactate clearance (8). This may account for the fact that "resting" levels of venous lactate commonly are elevated in such patients (6). ^{31}P-NMR studies have revealed an exaggerated fall in phosphocreatine relative to work load (1, 2, 10, 35). These findings are compatible with a low maximal rate of oxidative phosphorylation and an increased dependence upon anaerobic glycogenolysis and PCr hydrolysis to meet muscle energy needs in exercise (Figure 4).

In order to investigate further the physiological expression of the oxidative defect and the relationship between oxygen transport and oxygen extraction in respiratory chain disorders, we have measured cardiac output (acetylene rebreathing [36]) and have calculated systemic arteriovenous oxygen difference (a-v O_2 diff). Cardiac output in respiratory chain defects is essentially normal at rest, but with exercise increases excessively, relative to muscle metabolic rate (indicated by VO_2). The normal increase in cardiac output of 5-6 L for each L of increased oxygen uptake in exercise is indicative of a close, approximately 1:1 coupling of oxygen delivery and utilization. Each L of arterial blood normally transports approximately 200 ml of oxygen, and a 5- to 6-L increase in cardiac output is therefore necessary to transport 1 L of oxygen. In patients with respiratory chain abnormalities, despite normal hemoglobin levels, the slope of increase of cardiac output was approximately 3 times normal, consistent with a fundamental disturbance in oxygen transport. Correspondingly,

Human Respiratory Chain Disorders 257

Table 1 Maximal Cycle Exercise

	Work load (watts)	$\dot{V}O_2$ (ml/kg/min)	$\dot{V}E/\dot{V}O_2$	$\dot{V}E/\dot{V}CO_2$	RER	$\dot{Q}$ (ml/kg/min)	HR	A-vO$_2$ (ml/dl)	$\Delta\dot{Q}/\Delta\dot{V}O_2$	Lact (mM)	L:P
Control (n = 17)											
Mean	185	35	44	38	1.15	223	188	16.0	4.9	9.3	47.7
SD	55	6	6	6	0.06	32	8	1.9	0.7	2.2	11.4
Respiratory chain defects (n = 3)											
Mean	27	14	83	59	1.48	226	174	5.9	14.8	11.1	65.1
SD	20	4	34	15	0.25	61	8	0.2	1.4	1.6	19.2

Note. $\dot{V}O_2$, oxygen consumption; $\dot{V}E$, ventilation; $\dot{V}CO_2$, carbon dioxide production; RER, respiratory exchange ratio; $\dot{Q}$, cardiac output; HR, heart rate; A-vO$_2$, systemic arteriovenous O$_2$ difference; $\Delta\dot{Q}/\Delta\dot{V}O_2$, increase in cardiac output relative to the increase in oxygen uptake from rest to exercise; Lact, venous lactate; L:P, ratio of venous lactate to pyruvate.

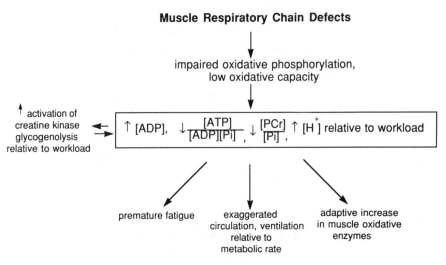

Muscle Respiratory Chain Defects

↓

impaired oxidative phosphorylation,
low oxidative capacity

↓

↑ activation of
creatine kinase
glycogenolysis
relative to workload

$\uparrow [ADP], \quad \downarrow \dfrac{[ATP]}{[ADP][Pi]}, \quad \downarrow \dfrac{[PCr]}{[Pi]}, \quad \uparrow [H^+]$ relative to workload

premature fatigue   exaggerated
circulation, ventilation
relative to
metabolic rate

adaptive increase
in muscle oxidative
enzymes

Figure 4. Schematic of local metabolic muscle abnormalities in patients with muscle respiratory chain defects. Possible relationships between these abnormalities and premature fatigue, altered cardiopulmonary regulation in exercise, and augmented mitochondrial biogenesis are indicated.

systemic arteriovenous oxygen difference increased minimally over resting levels, suggesting that the ability of working muscle to extract oxygen from circulating blood is profoundly impaired by respiratory chain defects. Maximal cardiac output in the patients was comparable to sedentary control subjects, consistent with the interpretation that oxygen extraction rather than oxygen delivery limits muscle oxidative metabolism *in vivo* in these patients. Similar disturbances in oxygen transport and oxygen extraction have been described experimentally with respiratory chain inhibitors such as amobarbital (31). The prominent tachycardia and sense of palpitations that accompany exercise in these patients presumably relate to the exaggerated cardiac output slope.

Typically, ventilation also is exaggerated relative to work load and metabolic rate in exercise. There is a steeper than normal rise in ventilation relative to $\dot{V}CO_2$ and $\dot{V}O_2$, a remarkably steep rise in the respiratory exchange rate (RER) relative to work load, and usually a supranormal RER with maximal exercise (3, 15; Table 1). In patients we have studied, RER in maximal exercise has ranged from 1.21-1.70 (normal 1.15 ± .06); and in a patient with complex I deficiency reported by Edwards and co-workers, the RER reached an incredible 3.3 (8).

The regulatory mechanisms involved in the exaggerated circulatory and ventilatory responses to exercise in these metabolic defects are incompletely understood. Increased "central command," that is, activation of brainstem cardiovascular and ventilatory centers in parallel with activation of motor units via the motor cortex and corticospinal tract, may be operative (9). However, the fact that cardiac output is normally coupled to metabolic rate in patients with muscular dystrophy (14), in whom a loss of functional muscle fibers likely is associated with increased motor unit recruitment (i.e., central command) at a given exercise work load, implies that other mechanisms participate. Reflex activation of brainstem cardiovascular centers, via thinly myelinated and unmyelinated afferent fibers that arise in skeletal muscle and are sensitive to metabolites produced during muscle contraction, is likely involved (27). A similar pattern of exaggerated cardiac output has been demonstrated in muscle energy defects that limit muscle oxygen utilization either by limiting the rate of production (e.g., muscle glycolytic defects) or oxidation of reducing equivalents; this fact implies that a normal capacity for muscle oxidative phosphorylation is crucial to normally link oxygen delivery and uptake in exercise. This hypothesis is supported by findings of impaired oxygen extraction in association with exaggerated blood flow, cardiac output, and ventilation under experimental conditions in which muscle oxidative metabolism is disturbed (24, 31).

Metabolic Milieu of Working Muscle in Respiratory Chain Defects

It is probable that the local metabolic state of active muscle is responsible for the premature muscle fatigue that is typical of these patients. ^{31}P-NMR determinations of high-energy phosphates in forearm muscle of affected patients at rest, during exercise, and during recovery have demonstrated metabolic abnormalities that may be relevant. It should be noted that reports of "mitochondrial myopathies" may include patients with biochemically well-defined respiratory chain defects as well as patients in whom biochemical information is lacking, incomplete, or indicative of other mitochondrial defects (1, 2).

At rest, muscle ATP levels are apparently near normal (2). However, muscle phosphocreatine (PCr) is low, and inorganic phosphate (P_i) may be elevated. Consequently, the phosphorylation potential ([ATP]/[ADP][P_i]), as calculated from the creatine kinase equilibrium (2) or estimated from the PCr/P_i ratio (1, 4), is characteristically subnormal, consistent with impaired oxidative phosphorylation. Correspondingly, calculated levels of free ADP are elevated (2). With exercise, there is little change in ATP. However, there is an exaggerated fall in the phosphorylation potential, as indicated by the PCr:P_i ratio, relative to work performed, indicative of attenuated capacity for oxidative phosphorylation (1, 2, 10, 35). After exercise, recovery of PCr typically is greatly delayed, consistent with the oxidative deficit. Curiously, the fall in muscle pH, as monitored by the chemical shift of P_i relative to PCr, is normal or even subnormal (1, 2), and the recovery of pH is rapid despite high and prolonged elevations of venous lactate. The basis of these pH findings is uncertain. Arnold and co-workers have suggested that accelerated extrusion of lactic acid from active muscle may be responsible (2). Alternatively, the buffering capacity of the muscle cell may be increased, possibly related to the increase in mitochondrial protein.

The link between these local metabolic abnormalities and premature muscle fatigue in muscle respiratory defects is incompletely understood, but elevations in inorganic phosphate, particularly elevations in diprotonated phosphate, have been implicated in the decline in contractile force in fatigued normal muscle (26, 37). In skinned fiber preparations, the accumulation of inorganic phosphate produces a fall in contractile force, which is potentiated by the accumulation of H^+ (5), presumably via inhibition of myosin ATPase. Similarly, in normal individuals the accumulation of diprotonated phosphate, as calculated from pH and P_i determinations by ^{31}P-NMR, has been shown to correlate with muscle fatigue in voluntary or electrically stimulated contractions (26).

Metabolic Milieu of Working Muscle: Implications for Muscle Adaptation

The exaggerated decline in the phosphorylation potential of working muscle that occurs as a result of respiratory chain defects may be instrumental in activating cardiopulmonary reflexes that normally are tightly geared to oxygen utilization in the terminal reaction of the respiratory chain, cytochrome c oxidase. Nuutinen and coworkers (31) identified a direct inverse correlation between $[ATP]/[ADP][P_i]$ and blood flow in cardiac muscle under circumstances in which oxygen utilization and delivery were normally matched (increased cardiac work and hypoxia). This linear relationship between blood flow and the phosphorylation potential was maintained during experimental inhibition of the respiratory chain with amobarbital, despite the fact that oxygen delivery and uptake were then dissociated so that blood flow was greatly exaggerated relative to muscle oxidative rate. An important role for the muscle phosphorylase potential in regulating blood flow was postulated. The metabolic factors that may directly link the muscle phosphorylation potential and blood flow are incompletely defined; however, a close proportionality between the decline in the phosphorylation potential and adenosine release has been demonstrated (17). These results therefore suggest that the normal tight link between myocardial oxygen uptake and blood flow is mediated by oxidative phosphorylation and imply that at a cellular level, the phosphorylation potential or closely related metabolites participate in regulating oxygen delivery.

Extrapolating these observations to working skeletal muscle suggests the following relationships. The block in oxidative phosphorylation in respiratory chain defects impairs oxygen extraction and the maximal rate of oxygen uptake ($\dot{V}O_2$max), resulting in an exaggerated fall in the phosphorylation potential relative to contractile work. The exaggerated drop in the phosphorylation potential promotes exaggerated systemic oxygen delivery, relative to the capacity of muscle to utilize oxygen at the level of cytochrome c oxidase, the terminal enzymatic reaction of the electron transport chain. The metabolic factors that might link the phosphorylation potential in working skeletal muscle and local and systemic oxygen delivery are uncertain; however, potential candidates include extracellular K^+, P_i, and adenosine (23).

The stimuli that trigger the increase in mitochondrial biogenesis typical of respiratory chain defects are not known, but the dissociation between habitual levels of contractile activity and levels of mitochondrial and oxidative enzyme synthesis suggests that local metabolic factors are operative. The role of mitochondria in oxidative metabolism is clear, and metabolites that reflect a cellular deficit in oxidative phosphorylation would represent physiologically economical regulatory signals. Thus, one may postulate that the relationship between contractile activity and mitochondrial biogenesis is a function of phosphorylation potential and time: the longer a given fall in the muscle phosphorylation potential is maintained, the greater the stimulus for synthesis of proteins involved in oxidative metabolism. Factors that modify the relationship between contractile activity and the phosphorylation potential could likewise alter the relationship between habitual physical activity and the synthesis of mitochondria and mitochondrial enzymes. Such a hypothesis could account for the augmented mitochondrial numbers and increased oxidative enzyme levels in muscle respiratory defects. A similar mechanism could account for the finding in some studies of higher levels of oxidative enzymes in the ischemic legs of physically active patients with unilateral claudication (20). Similarly, experimental iron deficiency, which lowers muscle cytochrome levels, has been shown to potentiate the exercise-induced increase in activity of representative Krebs cycle enzymes (38).

Summary

Human muscle respiratory chain defects are rare metabolic abnormalities that profoundly impair muscle oxidative capacity and characteristically produce intolerance of dynamic exercise, with rapid muscle fatigue. These defects disrupt the normal relationship between oxygen delivery and utilization in exercise and apparently disturb the normal relationship between habitual muscle contractile activity and mitochondrial biogenesis. These responses provide novel insights into the possible regulatory roles of muscle oxidative phosphorylation in the acute and chronic adaptations of skeletal muscle to exercise.

Acknowledgments

Dr. Gunnar Blomqvist provided invaluable support for the work related to this review. Research funds for this work were provided by the Veterans Administration; National Heart, Lung and Blood Institute Grant HL-06296; the Muscular Dystrophy Association; and the Harry S. Moss Heart Center. S.F. Lewis is the recipient of Research Career Development Award HL-01581.

References

1. Argov, Z.; Bank, W.J.; Maris, J.; Peterson, P.; Chance, B. Bioenergetic heterogeneity of human mitochondrial myopathies: phosphorus magnetic resonance spectroscopy. Neurology 37:257-262; 1987.

2. Arnold, D.L.; Taylor, D.J.; Radda, G.K. Investigation of human mitochondrial myopathies by phosphorus magnetic resonance spectroscopy. Ann. Neurol. 18:189-196; 1985.

3. Bogaard, J.M.; Busch, H.F.M.; Arts, W.F.M.; Heijsteeg, M.; Stam, H.; Versprille, A. Metabolic and ventilatory responses to exercise in patients with a deficient O_2 utilization by a mitochondrial myopathy. Adv. Exp. Med. Biol. 191:409-417; 1984.

4. Chance, B. Applications of ^{31}P NMR to clinical chemistry. Ann. N.Y. Acad. Sci. 428:318-332; 1984.

5. Cooke, R.; Pate, E. The effects of ADP and phosphate on the contraction of muscle fibers. Biophys. J. 48:789-798; 1985.

6. DiMauro, S.; Bonilla, E.; Zeviani, M.; Nakagawa, M.; DeVivo, D.C. Mitochondrial myopathies. Ann. Neurol. 17:521-538; 1985.

7. DiMauro, S.; Zeviani, M.; Servidei, S.; Bonilla, E.; Miranda, A.; Prelle, A.; Schon, E.A. Cytochrome oxidase deficiency: clinical and biochemical heterogeneity. Ann. N.Y. Acad. Sci. 488:19-32; 1986.

8. Edwards, R.H.T.; Wiles, C.M.; Gohil, K.; Krywawych, S.; Jones, D.A. Energy metabolism in human myopathy. In: Schotland, D.L., ed. Disorders of the motor unit. New York: John Wiley; 1982:715-735.

9. Eldridge, F.L.; Millhorn, D.E.; Waldrop, T.G. Exercise hyperpnea and locomotion: parallel activation from the hypothalamus. Science 211:844-846; 1981.

10. Eleff, S.; Kennaway, N.G.; Buist, N.R.M.; Darley-Usmar, V.M.; Capaldi, R.A.; Bank, W.J.; Chance, B. Proc. Natl. Acad. Sci. USA, 81:3529-3533.

11. Engel, A.G. Quantitative morphological studies of muscle. In: Engel, A.G.; Banker, B.Q., eds. Myology. New York: McGraw-Hill; 1986:1045-1079.

12. Gollnick, P.D.; Saltin, B. Skeletal muscle adaptability: significance for metabolism and performance. In: Peachey, L.D., ed. Handbook of physiology. Bethesda, MD: American Physiological Society; 1983:555-631. (Sect. 10).

13. Haller, R.G.; Cook, J.D.; Lewis, S.F. Impaired oxygen extraction by working muscle: a common denominator of mitochondrial myopathies. Neurology 39(S1):135; 1987.

14. Haller, R.G.; Lewis, S.F.; Cook, J.D.; Blomqvist, C.G. Hyperkinetic circulation during exercise in neuromuscular disease. Neurology 33: 1283-1287; 1983.

15. Haller, R.G.; Lewis, S.F.; Estabrook, R.W.; DiMauro, S.; Servidei, S.; Foster, D.W. Exercise intolerance, lactic acidosis and abnormal cardiopulmonary regulation in exercise associated with adult skeletal muscle cytochrome c oxidase deficiency. J. Clin. Invest. 84:155-161, 189.

16. Hayes, D.J.; Lecky, B.R.F.; Landon, D.N.; Morgan-Hughes, J.A.; Clark, J.B. A new mitochondrial myopathy—biochemical studies revealing a deficiency in the cytochrome b-c1 complex (complex III) of the respiratory chain. Brain 107:1165-1177; 1984.

17. He, M.-X.; Wangler, R.D.; Dillon, P.F.; Romig, G.D.; Sparks, H.V. Phosphorylation potential and adenosine release during norepinephrine infusion in guinea pig heart. Am. J. Physiol. 253:H1184-H1191; 1987.

18. Holt, I.J.; Harding, A.E.; Morgan-Hughes, J. Deletions of mitochondrial DNA in patients with mitochondrial myopathies. Nature 331:717-719; 1988.

19. Hoppel, C.L.; Kerr, D.S.; Dahms, B.; Roessmann, U. Deficiency of the reduced nicotinamide adenine dinucleotide dehydrogenase component of complex I of mitochondrial electron transport. J. Clin. Invest. 80:71-77; 1987.

20. Jansson, E.; Johansson, J.; Sylven, C.; Kaijser, L. Calf muscle adaptation in intermittent claudication. Side-differences in muscle metabolic characteristics in patients with unilateral arterial disease. Clin. Physiol. 8:17-29; 1988.

21. Kennaway, N.G.; Buist, N.R.M.; Darly-Usmar, V.M.; Papadimitriou, A.; DiMauro, S.; Kelley, R.; Capaldi, R.A.; Blank, N.K.; D'Agostino, A. Lactic acidosis and mitochondrial myopathy associated with deficiency of several components of complex III of the respiratory chain. Pediatr. Res. 18:991-999; 1984.

22. Land, J.M.; Morgan-Hughes, J.A.; Clark, J.B. Mitochondrial myopathy—biochemical studies revealing a deficiency of NADH-cytochrome b reductase activity. J. Neurol. Sci. 50:1-13; 1981.

23. Lewis, S.F.; Haller, R.G. The pathophysiology of McArdle's disease: clues to regulation in exercise and fatigue. J. Appl. Physiol. 61(2):391-401; 1986.

24. Liang, C.-S.; Hood, W.B., Jr. Afferent neural pathway in the regulation of cardiopulmonary responses to tissue hypermetabolism. Circ. Res. 38:209-214; 1976.

25. Martens, M.E.; Peterson, P.L,; Lee, C.P.; Nigro, M.A.; Hart, Z.; Glasberg, M.; Hatfield, J.S.; Chang, C.H. Kearns-Sayre syndrome: biochemical studies of mitochondrial metabolism. Ann. Neurol. 24:630-637; 1988.

26. Miller, R.G.; Boska, M.D.; Moussavi, R.S.; Carson, P.J.; Weiner, M.W. [31]P nuclear magnetic resonance studies of high energy phosphates and pH in human muscle fatigue. J. Clin. Invest. 81:1190-1196; 1988.

27. Mitchell, J.H.; Kaufman, M.P.; Iwamoto, G.A. The exercise pressor reflex: its cardiovascular effects, afferent mechanisms and central pathways. Annu. Rev. Physiol. 45:229-242; 1983.

28. Moreadith, R.W.; Batshaw, M.L.; Ohnishi, T.; Kerr, D.; Know, B.; Jackson, D.; Hruban, R.; Olson, J.; Reynafarje, B.; Lehninger, A.L. Deficiency in the iron-sulfur clusters of mitochondrial reduced nicotinamide-adenine dinucleotide-ubiquinone oxidoreductase (complex I) in an infant with congenital lactic acidosis. J. Clin. Invest. 74:685-697; 1984.

29. Morgan-Hughes, J.A. Defects of the energy pathways of skeletal muscle. In: Matthews, W.B.; Glaser, B.H., eds. Recent advances in clinical neurology. Edinburgh: Churchill Livingston; 1982:1-46.

30. Morgan-Hughes, J.A.; Darveniza, P.; Kahn, S.N.; Landon, D.N.; Sherratt, R.M.; Land, J.M.; Clark, J.B. A mitochondrial myopathy characterized by a deficiency in reducible cytochrome b. Brain 100:617-640; 1977.

31. Nuutinen, E.M.; Nishiki, K.; Erecinska, M.; Wilson, D.F. Role of mitochondrial oxidative phosphorylation in regulation of coronary blood flow. Am. J. Physiol. 243:H159-H169; 1982.

32. Olson, W.; Engel, W.K.; Walsh, G.O.; Einaugler, R. Oculocraniosomatic neuromuscular disease with "ragged-red" fibers. Arch. Neurol. 26:193-211; 1972.

33. Pette, D.; Klingenberg, M.; Bucher, T. Comparable and specific proportions in the mitochondrial enzyme activity pattern. Biochem. Biophys. Res. Commun. 7:425-429; 1962.

34. Petty, R.K.H.; Harding, A.E.; Morgan-Hughes, J.A. The clinical features of mitochondrial myopathy. Brain 109:915-938; 1986.

35. Radda, G.K.; Bore, P.J.; Gadian, D.G.; Ross, B.D.; Styles, P.; Taylor, D.J.;

Morgan-Hughes, J. ^{31}P NMR examination of two patients with NADH-CoQ reductase deficiency. Nature 295:608-609; 1982.

36. Triebwasser, J.H.; Johnson, R.L., Jr.; Burpo, R.P.; Campbell, J.C.; Reardon, W.C.; Blomqvist, C.G. Non-invasive determination of cardiac output by a modified acetylene rebreathing procedure utilizing mass spectrometer. Aviat. Space Environ. Med. 48:203-209; 1977.

37. Wilkie, D.R. Muscular fatigue: effects of hydrogen ions and inorganic phosphate. Fed. Proc. 45:2921-2923; 1986.

38. Willis, W.T.; Brooks, G.A.; Henderson, S.A.; Dallman, P.R. Effects of iron deficiency and training on mitochondrial enzymes in skeletal muscle. J. Appl. Physiol. 62(6):2442-2446; 1987.

Metabolic Dysfunction of Skeletal Muscle in the Diabetic Rat

R.A. John Challiss, Martin J. Blackledge, and George K. Radda
University of Leicester, Leicester and University of Oxford, Oxford, U.K.

A number of animal models of insulin-dependent diabetes mellitus (IDDM) have been developed that rely on either surgical or chemical depancreatectomy (10). Thus, a disease state similar to IDDM can be produced in rats by administration of the diabetogenic agent, streptozotocin (20), with the severity of the resulting disease being dose-related (12). Using animal models of IDDM, a large number of morphological, physiological, and biochemical changes have been documented to occur in skeletal muscle. In particular, changes in insulin sensitivity and responsiveness of glucose transport into skeletal muscle under basal conditions and during and after exercise have been extensively investigated (19, 21, 23, 24, 26). In addition, a number of quantitatively significant changes in the major energy-metabolizing pathways of skeletal muscle have been reported (9, 18), and the implications of an altered substrate utilization have been discussed (see 25 for review).

However, data pertaining to the significance of these observations to biomechanic and bioenergetic performance during exercise have received less attention. Phosphorus nuclear magnetic resonance spectroscopy (^{31}P-NMR) can be used to follow changes in phosphorus-containing metabolites and to monitor intracellular pH in skeletal muscle in vivo. In the present series of experiments, we have used ^{31}P-NMR to investigate whether bioenergetic changes occur in exercising skeletal muscle of diabetic animals and to correlate such changes with physiological performance. In addition, preliminary data are presented using a novel NMR technique (5) to obtain spatially resolved spectral information. This allows the question of whether fiber-specific metabolic changes occur in diabetic skeletal muscle in vivo to be addressed.

Experimental Design

Male Wistar rats (140-160 g) were injected (I.V.) with 50 mg/kg streptozotocin. At this dose a diabetic state can be produced, where plasma glucose is elevated (> 20 mM) and plasma insulin is reduced ($> 90\%$). Ketoacidosis, however, is modest; this reduces mortality and allows chronic changes in the untreated diabetic state to be investigated. Animals were diagnosed as diabetic after 48 hours and either were maintained untreated for the duration of the experiment or received twice-daily doses of insulin (Ultratard) to maintain optimal glycemic control. Changes in skeletal muscle were investigated 3 weeks after induction of diabetes. In all cases, the ankle flexor muscles were studied.

Animals were prepared for spectroscopic studies as previously described (5, 7); under anesthesia, electrodes were sewn into place on the left sciatic nerve, the leg was immobilized, and the distal tendon of the gastrocnemius muscle was ligated and attached to a force-displacement transducer. The animal was positioned in a perspex cradle, and NMR transmitter/receiver coils were placed into position. To allow quantitation of ^{31}P-NMR data, both the stimulated and contralateral ankle-flexor muscles were freeze-clamped after completion of the NMR examination. In addition, complementary "bench" experiments were performed to obtain more complete muscle metabolite and enzyme profiles (8).

We have used two spectroscopic methods to investigate muscle bioenergetics in the diabetic rat. The first method employs the simple "pulse-and-collect" technique described previously (6, 7), using a Helmholtz coil as transmitter and receiver. The dimensions of the coil were such that gastrocnemius, plantaris, and soleus muscles were within the sample volume.

The second method was the phase-modulated, rotating-frame imaging (PMRFI) technique, which allows localization of ^{31}P signals from flat longitudinal slices through the sample. This technique relies on a gradient B_1 excitation field in which spins experience a "flip-angle" dependent on their position in the B_1 field strength and the length of the transmitter pulse (see 4, 5). It is essential that the B_1 field gradient be linear in the reception region and that the B_1 isocontours be flat. Therefore, a double-coil system is used, consisting of a large surface coil transmitter (24-mm radius) and an electrically isolated, modified Helmholtz receiver coil (two circular loops of 10-mm radius, orthogonal to the transmitter coil). This allows collection of signal homogeneously from a region defined as 0.2–0.8 transmitter coil radii from the plane of the transmitter coil.

A set of free induction decays are collected, with the observation pulse width being incremented for each successive data acquisition. Thus, the nutational frequency at which the spin vector precesses assigns the position of the spin in the B_1 gradient. Optimization of signal collection is achieved by application of a phase pulse immediately after the incremental pulse (see 4). A two-dimensional Fourier transform of the data matrix produces a map of distance and chemical shift, representing spectra from a series of planar discs at various depths from the transmitter coil. The homogeneity of the receiver and the linearity of the B_1 transmitter gradient have been measured previously (3) and found to be adequate for 1-mm resolution.

Muscle contraction was caused by sciatic nerve stimulation at a supramaximal voltage (50-μs pulse width, 45 V). The knee and ankle joints were fixed such that contraction was isometric. For pulse-and-collect experiments, two stimulation frequencies were used; initially contraction was at 1 Hz for 24 min, followed by increasing the frequency to 5 Hz for the subsequent 12 min. For the PMRFI experiment, sciatic nerve stimulation was at 2 Hz. The PMRFI experiment was started approximately 20 min after initiation of stimulation, at which time intracellular pH and PCr, P_i, and ATP concentrations were constant.

Phosphocreatine, creatine, and ATP concentrations were determined in perchloric acid extracts from freeze-clamped muscles, using published high performance liquid chromatography (HPLC) methods (13). The chemically determined ATP was assumed to be entirely NMR-visible (see 17). Therefore, concentrations of other phosphorus-containing metabolites could be determined from fully relaxed ^{31}P-NMR spectra or by calculating correction factors (22) where spectra were collected under partially saturated conditions (pulse repetition time < 10 s). The free ADP concentrations were calculated from the creatine phosphokinase equilibrium, using an equilibrium constant of 1.66×10^9 M^{-1} (16). This assumes a free Mg^{2+} concentration of 1 mM for normal and diabetic muscle.

Bioenergetic Changes in Skeletal Muscle

Table 1 shows metabolite levels in ankle flexor muscles of insulin-treated diabetic (ITD) or untreated diabetic (UTD) and control (CON) animals. Generally, metabolite levels are similar in the 3 groups. The major change observed was a lower intracellular pH in the untreated diabetic animals. As a consequence of the lower pH, the calculated free ADP concentration was lower in muscle of UTD animals.

Table 2 shows the contractile performance of gastrocnemius muscle of UTD and CON animals during stimulation at 1 and 5 Hz. The decrease in initial twitch tension observed for the UTD group correlated with a 10-15% decrease in the ratio of gastrocnemius muscle weight to body weight. A significant decrease in the twitch tension development of UTD compared to CON animals was observed only at the end of the period of stimulation at 5 Hz.

Table 2 also shows the concentrations of ATP, PCr, and P_i and intracellular pH at these time-points during the stimulation protocol (for full time-course data, see 8). After 20 min stimulation at 1 Hz, intracellular pH and PCr concentration were significantly lower, and P_i concentration was significantly higher, in gastrocnemius muscle of UTD animals. This indicates that twitch tension is maintained by a greater reliance on glycolytic energy-producing mechanisms. At a stimulation frequency

Table 1 Metabolite Concentrations and Intracellular pH in Gastrocnemius and Plantaris Muscles at Rest

Metabolite (μmol/g of tissue)	CON n = 5	ITD n = 6	UTD n = 5
ATP	7.3 ± 0.7	7.4 ± 0.7	7.4 ± 0.2
PCr	34.2 ± 3.3	32.2 ± 3.6	30.8 ± 2.9
Creatine	6.2 ± 2.2	5.2 ± 1.9	3.8 ± 2.4
P_i	2.7 ± 0.7	2.9 ± 1.2	3.5 ± 1.3
PCr/(PCr + P_i)	0.91 ± 0.04	0.90 ± 0.02	0.89 ± 0.02
Glycogen	34.7 ± 4.0	35.1 ± 7.1	37.9 ± 6.7
pH_i	7.04 ± 0.05	7.02 ± 0.04	6.94 ± 0.05*
ADP_{free}[a]	10.3 ± 2.2	7.4 ± 2.1	5.2 ± 2.0*

Note. All values are presented as mean ± *SD* for *n* determinations. [a]nmol/g of tissue. [b]Statistical significance (Student's *t* test) is indicated as *p < .05 for UTD versus CON and ITD experimental groups.

Table 2   Biomechanical and Bioenergetic Performance of Diabetic (UTD) and Control (CON) Muscle During Stimulation at 1 and 5 Hz

| | | Time of stimulation | | |
		Rest	20 min at 1 Hz	10 min at 5 Hz
Twitch tension	CON	1.53 ± 0.18	1.76 ± 0.22	1.10 ± 0.18
(g/g body wt)	UTD	1.37 ± 0.27	1.31 ± 0.44	0.57 ± 0.22**
ATP	CON	7.27 ± 0.60	7.18 ± 1.05	6.89 ± 0.91
	UTD	7.42 ± 0.22	7.09 ± 0.63	6.40 ± 0.73
PCr	CON	28.1 ± 7.9	19.6 ± 3.3	8.6 ± 2.4
	UTD	27.1 ± 5.7	15.3 ± 2.0*	7.4 ± 1.3
P_i	CON	2.7 ± 0.7	9.8 ± 1.1	21.0 ± 2.8
	UTD	3.5 ± 1.3	13.0 ± 1.8*	20.4 ± 2.6
pH_i	CON	7.04 ± 0.06	6.96 ± 0.02	6.89 ± 0.05
	UTD	6.94 ± 0.05*	6.86 ± 0.05**	6.72 ± 0.06**

Note. Data were continuously acquired during muscle stimulation for 24 min at 1 Hz and 12 min at 5 Hz. Representative values taken from time courses are shown here. All values are mean ± SD for 5 experiments in each group. ATP, PCr, and P_i concentrations are given as μmol/g of tissue. Statistical significance (Student's t test) is indicated as $*p < .05$; $**p < .005$ for UTD versus CON experimental groups.

of 5 Hz, twitch tension is not maintained relative to control values and had declined to 42% of initial twitch tension, compared to a decline to 72% observed for the control group. Concentrations of PCr, P_i, and ATP were similar in the experimental group, but intracellular pH was significantly more acidic in the diabetic group. Consequently, the calculated free ADP concentration was decreased in the ankle flexor muscle of the diabetic animals (CON: 108 ± 15 (5)nmol/g; UTD: 65 ± 20 (5)nmol/g). There was no evidence of enhanced glycogen depletion in the diabetic group; gastrocnemius muscle glycogen concentration at the end of the stimulation protocol was 15.1 ± 4.8 (6)μmol glucosyl equiv./g (CON: 14.8 ± 7.4 (6)μmol glucosyl equiv./g). Thus, the reason for the fatigue observed in the diabetic muscle during stimulation at 5 Hz remains unresolved.

At the end of the 5 Hz stimulation period, ^{31}P-NMR spectra were acquired in 32-s blocks to allow the time-course of metabolic recovery to be investigated. Recovery was complete 20 min after termination of muscle stimulation, and a fully-relaxed spectrum was acquired at this point for comparison to spectra collected prior to initiating the muscle stimulation protocol. Analysis of full-recovery ^{31}P-NMR spectra revealed that ATP and PCr concentrations were not affected by the stimulation protocol in CON animals. However, significant ATP depletion occurred in the muscle of the diabetic group; this finding was confirmed by subsequent chemical analysis of freeze-clamped muscle samples. Gastrocnemius muscle ATP concentrations were 6.31 ± 0.75 (6) and 7.41 ± 0.46 (6)μmol/g for stimulated and contralateral muscles of diabetic rats, respectively ($p < 0.01$ for paired Student's t test).

Figure 1 shows the time course of PCr/(PCr + P$_i$) recovery for UTD and CON animals. Similar data were acquired for PCr, P$_i$, and intracellular pH recovery. Where necessary, sequential blocks of spectra were added to give 1-min time resolution with sufficient signal:noise ratio to allow confident quantitation. Curve-fitting routines revealed that PCr, P$_i$, and free ADP recovery rates were single exponentials, allowing first-order rate constants to be calculated; these values are presented in Table 3. As has previously been noted in human flexor digitorum superficialis muscle after exercise (2), metabolite recovery rates showed significant differences, with free ADP recovering at the fastest rate and PCr at the slowest in ankle flexor muscles of control animals. The rates of free ADP and PCr recovery were unaffected in the diabetic state (Table 3). However, the rate of P$_i$ recovery was significantly decreased, such that P$_i$ and PCr recovery rates were similar. The difference between the rates of P$_i$ and PCr recovery observed in the control group and previously reported in human studies (2, 22) implies that NMR-visible P$_i$ decreases transiently during the initial recovery phase. This as-yet-unexplained phenomenon does not appear to occur in skeletal muscle in the diabetic state.

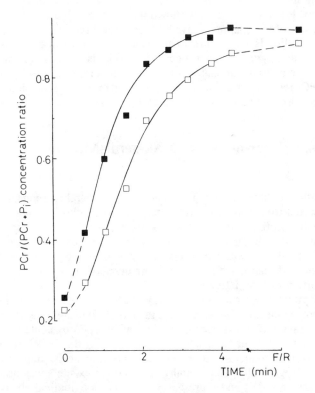

Figure 1.   Recovery of PCr/(PCr + P$_i$) after stimulation at 5 Hz in ankle flexor muscles of control (closed square) and diabetic (open square) rats. Data were collected to give 32-s time resolution. Mean values are shown for 6 determinations in each group. F/R represents data points acquired 20 min after termination of stimulation.

Table 3   Rates of PCr, P_i, and Free ADP Recovery After Muscle Stimulation at 1 and 5 Hz

	n	First-order rate constants (min^{-1})		
		Free ADP	P_i	PCr
CON	5	0.834 ± 0.136	0.516 ± 0.098**	0.390 ± 0.060***[+]
UTD	5	0.816 ± 0.239	0.256 ± 0.049***	0.269 ± 0.110***
p		NS	< .005	NS

Note. Values are mean ± SD for n determinations. Values were obtained by linear regression analysis of semilogarithmically transformed recovery data. Statistical significance for within-group variation (Student's t test for paired observations) is indicated as **p < .01; ***p < .005 for free ADP versus PCr and P_i; [+]p < .05 for PCr versus P_i.

As noted above, recovery rates of free ADP and PCr were not affected in the UTD group. Previously, we have shown that mitochondria isolated from gastrocnemius muscle of UTD animals have 30% decreased rates of pyruvate or glutamate oxidation (Challiss, Hayes, and Brosnan, unpublished results). It has also been previously shown that pyruvate dehydrogenase$_a$ activity is decreased in skeletal muscle in streptozotocin or alloxan diabetes (see 11). Therefore, it must be concluded that ADP and PCr recovery rates are not compromised by a 30% reduction in the capacity of skeletal muscle mitochondria to oxidize pyruvate.

Metabolic Heterogeneity in Skeletal Muscle

Investigations of heterogeneity in skeletal muscle have relied upon analysis of single fibers dissected from muscle biopsy material (15). Single-fiber analysis has shown that metabolite profiles differ markedly between fiber types and respond differently during muscle stimulation (14, 15). The ankle flexor muscle group shows a gradation of fiber types (1), with superficial muscle containing more than 75% type IIb fibers, whereas deeper muscle contains more than 50% type IIa fibers and a significant proportion of type I fibers.

We have previously shown the feasibility of acquiring spatially resolved ^{31}P-NMR spectra from the rat ankle flexor muscles in vivo (3, 5) using rotating-frame imaging techniques. Figure 2 shows spectral images of phosphorus-containing metabolites in ankle flexor muscle of a diabetic rat acquired using the PMRFI technique. Data sets were acquired either at rest (Figure 2a) or during steady state muscle stimulation at 2 Hz (Figure 2b). The spatially resolved composite slices used for quantitation are shown (I-IV) and represent 3- to 4-mm longitudinal slices through the muscle mass.

Preliminary quantitative data for the superficial (I) and deep (IV) muscle regions are shown in Table 4. Metabolite ratios are presented; it is not possible to measure absolute concentrations for two reasons: the anatomy of the rat leg causes a variable filling factor of the receiver coil, and the pulse repetition rate used (3 s) causes partial saturation of some of the compounds detected in the spectrum. P_i1ATP ratios are expressed with reference to the γ-ATP resonance, due to off-resonance effects distorting the spatial position of the β-ATP (3).

Intracellular pH increased from superficial to deep slices in control images of ankle flexor muscle at rest (5). A similar gradation was seen for diabetic animals; however, pH was significantly more acidic throughout the diabetic muscle image (Table 4). P_i/ATP increased from superficial to deep slices in both control and diabetic animals, whereas the gradation of $PCr/(PCr + P_i)$ seen in the control group was not evident in the diabetic group. No differences in P_i/ATP or $PCr/(PCr + P_i)$ between control and diabetic images were observed in resting muscle.

During muscle stimulation at 2 Hz, intracellular pH in diabetic animals was lower throughout the image than in control animals (Table 4). However, the pH gradation across the muscle was maintained in diabetic animals (slice I 6.89; slice IV 6.97). Generally, during stimulation $PCr/(PCr + P_i)$ was lower and P_i/ATP higher for

Table 4   Intracellular pH and Metabolite Ratios in Superficial and Deep Portions of the Ankle Flexor Muscles of Diabetic and Control Animals Determined In Vivo Using the PMRFI Technique

		Superficial (I)	Deep (IV)
At rest			
pH	CON	7.01 ± 0.02	7.09 ± 0.03
	UTD	6.90 ± 0.03*	6.95 ± 0.04*
$PCr/(PCr + P_i)$	CON	0.95 ± 0.01	0.88 ± 0.01[+++]
	UTD	0.94 ± 0.01	0.91 ± 0.01
P_i/ATP	CON	0.19 ± 0.02	0.38 ± 0.04[++]
	UTD	0.29 ± 0.06	0.45 ± 0.08[+]
2 Hz stimulation			
pH	CON	6.99 ± 0.02	7.03 ± 0.02[+]
	UTD	6.89 ± 0.02**	6.97 ± 0.02*[+++]
$PCr/(PCr + P_i)$	CON	0.60 ± 0.02	0.70 ± 0.02[++]
	UTD	0.54 ± 0.04	0.58 ± 0.03**
P_i/ATP	CON	1.41 ± 0.09	0.89 ± 0.11[+++]
	UTD	1.72 ± 0.23	1.66 ± 0.28*

Note. Values are calculated by triangulation of composite 3- to 4-mm longitudinal slices in regions I and IV, defined in Figure 2. Values are presented as mean ± SD for at least 4 separate experiments. Statistical differences between superficial and deep regions are given as [+]$p < .05$; [++]$p < .01$; [+++]$p < .005$. Differences between CON and UTD animals are given as *$p < .05$; **$p < .01$.

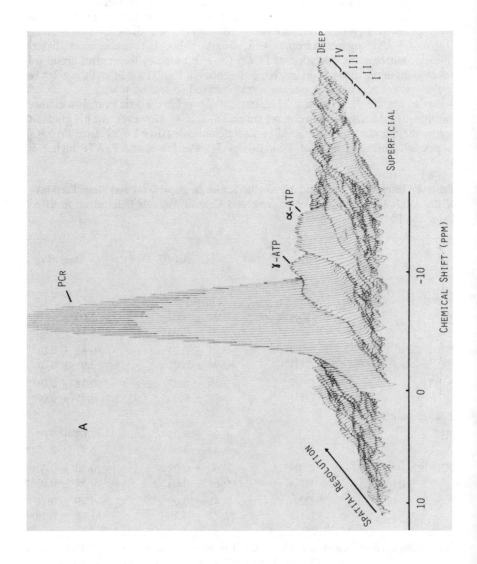

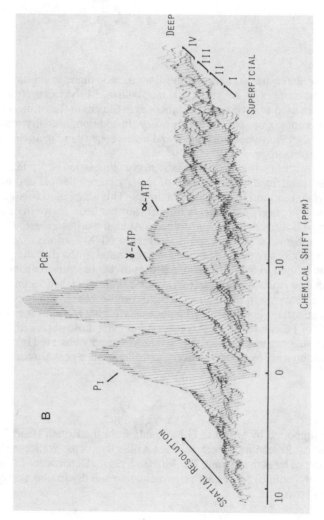

Figure 2. ³¹P-NMR stack plots of data from resting (A) and exercising (B) diabetic rat ankle flexor muscles. The regions I-IV were used for quantitation. Image B was collected during steady state stimulation (20 min after initiation of muscle contraction) at 2 Hz.

diabetic than for control animals. These effects were most marked in the deep muscle slices (Table 4), supporting previous reports that type IIa fibers are most severely affected in the diabetic state (9). These data support and extend the finding stated above, that at low work intensities where twitch tension is maintained, diabetic muscle has a greater dependency on glycolytic energy-producing mechanisms, with the deeper fibers of the ankle flexor muscles being more severely affected.

Summary

In these studies we have used a relatively mild, nonketotic diabetic animal model to investigate chronic changes in skeletal muscle metabolism. ^{31}P-NMR spectroscopic techniques have been used to investigate metabolism in the ankle flexor muscles at rest, during muscle contraction, and during recovery. In addition, spatially resolved metabolite levels and pH have been obtained, and heterogeneity in the ankle flexor muscles has been assessed.

At low work intensities (supramaximal sciatic nerve stimulation at 1 and 2 Hz), twitch tension was maintained at the expense of lower intracellular pH and higher rates of PCr utilization in muscle of diabetic animals. This adaptation to a greater dependence on glycolytic energy-producing mechanisms has been shown to be more marked in deep (type IIa) fibers in diabetic animals. At high work intensities (5 Hz), where oxidative mechanisms are required to operate at 80-90% of maximal rates to maintain ATP resynthesis, muscle fatigue is exaggerated in the diabetic group. This response may be due to the 30% decrease in pyruvate oxidative capacity observed in mitochondria isolated from gastrocnemius muscle of diabetic animals. In contrast, metabolic recovery in the immediate postexercise phase is only partially affected in the diabetic state. The rate of P_i disappearance during recovery is reduced; however, the rates of PCr and free ADP recovery approach those observed for the control group. This suggests that the decreased oxidative capacity observed in diabetic muscle does not compromise metabolic recovery in the immediate postexercise phase.

Acknowledgments

This work was supported by grants to G.K. Radda from the British Heart Foundation and the Medical Research Council. R.A.J. Challiss thanks the Wellcome Trust for financial support. The authors thank Dr. Mladen Vranic (Department of Physiology, University of Toronto) for his active participation and discussion during the initial stages of this work.

References

1. Armstrong, R.B.; Laughlin, M.H. Bloodflows within and among rat muscles as a function of time during high speed treadmill exercise. J. Physiol. (Lond.) 344:189-208; 1983.

2. Arnold, D.L.; Matthews, P.M.; Radda, G.K. Metabolic recovery after exercise and the assessment of mitochondrial function *in vivo* in human skeletal muscle by means of ^{31}P-NMR. Magn. Reson. Med. 1:307-315; 1984.

3. Blackledge, M.J.; Hayes, D.J.; Challiss, R.A.J.; Radda, G.K. One-dimensional rotating-frame imaging of phosphorus metabolites *in vivo*. J. Magn. Reson. 69:331-336; 1986.

4. Blackledge, M.J.; Rajagopalan, B.; Oberhaensli, R.D.; Bolas, N.; Styles, P.; Radda, G.K. Quantitative studies of human cardiac metabolism by ^{31}P rotating-frame NMR. Proc. Natl. Acad. Sci. USA 84:4283-4287; 1987.

5. Challiss, R.A.J.; Blackledge, M.J.; Radda, G.K. Spatial heterogeneity of metabolism in skeletal muscle *in vivo* studied by ^{31}P-NMR spectroscopy. Am. J. Physiol. 254:C417-C422; 1988.

6. Challiss, R.A.J.; Hayes, D.J.; Petty, R.F.H.; Radda, G.K. An investigation of arterial insufficiency in rat hindlimb: a combined ^{31}P-NMR and bloodflow study. Biochem. J. 236:461-467; 1986.

7. Challiss, R.A.J.; Hayes, D.J.; Radda, G.K. A ^{31}P-n.m.r. study of the acute effects of β-blockade on the bioenergetics of skeletal muscle during contraction. Biochem. J. 246:163-172; 1987.

8. Challiss, R.A.J.; Vranic, M.; Radda, G.K. Bioenergetic changes during contraction and recovery in diabetic rat skeletal muscle. Am. J. Physiol. 256:E129-E137; 1989.

9. Chen, V.; Ianuzzo, C.D. Metabolic alterations in skeletal muscle of chronically streptozotocin-diabetic rats. Arch. Biochem. Biophys. 217:131-138; 1982.

10. Fischer, L.J. Drugs and chemicals that produce diabetes. Trends Pharmacol. Sci. 6:72-75; 1985.

11. Fuller, S.J.; Randle, P.J. Reversible phosphorylation of pyruvate dehydrogenase in rat skeletal muscle mitochondria: effects of starvation and diabetes. Biochem. J. 219:635-646; 1984.

12. Ganda, O.P.; Rossini, A.A.; Like, A.A. Studies on streptozotocin diabetes. Diabetes 25:595-603; 1976.

13. Harmsen, E.; DeTombe, P.P.; DeJong, J.W. Simultaneous determination of myocardial adenine nucleotides and creatine phosphate by high performance liquid chromatography. J. Chromatogr. 230:131-136; 1982.

14. Hintz, C.S.; Chi, M.M.-Y.; Fell, R.D.; Ivy, J.L.; Kaiser, K.K.; Lowry, C.V.; Lowry, O.H. Metabolite changes in individual rat muscle fibers during stimulation. Am. J. Physiol. 242:C218-C228; 1982.

15. Hintz, C.S.; Chi, M.M.-Y.; Lowry, O.H. Heterogeneity in regard to enzymes and metabolites within individual muscle fibers. Am. J. Physiol. 246:C288-C292; 1984.

16. Lawson, J.W.R.; Veech, R.L. Effects of pH and free Mg^{++} on the K_{eq} of the creatine kinase reaction and other phosphate hydrolases and transferases. J. Biol. Chem. 254:6528-6537; 1979.

17. Meyer, R.A.; Kushmerick, M.J.; Brown, T.R. Application of ^{31}P-NMR spectroscopy to the study of striated muscle metabolism. Am. J. Physiol. 242: C1-C11; 1982.

18. Noble, E.G.; Ianuzzo, C.D. Influence of training on skeletal muscle enzymatic adaptations in normal and diabetic rats. Am. J. Physiol. 249:E360-E365; 1985.

19. Ploug, T.; Galbo, H.; Richter, E.A. Increased muscle glucose uptake during contractions: no need for insulin. Am. J. Physiol. 247:E726-E731; 1984.

20. Rerup, C.C. Drugs producing diabetes through damage of the insulin secreting cells. Pharmacol. Rev. 22:485-518; 1970.

21. Richter, E.A.; Ploug, T.; Galbo, H. Increased muscle glucose uptake after exercise: no need for insulin during exercise. Diabetes 34:1041-1048; 1985.

22. Taylor, D.J.; Bore, P.J.; Styles, P.; Gadian, D.G.; Radda, G.K. Bioenergetics of intact human muscle. A ^{31}P-nuclear magnetic resonance study. Mol. Biol. Med. 1:77-94; 1983.

23. Wallberg-Henriksson, H.; Holloszy, J.O. Contractile activity increases glucose uptake by muscle in severely diabetic rats. J. Appl. Physiol. 57:1045-1049; 1984.

24. Wallberg-Henriksson, H.; Holloszy, J.O. Activation of glucose transport in diabetic muscle: responses to contraction and insulin. Am. J. Physiol. 249: C233-C237; 1985.

25. Wasserman, D.H.; Vranic, M. Interaction between insulin and counter-regulatory hormones in control of substrate utilisation in health and diabetes during exercise. Diabetes Metab. Rev. 1:359-384; 1986.

26. Young, D.A.; Wallberg-Henriksson, H.; Sleeper, M.D.; Holloszy, J.O. Reversal of the exercise-induced increase in muscle permeability to glucose. Am. J. Physiol. 253:E331-E335; 1987.

PART VI

Determinants of Extramuscular Substrate Utilization During Exercise

Hormonal Mechanisms That Act to Preserve Glucose Homeostasis During Exercise: Two Controversial Issues

M. Vranic and H.L.A. Lickley
University of Toronto, Toronto, Ontario, Canada

In order to meet increased energy demands during exercise, there are four energy depots available: liver and muscle glycogen, and esterified fat stored in both adipocytes and muscle (9, 12). Nervous and endocrine systems regulate fuel fluxes from these energy depots to optimize exercise performance with respect to its intensity and duration. Although fat represents potentially a much larger energy store than carbohydrates, there is a much tighter control of glucose homeostasis than of fatty acid homeostasis. The reason for this is that neuroendocrine factors control both glucose production by the liver and glucose uptake by the muscle, and muscle glycogenolysis. On the other hand, the neuroendocrine control of FFA fluxes is limited to FFA production by the adipocyte. We have postulated that under most conditions, the interaction of glucagon and insulin controls mobilization of glucose by the liver, whereas the interaction between epinephrine and insulin controls the uptake of glucose by the muscle (Figure 1). The brain plays an essential role in these regulations. During rest, the brain responds only to a large decrease in plasma glucose, whereas during exercise, minimal changes in plasma glucose elicit an excessive release of epinephrine (34). During exercise, the brain is also very sensitive to small changes in oxygen delivery, so that slight hypoxia can result in near-maximal releases of all counterregulatory hormones (35). It is not the purpose of this paper to review the literature covering this topic because it has been covered extensively in recent reviews (6, 11, 16, 29, 38, 40). The emphasis of this paper is to summarize results of our most recent experiments.

In the past few years, a number of controversies have arisen concerning the regulation of fuel fluxes during exercise. In this paper we will address two of these. First, is insulin an essential regulator of glucose uptake and metabolism during exercise? Second, is there a redundancy in control systems that regulate glucose fluxes, and is glucagon as important a regulator in glucose production in man as in animals?

Is Insulin an Essential Regulator of Glucose Uptake and Metabolism During Exercise?

Soon after the discovery of insulin, it was observed that exercise induces hypoglycemia in diabetics. It was assumed by many that muscular contraction per se can

279

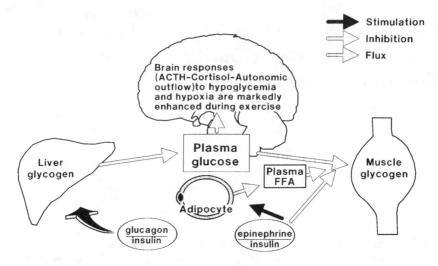

● Interaction between GLUCAGON, EPINEPHRINE and INSULIN determines
the fuel contribution of liver and muscle glycogen to exercising muscle
● Brain glucopenia shifts the balance toward muscle glycogenolysis

Figure 1. The interaction between the brain, liver, muscle, and fat cells in control of glucose homeostasis.

increase glucose uptake even in the absence of insulin. Initially, experiments performed in situ (with perfused rat hindquarters) suggested that some insulin is needed during muscular contraction to increase glucose uptake adequately (1). However, recent evidence suggests that this may not be the case (14, 20, 21, 22, 31). These experiments indicate that even in the total absence of insulin, there is a complete or almost complete increase in glucose uptake during muscular contractions. The potential problem with some in situ experiments is that oxygen delivery to the muscle may not be physiological. This is important because the in vivo experiments have shown that even a marginal decrease of oxygen delivery can greatly increase glucose uptake by the muscle, irrespective of hormonal interactions that normally control this process (35). It is also difficult to provide definitive proof that there is no remaining insulin bound to the muscles. Finally, the possibility has not yet been explored whether insulin-like growth factors (IGF 1 or 2), normally present in tissues, could replace some insulin effects in the absence of insulin. The main difference between some in situ and in vivo experiments is that the perfusion media (unless blood is used) do not contain the physiological mixture of substrates, minerals, and hormones that normally perfuse a muscle. In addition, during exercise in vivo, there is excessive release of hormones and substrates, which interfere with glucose uptake by the muscle.

The importance of insulin in regulating glucose fluxes was first demonstrated in depancreatized dogs (15, 28). Depancreatized dogs were used for two main reasons. Dogs are a unique species in having an abundant source of glucagon 3500 present in the oxyntic mucosa of the stomach (5, 30). This purified stomach glucagon has the same in vivo and in vitro effects as pancreatic glucagon (5, 23) and is synthesized from precursor amino acids in the mucosa (8). AV balance studies have also demonstrated that the stomach secretes glucagon almost exclusively, whereas the rest of the GI tract secretes glucagon-like peptides (19). Thus, the depancreatized dog is a unique model of selective insulin deficiency, and in contrast to humans, insulin replacement can be administered intraportally when needed. Without intraportal insulin replacement, a proper balance between the liver and periphery with respect to insulinization cannot be achieved.

The work in dogs (Figure 2) demonstrated that glucose homeostasis can be maintained only when insulin infusion is kept constant. With insulin deficiency there is only a marginal increase in glucose metabolic clearance, and metabolic control deteriorates with exercise. With subcutaneous insulin injection, hyperinsulinemia is encountered for three reasons: There is basal hyperinsulinemia because insulin treatment is aimed at maintaining adequate insulin levels in portal blood; insulin release into blood cannot be decreased, as observed physiologically; exercise accelerates insulin release from the subcutaneous depot unless this release is already at its maximum (15). This explains why exercise decreases plasma glucose. The insulin excess mainly prevents an increase of glucose production, but it also can lead to excessive glucose utilization. Similar experiments in humans corroborated the data in dogs (43). In addition, it was shown that exercise leads to lowering of plasma glucose in NIDDM because in NIDDM, in contrast to normal individuals, insulin secretion was not suppressed during exercise (18).

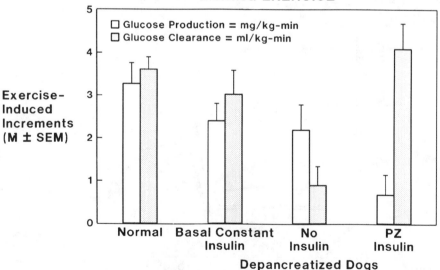

Figure 2. Exercise-induced average increments (M ± SEM) in glucose production and metabolic clearance. Glucose production and metabolic clearance were measured in depancreatized dogs either maintained on an infusion of insulin (230 μU/kg/min) or deprived of insulin. (Modified from 15.)

282 Vranic and Lickley

More recently (42), the critical role of insulin during exercise in IDDM was further explored. When plasma glucose was maintained at only 20 mg above normal by constant insulin infusion, glucose turnover was increased by 20% in the basal state. During exercise, the increase in lactate doubled. With an adequate correction in insulin infusion, basal glucose turnover and the lactate response to exercise fully normalized (Figure 3). The excessive response of lactate emphasizes the importance of insulin in maintaining glucose oxidation, when in the muscle neither glucose uptake nor glycolysis is increased. Thus, there is no question that in vivo insulin plays a pivotal role not only in the control of glucose production but also in the control of glucose uptake by the muscle. The question remains, however, whether the primary role of insulin in control of glucose metabolism in the muscle is direct or indirect. Figure 4 illustrates that insulin and catecholamines interact in the control of

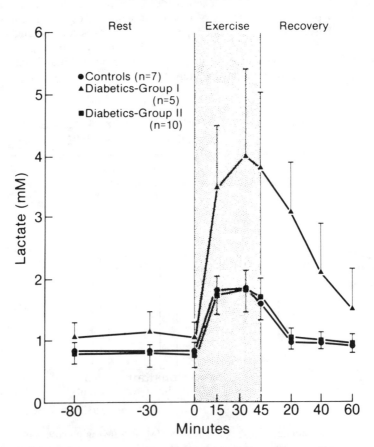

Figure 3. The effect of exercise (55% V̇O₂max) on plasma lactate in 7 controls and in insulin-infused IDDM. Square, 10 patients with plasma glucose identical to controls (90 mg%); triangle, 5 patients with plasma glucose at 110 mg%. (Modified from 42 and 44.)

CATECHOLAMINE–INSULIN INTERACTION IN EXERCISE

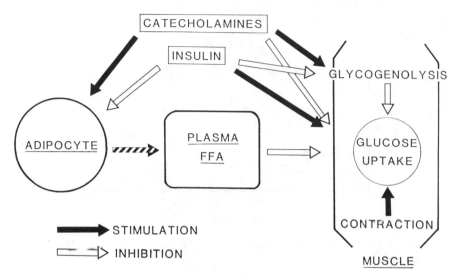

Figure 4.   Interaction between catecholamines and insulin in control of glucose uptake.

glycogenolysis in the muscle, in the control of glucose transport, and in the control of glycolysis by the adipocyte. Beta blockers can block all these effects of catecholamines. Therefore, in order to delineate the importance of insulin, beta blockade was applied to dogs that had either some residual insulin (alloxan diabetes) or were fully deprived of insulin (depancreatized).

Figure 5 illustrates that in the presence of some insulin, beta blockade could fully restore the increase of glucose metabolic clearance observed in normal dogs during exercise (37, 38). This could indicate that the main role of insulin during exercise is to counterbalance the effects of catecholamines. If that is true, either insulin is not needed, or a small amount of insulin will suffice. Figure 6 (3) illustrates the effect of beta blockade in depancreatized dogs. Metabolic clearance was calculated by correcting total glucose clearance for glycosuria, which was measured at frequent intervals during exercise. Surprisingly, beta blockade had no effect on glucose clearance. In contrast, however, beta blockade had a pronounced effect on plasma concentration of lactate, glycerol, and fatty acids (Figure 7). Thus, some effects of catecholamines on both muscle and adipocytes were blocked. Figure 8 summarizes the data observed in partially and totally insulin-deprived dogs, illustrating the relationship between the concentration of plasma FFA and metabolic glucose clearance (MCR). It appears that the glucose–fatty acid cycle is important in the control of glucose metabolism in the working muscle. It could be that the main effect of beta blockade on glucose uptake in the muscle was to suppress lipolysis and thereby FFA oxidation in the muscle, so that MCR increased even when the amount of insulin is very small. In contrast, in total insulin deficiency, although the suppression of fatty acids was of the same magnitude as in alloxan diabetic dogs,

Effect of exercise ± β-blockade in partial insulin deficiency

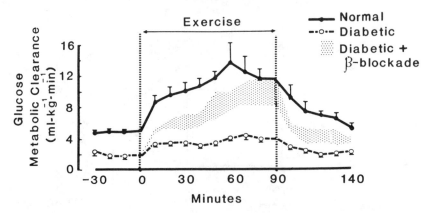

Figure 5. Effect of exercise in normal and alloxan-diabetic dogs with or without beta-blockade. (Modified from 37.)

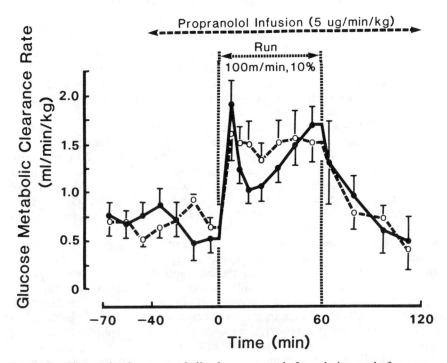

Figure 6. Changes in glucose metabolic clearance rate before, during, and after exercise with (dashed line) and without (solid line) concomitant propranolol infusion in depancreatized dogs deprived of insulin injection for 48 hours. (Modified from 3.)

Effect of β–Adrenergic Blockade in Exercising Insulin-Deficient Dogs

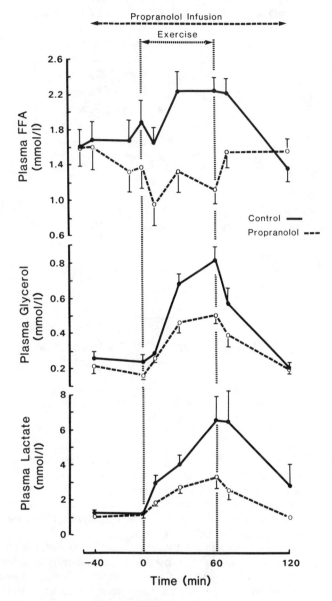

Figure 7.   Effect of exercise with or without beta-blockade (propranolol) in depancreatized dogs deprived of insulin for 48 hours. (Modified from 3.)

the concentration of fatty acids remained above a critical threshold level. We concluded that the glucose–fatty acid cycle works only when plasma FFA are below 1.5 mmol/L. If this is correct, then a more complete suppression of FFA oxidation could increase glucose clearance even in the total absence of insulin. This, however,

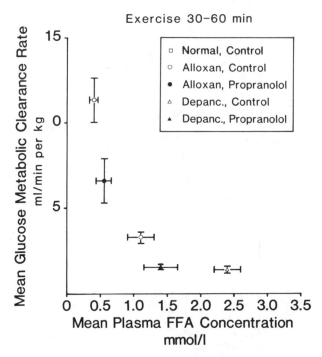

CORRELATION BETWEEN FFA CONCENTRATION
AND METABOLIC GLUCOSE CLEARANCE

Exercise 30–60 min

Mean Glucose Metabolic Clearance Rate
ml/min per kg

□ Normal, Control
○ Alloxan, Control
● Alloxan, Propranolol
△ Depanc., Control
▲ Depanc., Propranolol

Mean Plasma FFA Concentration
mmol/l

Figure 8. Relationship between mean FFA and mean glucose metabolic clearance rate
during 30-60 min of running exercise in dogs under five different conditions (see
legend). The panel depicts mean values ± SEM. (Modified from 3.)

still remains to be demonstrated. Presently, our working hypothesis is that the main
role of insulin during exercise is an indirect one: to restrain lipolysis in adipocytes
and thereby the oxidation of fatty acids in the muscle (glucose-FFA cycle) (7). Without
this restraint, catecholamines, which are always elevated during exercise, will maintain the flux of fatty acids at such high levels that metabolic clearance of glucose
can be increased in the muscle only marginally.

The in situ experiments (4) we recently performed also support the idea that very
little, if any, insulin is needed to directly control carbohydrate metabolism in the
muscle during exercise. Three groups of streptozotocin-diabetic rats were studied.
Experiments were performed 3 weeks after the induction of diabetes. Some rats were
left without any treatment, others were well controlled with insulin injections, and
in still others insulin treatment was withheld for 3 days before the study. Bioenergetic
changes during contraction and recovery in diabetic rat skeletal muscle were studied
by phosphorus magnetic resonance (^{31}P-NMR) spectroscopy and by conventional
biochemical methods performed in muscle samples obtained at sacrifice. The advantage of NMR technique was that it was possible to obtain frequent biochemical data
during muscle contraction without invasive techniques. These measurements included

inorganic phosphorus, phosphocreatine, and pH. In the group that did not receive any insulin, at low muscle-work intensity, contractile performance was maintained by an increased reliance on glycolytic mechanisms of ATP resynthesis. At high working intensity, the decreased rate of pyruvate utilization (defect of the enzyme pyruvate dehydrogenase) could no longer be overcome by an increased glycolytic rate, and force failure occurred. During recovery, however, resynthesis of phosphocreatine normalized. Surprisingly, all the biochemical parameters measured in rats without insulin injection for 3 days were normal. This reinforces the suggestion that the small amount of insulin (10% normal) found in streptozotocin-diabetic rats is sufficient to control muscle metabolism. We feel that this is because during in situ contraction of one muscle (gastrocnemius), there is no increased release of catecholamines or stimulation of lipolysis in the adipocytes. Thus, insulin is not needed to counterbalance the effects of increased counterregulation. Furthermore, because both diabetic, insulin-deprived groups had the same alteration in substrate delivery (glucose, fatty acids, ketone bodies), the difference in contractile performance between acutely and chronically diabetic rats is likely to be due to a chronic metabolic impairment within the skeletal muscle rather than as a consequence of altered substrate delivery. In contrast to the events during muscular contraction, the rate of glycogen resynthesis is decreased by hypoinsulinemia of either chronic or acute duration.

In conclusion, the data in vivo clearly demonstrate that insulin is a pivotal regulator of carbohydrate metabolism both in the liver and in muscle, not only in rest but also during exercise. The main control of muscle metabolism, however, could be through an indirect pathway. Data in vitro suggest that the main role of insulin may be to regulate lipolysis and, thereby, FFA oxidation in muscle. Through the glucose–fatty acid cycle, the oxidation of fatty acid in the muscle could then also regulate glucose uptake. At the present time, it is not known whether regulation of glucose metabolism in the muscle is normal even in the total absence of insulin, if all the effects of counterregulation are completely blocked.

Is There a Redundancy in Control Systems That Regulate Glucose Fluxes?

As described elsewhere in detail (40), nervous and endocrine systems regulate fuel fluxes from energy depots to optimize exercise performance with respect to its intensity and duration. It has been suggested (10) that there is redundancy in the control systems that regulate glucose fluxes because deficiency of one system does not necessarily lead to overt hypoglycemia. We will attempt to demonstrate that the different control systems are not necessarily redundant but that prevention of overt hypoglycemia may occur at the expense of a shift of fuel fluxes. For example, when dogs were exercised, glucagon secretion was suppressed by somatostatin, and glucose production by the liver decreased, but the hypoglycemia that ensued was only transient (13, 34). This transient hypoglycemia, however, resulted in increased epinephrine secretion. This led to an increase in glycogenolysis and a decrease in glucose uptake by the peripheral tissues. Thus, overt hypoglycemia was prevented at the expense of increased muscle glycogenolysis. The shift of stored fuel utilization from liver to muscle is not optimal for endurance exercise. Two lines of evidence

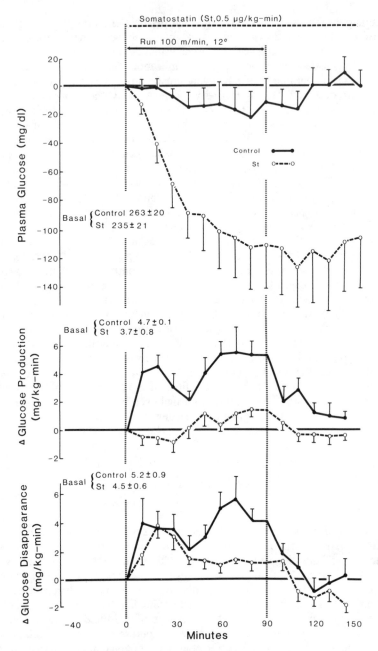

Figure 9. Effects in alloxan-diabetic dogs of exercise alone (control) or exercise and somatostatin (St) on changes in plasma glucose, rate of hepatic glucose production, and rate of glucose disappearance. Data are shown as deviations (Δ) from basal values. Exercise and somatostatin infusion were begun at $t = 0$. Vertical bars, *SE*; $n = 6$ for both protocols. (Reproduced from 34 with permission.)

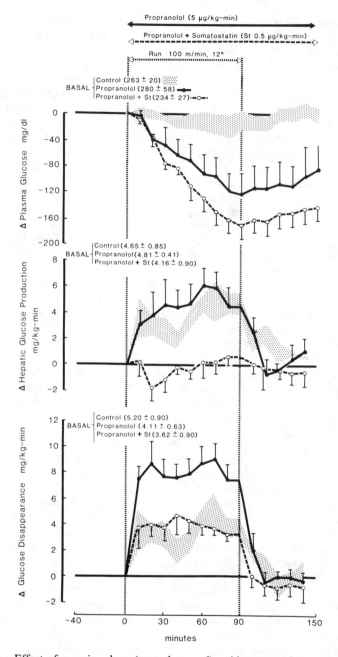

Figure 10. Effect of exercise alone (control, $n = 6$), with propranol ($n = 6$), or with propranol + somatostatin ($n = 5$) in alloxan-diabetic dogs on changes in plasma glucose, rate of hepatic glucose production, and rate of glucose disappearance. Data shown as deviations (Δ) from basal values. Exercise and infusions were begun at $t = 0$. Stippled area: mean $\pm$ *SE* for exercise alone; vertical bars: *SE*. (Reproduced from 35 with permission).

demonstrated that this shift was due to glucagon-epinephrine interaction. First, when plasma glucose concentration was maintained with a euglycemic glucose clamp, the release of epinephrine and glucose uptake by the muscle was normalized, whereas suppression of glucose production was even more marked (34). Second, when glucagon concentration was restored by glucagon infusion given concurrently with somatostatin, glucose production by the liver was normalized (13). The pivotal role of the glucagon:insulin ratio in the control of glucose production during exercise was demonstrated through a very close linear correlation between the two parameters.

The dog has also been used to study the metabolic role of the exercise-induced fall in insulin, independent of glucagon (32). One advantage is that the two pancreatic hormones can be infused into the portal vein, thereby alleviating the problem caused by introducing insulin peripherally (10, 24, 41). When insulin was infused intraportally at the onset of exercise in order to prevent its fall, the increase in glucagon was blunted. The failures of insulin to fall and glucagon to rise led to a 78% reduction in tracer-determined glucose output. When the fall in insulin was prevented and glucagon levels were restored by an intraportal infusion of this hormone, glucose production was still only 45% of the normal response, but the gluconeogenic conversion rate and efficiency were normalized (39). Thus, the fall in insulin facilitates the rise of glucagon, and normal changes in insulin and glucagon are necessary for the control of glucose production. Furthermore, the fall in insulin controls liver glycogenolysis, whereas the rise in glucagon is critical for both the increase in gluconeogenesis and glycogenolysis.

There was no correlation between epinephrine and glucose production by the liver; therefore, it appeared that the main role of the catecholamines was to decrease peripheral glucose uptake. It is remarkable that even a small variation of plasma glucose during exercise induced a major increase in epinephrine release (34). This illustrates the notion that the adrenomedullary system represents an even more important safeguard in exercise than at rest.

In humans, in contrast to dogs, plasma glucagon increases only during hypoglycemic or exhaustive exercise. The hypoglycemic effect of acute glucagon suppression during exercise was also demonstrated in humans (2). However, the glucagon:insulin ratio increases with exercise also in humans because of the suppression of insulin secretion. Therefore, the question has been asked whether change in the glucagon:insulin ratio is essential for the control of glycemia during exercise in humans. The problem is that the peripheral measurements of glucagon and insulin do not necessarily reflect changes of these hormones in portal blood (26). Increases in glucose production have been seen in depancreatized dogs (28) and in Type I diabetics when changes of this ratio measured in peripheral blood were not detectable (42). To overcome this problem, a bihormonal insulin-glucagon clamp was applied during light (40% $\dot{V}O_2$max) (41) and moderate (60% $\dot{V}O_2$max) (10) exercise. In the former case, it was concluded that hypoglycemia occurred invariably when the change in this ratio was prevented. In the latter, a change in this ratio was important only if there were concurrent alpha and beta adrenergic blockades. Furthermore, it appears that increments of glucagon, but not decrements of insulin, play a major role in the secondary line of defense against hypoglycemia during exercise (27). Presently, it is not clear whether the sharp divergence of results (10, 41) is due only to the intensity of exercise or to the methodology related to the bihormonal clamp applied through a peripheral route that is not physiological, because the important portoperipheral insulin gradient is lost and the concentration of hormones perfusing the liver is unknown.

In diabetes the effect of glucagon suppression is readily demonstrable (36). In alloxan-diabetic dogs during exercise, glucagon suppression so virtually abolished the rise in glucose production that plasma glucose promptly fell (Figure 9). Because basal glucose concentration was elevated, there was no hypoglycemia during exercise; therefore, it was not necessary to establish a glucose clamp in order to assess the impact of glucagon suppression. It was very interesting to observe that as plasma glucose declined, the excessive release of catecholamines and cortisol normalized. It would thus appear that hyperglycemia, and not only hypoglycemia, leads to excessive counterregulation. Because amelioration of hyperglycemia was associated with normalization of the counterregulatory response, it could be that hyperresponsiveness of those hormones was related to osmotic effects from glucose.

We wanted to see whether beta-blockade would result in decreased hepatic glucose production in diabetic dogs, and also whether or not there is a synergistic effect between glucagon suppression and beta-blockade in alloxan-diabetic dogs (37). Beta-blockade was effective because the response of lactate to exercise was diminished and the FFAs were suppressed below basal. However, these effects of beta-blockade were not altered by the somatostatin-induced suppression of glucagon. Figure 10 illustrates that the combined suppression of glucagon and beta-blockade resulted in a more marked decrease in plasma glucose. Interestingly, however, glucose output by the liver was affected only by glucagon suppression, whereas metabolic glucose clearance (mainly in the muscle) was affected only by beta-blockade. Thus, it appears that in the diabetic dogs, glucagon affects only the liver, and catecholamines only peripheral glucose uptake. Similar conclusions have also been reached in exercising Type I diabetics (25).

The important role of glucagon and lack of importance of catecholamines in control of hepatic glucose production in health and diabetes, where some residual insulin is still present, dramatically changes in a state of total deprivation. Thus, in depancreatized dogs (3), as also observed previously (28), glucagon levels did not rise; they decreased moderately during exercise, and catecholamines were shown to be important regulators of hepatic glucose production. Thus, in the absence of insulin, as also observed in resting dogs (17), glucagon may not be of primary importance for the control of glucose production.

In conclusion, our work suggests that excessive release of epinephrine can replace glucagon lack in the maintenance of glucose homeostasis, but the two glucoregulatory mechanisms are different and, therefore, not redundant. Glucagon-insulin interaction mainly controls the liver, whereas catecholamine-insulin interaction controls glucose uptake, probably mainly through indirect mechanisms.

References

1. Berger, M.; Hagg, S.; Ruderman, N.B. Glucose metabolism in perfused skeletal muscle: interaction of insulin and exercise on glucose uptake. Biochem. J. 146: 231-238; 1975.

292   Vranic and Lickley

2. Bjorkman, O.; Felig, P.; Hagenfeldt, L.; Wahren, J. Influence of hypoglucagonemia on splanchnic glucose output during leg exercise in man. Clin. Physiol. 1:43-57; 1981.

3. Bjorkman, O.; Miles, P.; Wasserman, D.; Lickley, L.; Vranic, M. Regulation of glucose turnover during exercise in pancreatectomized, totally insulin deficient dogs: effects of beta-adrenergic blockade. J. Clin. Invest. 81:759-767; 1988.

4. Challiss, R.A.J.; Vranic, M.; Radda, G.K. Bioenergetic changes during contraction and recovery in diabetic rat skeletal muscle. Am. J. Physiol. 256: E129-E137, 1989.

5. Doi, K.; Prentki, M.; Yip, C.; Muller, W.; Jeanrenaud, B.; Vranic, M. Identical biological effects of pancreatic glucagon and a purified moiety of canine gastric glucagon. J. Clin. Invest. 63:525-531; 1979.

6. Galbo, H. Hormonal and metabolic adaptation to exercise. Stuttgart/New York: George Thieme Verlag; 1983.

7. Garland, P.B.; Newsholme, E.A.; Randle, P.J. Regulation of glucose uptake by muscle: 9. Effects of fatty acids and ketone bodies, and of alloxan-diabetes and starvation on pyruvate metabolism and on lactate/pyruvate and L-glycerol 3-phosphate/dihydroxyacetone phosphate concentrations in rat heart and rat diaphragm muscles. Biochem. J. 93:665-678; 1984.

8. Hatton, T.W.; Yip, C.C.; Vranic, M. Biosynthesis of glucagon (IRG3500) in canine gastric mucosa. Diabetes 34:38-46; 1985.

9. Hermansen, L.; Hultman, E.; Saltin, B. Muscle glycogen during prolonged severe exercise. Acta Physiol. Scand. 71:129-139; 1967.

10. Hoelzer, D.R.; Dalsky, G.P.; Clutter, W.E.; Shah, S.D.; Holloszy, J.O.; Cryer, P.E. Glucoregulation during exercise hypoglycemia is prevented by redundant glucoregulatory systems, sympathochromaffin activation and changes in islet hormone secretion. J. Clin. Invest. 77:212-221; 1986.

11. Horton, E.S. Exercise and physical training: effects on insulin sensitivity and glucose metabolism. In: DeFronzo, R.A., ed. Diabetes/metabolism reviews. J. Wiley; 1986:1-17. (Vol. 2).

12. Issekutz, B. Effects of glucose infusion on hepatic and muscle glycogenolysis in exercising dogs. Am. J. Physiol. (Endocrinol. Metab.) 240:451-457; 1981.

13. Issekutz, B.; Vranic, M. Role of glucagon in the regulation of glucose production in exercising dogs. Am. J. Physiol. 238:E13-E20; 1980.

14. James, D.E.; Kraegan, E.W.; Chisholm, D.J. Muscle glucose metabolism in exercising rats: comparison with insulin stimulation. Am. J. Physiol. 248: E575-D580; 1985.

15. Kawamori, R.; Vranic, M. Mechanism of exercise-induced hypoglycemia in depancreatized dogs maintained on long-acting insulin. J. Clin. Invest. 59: 331-337; 1977.

16. Kemmer, F.W.; Berger, M. Therapy and better quality of life: the dichotomous role of exercise in diabetes mellitus. In: DeFronzo, R.A., ed. Diabetes/ metabolism reviews. J. Wiley, Inc.; 1986:53-68. (Vol. 2).

17. Lickley, H.L.A.; Kemmer, F.W.; Doi, K.; Vranic, M. Glucagon suppression improves glucoregulation in moderate but not chronic severe diabetes. Am. J. Physiol. 245:E424-E429; 1983.

18. Minuk, H.L.; Vranic, M.; Marliss, E.B.; Hanna, A.K.; Albisser, A.M.; Zinman, B. Glucoregulatory and metabolic response to exercise in obese, non-insulin dependent diabetes. Am. J. Physiol. 240:E458-E464; 1981.

19. Muller, W.A.; Girardier, L.; Seydoux, J.; Berger, M.; Renold, A.E.; Vranic, M. Extrapancreatic glucagon and glucagon-like immunoreactivity in depancreatized dogs: a quantitative assessment of secretion rates and anatomical delineation of sources. J. Clin. Invest. 62:124-132; 1978.

20. Nesher, R.; Karl, I.E.; Kipnis, K.M. Dissociation of the effect(s) of insulin and contraction on glucose transport in rat epitrochlearis muscle. Am. J. Physiol. 249:C226-C232; 1985.

21. Ploug, T.; Galbo, H.; Richter, E.A. Increased muscle glucose uptake during contraction: no need for insulin. Am. J. Physiol. (Endocrinol. Metab.) 247: 726-731; 1984.

22. Richter, E.A.; Ploug, T.; Galbo, H. Increased muscle glucose uptake after exercise. No need for insulin during exercise. Diabetes 34:1041-1048; 1985.

23. Ross, G.; Lickley, H.L.A.; Vranic, M. Extrapancreatic glucagon in control of glucose turnover in depancreatized dogs. Am. J. Physiol. 234(2):E213-E219; 1978.

24. Shilo, S.; Sotsky, M.; Shamoon, H. Effect of plasma insulin on glucose kinetics in exercising non-diabetic and Type I diabetic man. Diabetes 36(Suppl. 1):16A; 1987.

25. Simonson, D.C.; Koivisto, V.; Sherwin, R.S.; et al. Adrenergic blockade alters glucose kinetics during exercise in insulin-dependent diabetics. J. Clin. Invest. 73:1648-1658; 1984.

26. Sirek, A.; Vranic, M.; Sirek, O; Vigas, M.; Policova, A. The effect of growth hormone on acute glucagon and insulin release. Am. J. Physiol. 237:E107-E112; 1979.

27. Tuttle, K.R.; Marker, J.C.; Dalsky, G.P.; Schwartz, N.S.; Shah, S.D.; Clutter, W.E.; Holloszy, J.O.; Cryer, P.E. Glucagon, not insulin, may play a secondary role in defense against hypoglycemia during exercise. Am. J. Physiol. 254:E713-E719; 1988.

28. Vranic, M.; Kawamori, R.; Pek, S.; Kovacevic, N.; Wrenshall, G. The essentiality of insulin and the role of glucagon in regulating glucose utilization and production during strenuous exercise in dogs. J. Clin. Invest. 57:245-255; 1976.

29. Vranic, M.; Lickley, H.L.A.; Davidson, J.K. Exercise and stress in diabetes mellitus. In: Davidson, J.K., ed. Clinical diabetes mellitus: a problem oriented approach. New York: Thieme-Stratton, Inc.; 1986:172-205.

30. Vranic, M.; Pek, S.; Kawamori, R. Increased "glucagon immunoreactivity" in plasma of totally depancreatized dogs. Diabetes 23:905-912; 1975.

31. Wallberg-Henriksson, H.; Holloszy, J.O. Contractile activity increases glucose uptake by muscle in severely diabetic rats. J. Appl. Physiol. 57:1045-1049; 1984.

32. Wasserman, D.H.; Goldstein, R.; Donahue, P.; Passalaqua, S.; Lacy, D. Importance of the exercise-induced fall in insulin to the regulation of hepatic carbohydrate metabolism. Diabetes 36(Suppl. 1):39A; 1987.

33. Wasserman, D.H.; Lacy, D.B.; Goldstein, R.; Williams, P.; Cherrington, A.D. Role of the exercise-induced fall in insulin independent of the effects of glucagon (abstract). Med. Sci. Sports Exerc. 20:84; 1988.

34. Wasserman, D.H.; Lickley, H.L.A.; Vranic, M. Interactions between glucagon and other counterregulatory hormones during normoglycemic and hypoglycemic exercise. J. Clin. Invest. 74:1404-1413; 1984.

35. Wasserman, D.H.; Lickley, H.L.A.; Vranic, M. Effect of hematocrit reduction on hormonal and metabolic responses to exercise. J. Appl. Physiol. 58: 1257-1262; 1985.

36. Wasserman, D.H.; Lickley, H.L.A.; Vranic, M. Important role of glucagon during exercise in diabetic dogs. J. Appl. Physiol. 59:1272-1281; 1985.

37. Wasserman, D.H.; Lickley, H.L.A.; Vranic, M. Role of beta-adrenergic mechanisms during exercise in poorly controlled insulin deficient diabetes. J. Appl. Physiol. 59:1282-1289; 1985.

38. Wasserman, D.H.; Vranic, M. Interaction between insulin and counterregulatory hormones in control of substrate utilization in health and diabetes during exercise. In: DeFronzo, R.A., ed., Diabetes/metabolism reviews. J. Wiley & Sons, Inc.; 1986:159-183. (Vol. 1).

39. Wasserman, D.H.; Vranic, M. Exercise and diabetes. In: Alberti, K.G.M.M.; Krall, L.P., eds. The diabetes annual/3. Amsterdam: Elsevier; 1987:527-559.

40. Wasserman, D.H.; Vranic, M. Exercise and diabetes. In: Alberti, K.G.M.M.; Krall, L.P., eds. The diabetes annual/4. Amsterdam: Elsevier; p. 116-142, 1988.

41. Wolfe, R.R.; Nadel, E.R.; Shaw, J.H.F.; Stephenson, L.A.; Wolfe, M. Role of changes in insulin and glucagon in glucose homeostasis in exercise. J. Clin. Invest. 77:900-907; 1986.

42. Zinman, B.; Marliss, E.B.; Hanna, A.K.; Minuk, H.L. Vranic, M. Exercise in diabetic man: glucose turnover and "free" insulin responses after glycemic normalization with intravenous insulin. Can. J. Physiol. Pharmacol. 60: 1236-1240; 1982.

43. Zinman, B.; Murray, F.T.; Vranic, M.; Albisser, A.M.; Leibel, B.S.; McClean, P.A.; Marliss, E.B. Glucoregulation during moderate exercise in insulin treated diabetics. J. Clin. Endocrinol. Metab. 45:641-652, 1977.

44. Zinman, B.; Stokes, E.F.; Albisser, A.M.; Hanna, A.K.; Minuk, H.L.; Stein, A.N.; Leibel, B.S.; Marliss, E.B. The metabolic response to glycemic control by the artificial pancreas in diabetic man. Metabolism 28:511-518; 1979.

Glucose Transport in Skeletal Muscle

Arend Bonen, John C. McDermott, and Meng H. Tan
Dalhousie University, Halifax, Nova Scotia, Canada

Skeletal muscle is the major user of glucose; by mass, muscle is the most important repository for this carbohydrate (i.e., 70% of the total glycogen), and most of the radiolabeled glucose accumulates in this tissue within a few hours after its administration. Glucose metabolism also provides a considerable proportion of the energy needs of skeletal muscle at rest and during exercise. The focus of this review will be to examine glucose utilization by skeletal muscle and to consider the possible mechanisms responsible for alterations in the use of this substrate. In this context insulin is also extremely important because it contributes to the uptake and metabolism of glucose in muscle and is always present in the healthy organism. However, we will also consider the idea that glucose uptake in skeletal muscles may be regulated by their activity patterns.

Glucose Utilization During Exercise

When skeletal muscle metabolism is increased, as during exercise, glucose uptake is increased (i.e., increased blood flow × increased a-$\bar{v}$ difference), and this can be further stimulated when glucose is ingested during mild exercise (1).

Studies with ^{13}C-glucose have shown that the rate of metabolism of this substrate increases progressively up to 64% $\dot{V}O_2$max (68) (Figure 1). A 100-g load of glucose is nearly 50% recovered as CO_2 after 90 min of exercise at 64% $\dot{V}O_2$max (68). Yet, even at higher intensities of exercise (80% $\dot{V}O_2$max), glucose can seemingly deliver almost as much substrate as endogenous muscle glycogen (13). Only when exercise levels are very intense (100% $\dot{V}O_2$max) does glucose appear to accumulate excessively within a muscle (45). Apparently, glucose and other blood-borne substrates become progressively less important for muscle as the intensity of muscle contractility increases (89). Interestingly, during moderate exercise (45% $\dot{V}O_2$max), it seems to matter little exactly when glucose is ingested because similar amounts are oxidized if glucose is consumed during exercise or 3 hours before exercise (39, 51) (Figure 1).

A number of studies have suggested that insulin and contractility act independently to stimulate glucose uptake. For example, when glucose is ingested prior to exercise, the resultant increase in insulin is designed to clear glucose from the circulation. However, when exercise commences while insulin levels are still elevated, an accelerated efflux of glucose from plasma occurs (10, 19). It is now known that contractility and insulin stimulate glucose uptake in an additive manner (see below).

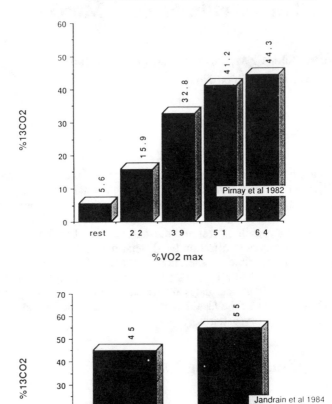

Figure 1. Oxidation of ¹³C-glucose during 90 min of exercise at different intensities (upper panel), and similar oxidation rates of glucose during moderate exercise when glucose is ingested 3 hours before or immediately before exercise (drawn from data in refs. 39, 68).

Glucose Uptake in Skeletal Muscle

In the past 5 years, considerable attention has been devoted to studying the regulation of glucose uptake in muscle. Attention has focused on differences in glucose uptake and metabolism among skeletal muscles, autoregulation of glucose uptake, glucose uptake kinetics in contracting muscles, and mechanistic aspects of the insulin receptor signal transduction, namely, insulin binding to its receptor, receptor protein kinase activity, and glucose transporter mobility and characteristics.

Our observation that the inherent glucose uptake capacities of skeletal muscles differ widely (13) has been observed by others as well, both in vivo (34, 37) and in situ (71) (Figure 2). Specifically, the insulin sensitivity and insulin responsiveness of oxidative muscles at rest is greater than in glycolytic types of muscle. In vivo the rate of glucose uptake at rest in the soleus is 2- and 8-fold greater than in red and white gastrocnemius, respectively (37, 38).

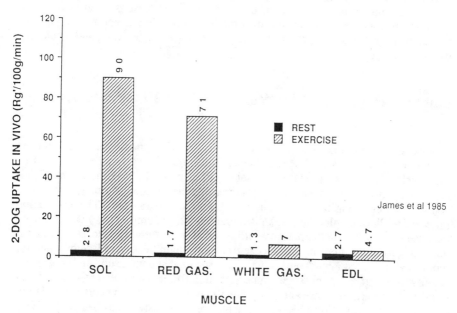

Figure 2. Heterogeneity of 2-deoxy-d-glucose uptake in skeletal muscle in conscious resting and exercising rats (drawn from data in ref. 38).

When muscle activity is increased by exercise, a greater absolute increase in glucose uptake is found in soleus, a slow-twitch oxidative (SO) muscle, than in fast-twitch oxidative glycolytic (FOG) and fast-twitch glycolytic (FG) muscles (14). This, however, may reflect differences in the types of muscles recruited during exercise as well as a disproportionate reliance on this substrate among exercising muscles.

The reasons for these inherent glucose uptake differences are not entirely clear. In part, these differences are mirrored by differences in insulin binding among muscles (7) and differences in glucose transporter availability in the absence of insulin (unpublished data) among muscles. Several studies indicate that increments in blood-flow within a muscle increase its glucose uptake (17, 76). However, James et al. (37) have argued that coincident differences in blood flow and glucose uptake among different types of muscles are just that—coincidences—because alterations in blood flow did not proportionately alter changes in glucose uptake among muscles.

Other factors besides blood flow can also change glucose uptake. For example, when muscle has been electrically stimulated, the heterogeneity in glucose uptake among muscles is less pronounced, and glucose uptake increases, despite the fact that flow rates of perfusates were identical in control and electrically stimulated muscles (72, 73). This indicates that there are changes within the muscle membrane that are provoked by contractile activity. We speculate that such changes are most likely changes in the number and/or the activities of the glucose transporter (GT) that are required to facilitate the transport of glucose across the muscle membrane.

Whatever the mechanisms involved, it is clear that exercise presents a very strong stimulus for taking up glucose in muscle, one that is at least as great as that provided by maximal levels of insulin in some instances. Understanding the putative mechanisms involved may provide an explanation for this interesting and potentially useful phenomenon.

Glucose Transport Kinetics in Muscle: Vmax and Km

In isolated muscle (52, 64, 70) and in humans (29, 97), glucose transport has been shown to follow Michaelis-Menten kinetics. It has also been generally accepted that the effects of insulin on glucose disposal are to increase the maximum rate of glucose transport (Vmax), presumably by increasing the number of glucose transporters, without observing any changes in the Km for glucose transport. The observation in recent studies that glucose uptake is increased after exercise (14, 72) and during exercise (65, 69, 92) in the presence of insulin at nonsaturating glucose concentrations suggested that the Km for glucose transport might be lowered. Subsequently, Ploug et al. (70), though not others (65), have shown that both insulin and contractile activity lowered the Km in skeletal muscle. Similarly, it is now also recognized that in fat cells, insulin increases not only the Vmax of glucose transport (56, 86) but also lowers the Km (96), when experiments are rigorously controlled (86). These changes in Km and Vmax also appear to be consonant with recently identified changes in GT activity (i.e., changes in GT cooperativity, affinity, and translocation) (30).

In marked contrast, studies in humans under hyperinsulinemic conditions (forearm muscle) (97) and in perfused rat muscle under hyperinsulinemic and hyperglycemic conditions (52) indicated that there can be an increase in both Km and Vmax. This increase in Km was interpreted as a shift in the rate-limiting step from glucose transport to glucose disposal rather than a decrease in the affinity of the glucose transport system for glucose. Thus, under pathophysiological conditions (hyperinsulinemia or hyperglycemia), there may be a shift in the rate-limiting step from glucose transport to glucose disposal.

Muscle Contractility and Glucose Transport

Work by Berger, Hagg, and Ruderman (5) and Vranic et al. (88) indicated that glucose uptake in muscle could be augmented only by the presence of small quantities of insulin. More recently, this dogma has been seriously challenged, because glucose uptake was increased after exercise even in the absence of insulin (14, 72). Work by several groups using different approaches have all shown that contractile activity increases glucose uptake and that insulin per se is not required for this purpose (65, 69, 73, 92). Furthermore, it was also shown that the effects of insulin and contractile activity on glucose uptake are additive (65, 73, 91) (Figure 3). This additive effect of insulin and contractility suggests strongly that independent

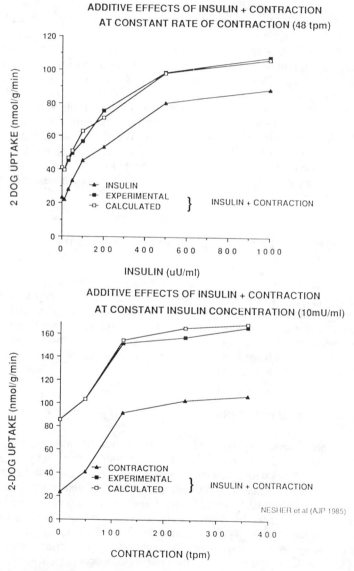

Figure 3. Additive effects of insulin and contractile activity on glucose uptake in epitrochlearis muscle in vitro (drawn from data in ref. 65).

mechanisms are involved in stimulating glucose transport. Presumably, both insulin and contractility recruit GTs because the effects of both of these stimuli on glucose uptake in muscle are blocked by cytochalasin B (65) (see below for further discussion).

In most studies to date, contractile activity is also accompanied by a concomitant glycogen loss. It had been thought that glycogen loss accounted for the increase in glucose uptake after exercise (100), but recent work fails to support this idea because glucose uptake declines rapidly even when glycogen synthesis is not occurring (70, 99). The augmented rate of glucose uptake after exercise returns to basal glucose uptake rates at quite different time courses in soleus (26 min) and red gastrocnemius (69 min) (70) and seems to be delayed further in the presence of insulin (99).

The differences in these time courses raise interesting questions about the underlying mechanism(s) provoking these differences in metabolically heterogeneous skeletal muscles. One suggestion is that insulin retards the rate of translocated GTs recycling back to intracellular "storage" sites (99). This, however, is unlikely to account for differences among muscles, particularly because soleus muscle is much more insulin-sensitive than other muscles but exhibits the most rapid renormalization of glucose uptake after exercise (see above). The translocation hypothesis for GTs may be but one mechanism that permits augmented glucose uptake; changes in affinity and cooperativity are now also documented for GT (30). These factors may be significant in skeletal muscles because they are not necessarily insulin-dependent (31).

Mechanisms for Increasing Glucose Transport

It is well accepted that the action of insulin is initiated by the binding of this hormone to its receptor, followed thereafter by a cascade of responses beyond the receptor. Currently, the first action beyond insulin binding seems to be the activation of the protein tyrosine kinase of the β subunit of the receptor, followed thereafter by the mobilization (translocation or affinity changes) in the glucose transporter. An additional phenomenon is the stimulatory effect of low levels of glucose on glucose transport into muscle (autoregulation).

Autoregulation of Glucose Uptake

The idea that glucose regulates its own uptake has recently been described. Prolonged incubation (3-5 hours) of intact soleus or epitrochlearis muscles, skeletal myocyte, and myotubes with low levels of glucose (< 3 mM) increased 2-DOG and 3-O-MG uptake (by increasing its Vmax), so that the addition of even supramaximal quantities of insulin (0.1-100 nM) failed to increase glucose uptake (75, 98). A threshold or set point seems to exist at about 3.0-4.5 mM glucose. At this point the lowering of the glucose increases uptake by 25-35%, whereas increasing the incubating glucose lowers the transport by about 1-3% per additional millimole of glucose (75). Insulin stimulation of the transport system occurs only in this "downregulated" mode. Thus, glucose and insulin appear to compete for some of the same fraction of the glucose transport that can be regulated (75, 98).

The mechanisms for this hypoglycemic-induced effect are not clear. Protein synthesis seems to be involved because cycloheximide blocked 65% of the increased glucose transport at low glucose concentrations (98). This may involve an inhibition of the synthesis of new glucose transporters (GT) from high-density microsomal fractions because plasma membrane GTs are not affected by cycloheximide (58, 59). It would appear, therefore, that low levels of glucose provide a signal for the mobilization of glucose transporters. With the cloned β-cell line HIT-T15, glucose transporters have been suggested to behave as a glucose sensor (2). A similar function appears to be present in skeletal muscle.

Insulin Binding and Glucose Transport

The binding of insulin to its receptor initiates a cascade of biological responses. This receptor is a tetramer with two extracellular-subunits (135,000 Da) containing the hormone binding sites and two β-subunits (90,000 Da), which exhibit ATP binding activity and tyrosine kinase activity on their cytosolic domains (21, 42).

A dominant theme in the 1970s was that insulin binding to its receptor could account for insulin action beyond the receptor. Therefore, exercise-induced increments in glucose uptake were attributed to increments in insulin binding (53). With the introduction of the in vitro, isolated muscle preparation for insulin binding (55), it became possible to study concomitantly the insulin bound to a muscle and its glucose uptake. We applied these procedures to study whether the effects of acute alterations in glucose uptake and metabolism were accompanied by concomitant alterations in insulin binding to skeletal muscles.

With mice we observed that after nonexhaustive exercise, glucose uptake and rates of glycolysis and glycogenesis were increased in soleus and EDL muscles, but insulin binding was not altered (14). After exhaustive exercise similar increments occurred in glucose uptake and metabolism, but insulin binding remained unaltered in the soleus and decreased in the EDL (11) (Figure 4). Conversely, we were able to reduce glucose uptake and metabolism with corticosterone while not altering insulin binding (84).

We also developed a procedure to measure insulin binding in human muscle (9). When we used exercise protocols that were known to increase glucose uptake, we found that insulin binding remained unaltered after moderate exercise (60 min, < 60% $\dot{V}O_2$max) and very markedly decreased (40-50% reductions) immediately after and for 60 min after heavy exercise (60 min, 69-85% $\dot{V}O_2$max) (12) (Figure 5). Similar decrements were observed in insulin bound to monocytes after heavy exercise; this was attributed to an unknown, dialyzable factor in the serum of exercised individuals (60). Collectively, these data suggest that acute alterations in glucose uptake in exercising skeletal muscles cannot be accounted for by changes in insulin binding to its receptor.

Insulin Receptor Kinase Activity and Glucose Transport

The discovery of insulin-stimulated tyrosine kinase activity (protein tyrosine kinase EC 2.7.1.112) on the insulin receptor β-subunit led to the proposal that insulin's various biological effects may be mediated via the kinase activity of its receptor (42).

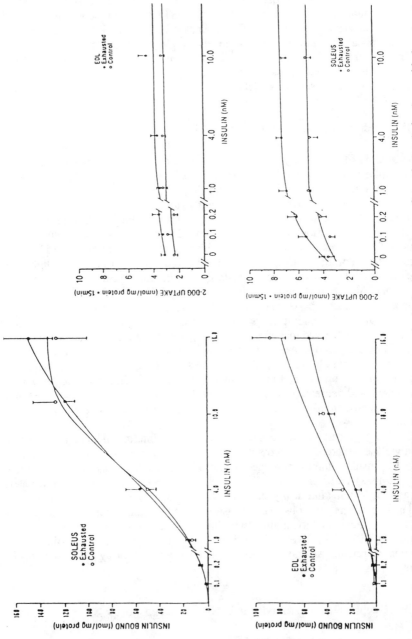

Figure 4. Increased uptake of 2-DOG in muscle from exercised mice in the absence of any change (soleus), or with decrements (EDL), in insulin binding (11).

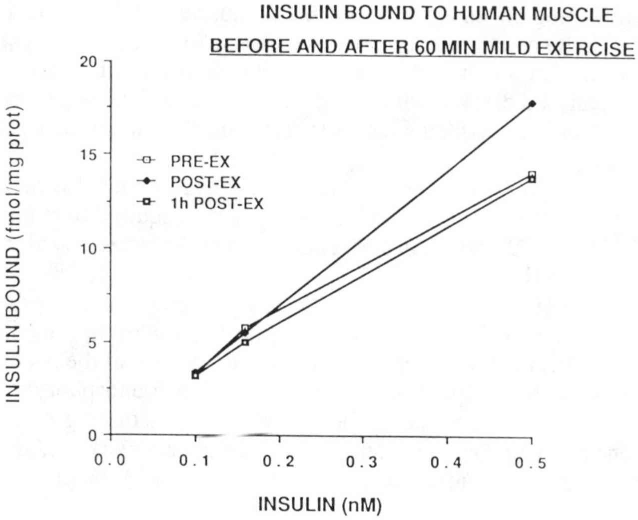

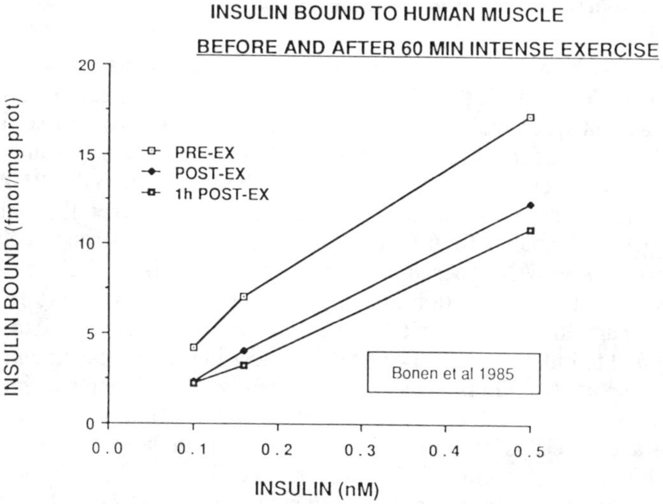

INSULIN BOUND TO HUMAN MUSCLE
BEFORE AND AFTER 60 MIN MILD EXERCISE

INSULIN BOUND TO HUMAN MUSCLE
BEFORE AND AFTER 60 MIN INTENSE EXERCISE

Bonen et al 1985

Figure 5. Unaltered insulin binding in human skeletal muscle after 1 hour of mild exercise (<60% VO₂max) and decrements in insulin binding after 1 hour of intense exercise (69-85% VO₂max) (12).

Yet, despite considerable evidence for autophosphorylation of the receptor and subsequent phosphorylation of other substrates by the receptor, in various tissues including skeletal muscle (15, 32, 54), little consistent evidence is available to demonstrate that phosphorylation is *the* signal to convey the postreceptor effects of insulin. In insulin-resistant obese mice, soleus muscle glucose uptake is known to be reduced. In addition, insulin receptor tyrosine kinase activity for phosphorylating itself and exogenous substrates is also lowered, suggesting that this kinase activity is central to maintaining normal glucose uptake in muscle. Yet, in trained animals a lower tyrosine kinase activation occurred in response to insulin than in sedentary animals (23), despite the known increments in glucose uptake in trained muscles (22, 85, also unpublished data). Such discrepant results cast doubt on whether protein kinase activation is an essential step for signaling the effects of insulin after it has bound to the receptor.

Similar disagreements on the receptor kinase function are found elsewhere. Some studies indicate that protein tyrosine kinase activity is not required to stimulate glucose uptake (26, 41, 61, 79), whereas others demonstrate that protein tyrosine kinase activity of the receptor is required for glucose transport (18, 24, 28). The belief that the insulin stimulates the tyrosine-specific autophosphorylation of the insulin receptor on its β-subunit, which then results in the activation of its exogenous protein kinase activity, has not been borne out. Insulin stimulation of the insulin receptor kinase can occur in the complete absence of β-subunit autophosphorylation (62). It appears that the quest for determining the signal(s) for transmitting insulin action after this hormone has bound to its receptor is exceedingly complex, and the current experimental tools may be inadequate (see 74).

Glucose Transporters (GT) and Glucose Transport

Attention is now being focused on the role of the GT in skeletal muscle. To date, most of our knowledge about the GT is derived from studies on adipocytes and red blood cells. Recent work indicates that the GT mRNA is a 2.8-kilobase transcript that is quite homologous in all rat and human insulin-insensitive and insulin-sensitive tissues examined, except the liver. The relative abundance in GT mRNA differs among tissues (25). The greater than 97% sequence identity of over 492 amino acids between rat (6) and human GTs (63) in cDNA probe suggests a strong evolutionary conservation of GT activity. These results suggest that it is likely that the GTs from most tissues, except liver, function in a similar manner. Yet, Wang (93) has proposed that there are different GTs in adipocytes and muscle. Obviously, experimental proof is required to link the tissue specific differences in GT to concomitant changes in glucose transport. Only in this manner can it be discovered whether the putative differences or similarities of GTs in different tissues are biologically important.

At any instant the GT is presumed to possess only a single glucose binding site. Work with nontransported glucose derivatives in red blood cells indicates that the orientation of glucose is preserved during translocation: the C-1 end of the sugar interacts with the transporter at the external face, and the C-6 end interacts at the cytoplasmic face (3). By measuring glucose transport activity of reconstituted liposomes, Kono et al. (49) have provided evidence that changes in cytochalasin B binding correspond to changes in the distribution of GTs. The number of GTs in plasma membranes prepared from isolated rat adipocytes can be determined by quantifying the specific binding of cytochalasin B to the membranes.

Current knowledge about the GT indicates (a) that it is a glycoprotein (44), (b) that insulin promotes the translocation of the GT from an intracellular site to the plasma membrane (20, 83), and (c) that this is an energy-dependent process (50). Karnieli et al. (43) demonstrated elegantly (a) the reciprocal effects of insulin on GT loss from the low-density microsomes to their appearance in the plasma membrane ($T_{1/2}$ of 2.5 min) and (b) the reciprocal reversal of these steps in the presence of anti-insulin antibody ($T_{1/2}$ of 9 min). Thus, in the adipocytes there is convincing evidence that insulin increases the number of GTs in plasma membranes via a rapid, energy-dependent translocation of the GTs from a specific intracellular pool. The appearance of GTs preceded the appearance of increased glucose transport activity ($T_{1/2}$ of 4 min) by 1.5 minutes (43).

Recently, it has been shown that there are two forms of GT, an immature form that is insulin-insensitive to translocation in fat cells and an insulin-sensitive form that is translocated from the low-density microsomal pool to the membrane. The immature form is located only in the high-density microsomal pool, suggesting that it is synthesized in the endoplasmic reticulum to be transformed to insulin-sensitive GT in the low-density microsomal pool by the addition of charged sugar residues (35, 58, 59).

It was recently found that glucose transport can be dissociated from GTs in the plasma membrane. For example, isoproterenol reduces 3-O-MG transport in fat cells without altering the number of GTs in the plasma membranes (40) (Figure 6). Similarly, cycloheximide reduces GTs by 50% in the plasma membrane while glucose

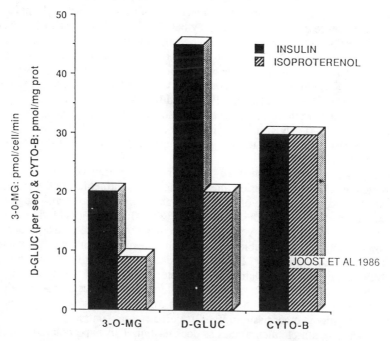

Figure 6.   Dissociation between glucose transport and the number of glucose transporters in the plasma membrane of rat adipocytes (drawn from data in ref. 40).

transport in these membranes is not altered (4). This suggests that GT numbers alone in the plasma membrane do not fully account for glucose transport rates. Recent evidence of changes in GT affinity and cooperativity that occur in the presence of insulin must also be considered (30).

Glucose Transporters and Skeletal Muscle

The known sequence of the GT (6, 63) conveys little information about the physiological role of GTs, particularly in skeletal muscle, in which glucose transport is rapidly activated with contractility in the absence of insulin and in the absence of changes in insulin binding (see above). Therefore, pertinent questions are (a) whether it is reasonable to expect that the GTs might also be mobilized independently of insulin binding to its receptor, and (b) whether there are differences in GT in oxidative and glycolytic types of skeletal muscle. We believe that persuasive circumstantial evidence does indeed suggest that (a) GT are mobilized in the absence of insulin, (b) GT affinity and activity may be altered by contractile activity, and (c) there are likely GT differences among FT and ST types of muscles.

Measurement of GTs, via cytochalasin B binding, in skeletal muscle has been accomplished with great difficulty by several investigators (46, 47, 94, 95). From this work with ^{3}H-cytochalasin B binding to quantify the GTs, skeletal muscle plasma membranes exhibited the following characteristics: (a) D-glucose inhibitable ^{3}H-cytochalasin B binding; (b) time-dependent cytochalasin B inhibition of D-glucose (not L-glucose) uptake by plasma membranes; (c) saturable ^{3}H-cytochalasin B binding in the presence of excess unlabeled cytochalasin B (10 μM); and (d) saturable binding increasing proportionally with increasing membrane protein in the binding assay (46, 48, 94). The transporter in muscle has been identified as a polypeptide with a mobility (SDS polyacrylamide electrophoresis) corresponding to a molecular weight of 45,000-50,000. We have found that GT differences exist between different types of skeletal muscles that parallel their differences in glucose uptake (Figure 7). Apparent translocation from intracellular pools to the plasma membrane has also been shown (46, 94). Thus, it is this insulin-induced increase in GT in the plasma membranes that is thought to initiate glucose uptake in muscle at rest after insulin has bound to its receptor.

The GT translocation hypothesis may or may not be important when skeletal muscle is contracting and for some period after contraction. Contractile activity stimulates glucose uptake in the absence of insulin (see above), and this remains augmented for some time after contractions have ceased (27, 70). Also, glycolytic muscle is quite unresponsive to insulin, yet its ability to increase glucose uptake, when contracting, can be quite remarkable (72). At such times insulin binding is not altered or even decreased in muscle (12, 14). These data suggest that the increase in glucose transport cannot be explained by a greater activation of the insulin signal.

This, however, does not imply that GT translocation is not occurring, merely that insulin is likely not involved, because insulin-mimetic agents and drugs can also affect GT mobility in other tissues (36, 80). Furthermore, contractile activity hyperpolarizes skeletal muscle membranes as does insulin. This hyperpolarization alone rapidly ($\leqslant$ 1 s) increases glucose transport in muscle (101, 102) and may therefore also initiate GT translocation in an insulinlike manner. Glucose uptake is increased

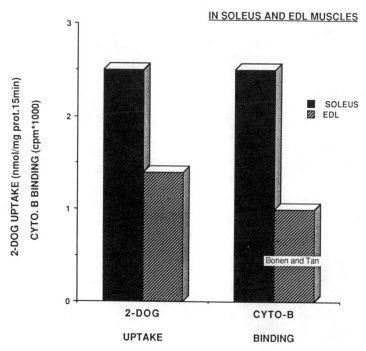

Figure 7. Heterogeneity of glucose transporters and 2-DOG uptake in skeletal muscle (unpublished data).

by hyperpolarization and can be further increased by the addition of insulin (57) (Figure 7), a situation that is similar to the additive effects of contractile activity and insulin on glucose uptake in whole muscle (65).

An alternative or concomitant means to increase glucose transport may involve changing the affinity of the GT. Certainly, there has been some question as to whether GT translocation is the only mechanism involved in stimulating glucose transport. In fat cells 3-O-MG transport is increased 10- to 20-fold, whereas the insulin-induced increase in GT is only 4-fold (81). Similarly, in skeletal muscle only a 2-3 fold increase of GTs has been noted in the presence of insulin, when in fact a much greater increase in glucose transport occurred (i.e., 5-fold) in such muscle (46). Therefore, it has been suggested that GT may undergo conformational changes when they are brought to the membrane. Indeed, in rat brown adipose tissue, insulin increases the Hill coefficient of plasma membrane GT for cytochalasin B from 1.1 to 2.2, indicating the presence of positive cooperativity among transporters; a decrease in the Kd (apparent dissociation constant) of GT to cytochalasin B indicated an increase in the affinity of plasma membrane GT (30) (Figure 8). Interestingly, in the absence of insulin, analogous changes have been found in GT of brown adipose tissues in cold-acclimated rats (31). Thus, not only is the translocation of GT altered but so

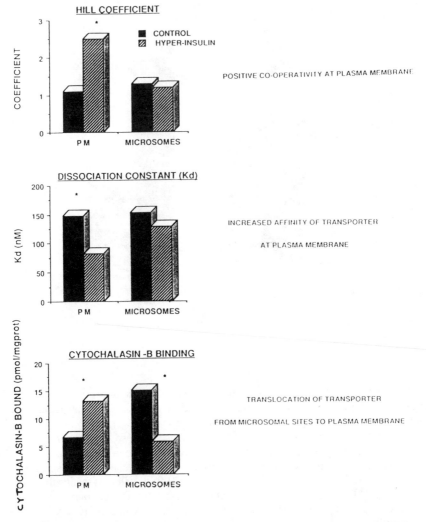

Figure 8. Effects of insulin on properties of glucose transporters in rat brown adipose tissues (drawn from data in ref. 30).

are the properties and behavior of GT, either by insulin or noninsulin factors (e.g., cold exposure).

We speculate that in contracting skeletal muscle, both translocation of GT and changes in GT affinity may occur because of the recent demonstration by Ploug et al. (70) that both Vmax and Km of 3-O-MG transport are altered in contracting skeletal muscle. Furthermore, the observation that GT in skeletal muscles are primarily associated with the transverse tubules, which constitute about 70-80% of the total surface of the muscle membrane, might suggest that this location of GT provides for an efficient distribution of glucose into muscle. Alternatively, it has been suggested that the GTs located here are of minor importance and are nascent (16), implying that these may be recruited when muscles begin to contract. Experimental evidence is required to elucidate these possibilities. Finally, the augmented glucose transport after exercise disappears rapidly in the absence of insulin (70), but at different rates in soleus and RG. This at least suggests that GT mobility, GT affinity, and/or GT cooperativity may differ among muscles, presuming that the experimental treatment involved (anaesthesia) is not dictating such observations.

Muscle Activity as the Stimulus for Glucose Uptake

A unifying physiological phenomenon in skeletal muscle, whatever the biochemical mechanisms, that seems to account for rapid and chronic changes in glucose uptake by muscle is the activity pattern of that muscle. Thus, in general, when muscle activity is increased, glucose uptake is also increased, and when muscle activity is reduced, glucose uptake is also reduced. This idea is supported by experimental models of muscle hypoactivity and muscle hyperactivity.

Decreasing Muscle Activity

When muscle activity is reduced by anaesthesia, a large decrease in glucose utilization occurs in postural muscles (soleus and adductor longus) but not in nonpostural muscles (EDL, tibialis anterior, epitrochlearis) (37, 67). Limb immobilization progressively lowers glucose uptake with time (66). Similarly, denervation rapidly reduces glucose uptake in soleus (−49%) and plantaris (−58%) by 3 hours after surgery, whereas no effects on glucose uptake were observed in the gastrocnemius muscle in the first 24 hours after surgery (87). Others have also shown that glucose uptake and utilization are reduced after denervation in soleus, epitrochlearis, and diaphragm (82). With prolonged denervation glucose uptake was also lowered in denervated plantaris and gastrocnemius, which lost their responsiveness to insulin, as did the soleus (87). The only model that runs counter to the idea that glucose uptake is reduced with reduced muscle activity is the hindlimb suspension model. Short-term (6 days) or long-term (28 days) hindlimb suspension increases glucose uptake in soleus muscle but not in the EDL (8, 33).

Increasing Muscle Activity

When activity in soleus and EDL muscle is increased either by stretch (78), or by compensatory activity in the diaphragm, glucose uptake is increased (82). Muscular exercise also increases the glucose transport (3-O-MG) in diabetic skeletal muscle (90). With chronic muscle activity, such as provided by exercise training, glucose uptake is increased in the trained muscles (22, 85). Recent work in this laboratory suggests that the effects of training are not due simply to the effects of the last exercise bout because glucose metabolism remain greater in trained animals for up to 96 hours after the last exercise bout (unpublished data).

These data suggest strongly that the activity level of a muscle is probably a primary determinant of muscle glucose uptake and utilization, with insulin providing an additional regulatory role that is additive to the effects provoked by contractile activity or inactivity. Insulin is clearly required to sustain intramuscular enzymatic activities (91) for postreceptor glucose disposal. Thus, in muscle, activity level may well be the primary determinant for glucose transport across the membrane.

Summary

The recent observations on glucose transport in skeletal muscle do correlate reasonably with the observations on GT activity. For example, the increase in Vmax of glucose transport during contraction may be explained in terms of the hypothesis that translocation brings more GT to the membrane. The reduction in glucose Km suggests strongly that the GT affinity is increased, and it corresponds to other data for the GTs in which the Hill coefficient increases and the Kd decreases (30). These alterations in the properties of GT support current thinking that translocation is not the only means to increase glucose transport. Furthermore, the postexercise increase in glucose transport is maintained by low levels of insulin in vivo (99) and requires maintenance of protein synthesis; this corresponds to the idea that new GTs are synthesized in the high-density microsomal fraction of the cell. The additive stimulation of insulin and contraction on glucose transport suggest that this requires independent mechanisms, possibly involving the additional recruitment of intracellular GTs or nascent surface GTs by contraction, or involving altering the properties of GTs located at the plasma membrane. The idea of inactive GTs in the membrane may also manifest itself as a decrease in the Km for glucose transport when and if nascent GTs are activated. These nascent GTs might be those GTs found in the transverse tubules of skeletal muscle (16). Recent observations that glucose transport can be dissociated from the number of GTs in the plasma membrane (4, 40) suggest that mechanisms other than GT translocation require further investigation as having a major role in facilitating glucose transport.

Clearly, skeletal muscle is a dynamic tissue in which glucose transport is rapidly altered in response to the muscle's activity. As such, it represents an excellent system in which to investigate putative roles for various mechanisms believed to alter glucose transport.

References

1. Ahlborg, G.; Felig, P. Influence of glucose ingestion on fuel-hormone response during prolonged exercise. J. Appl. Physiol. 41:683-688; 1976.

2. Ashcroft, S.J.H.; Stubbs, M. The glucose sensor in HIT cells is the glucose transporter. FEBS Lett. 219:311-315; 1987.

3. Baldwin, S.A.; Lienhard, G.E. Glucose transport across plasma membranes: facilitated diffusion systems. Trends in Biochem. Sci. 6:208-211; 1981.

4. Baly, D.L.; Horuk, R. Dissociation of insulin-stimulated glucose transport from the translocation of glucose carriers in rat adipose cells. J. Biol. Chem. 262:21-24; 1987.

5. Berger, M.; Hagg, S.A.; Goodman, M.N.; Ruderman, N.B. Glucose metabolism in perfused skeletal muscle. Effects of starvation, diabetes, fatty acids, acetoacetate, insulin and exercise. Biochem. J. 158:191-202; 1976.

6. Birnbaum, M.J.; Haspel, H.C.; Rosen, O.M. Cloning and characterization of a cDNA encoding the rat brain glucose-transporter protein. Proc. Natl. Acad. Sci. USA 83:5784-5788; 1986.

7. Bonen, A.; Clune, P.A.; Tan, M.H. Chronic exercise increases insulin binding in muscles but not liver. Am. J. Physiol. 251:E196-E203; 1986.

8. Bonen, A.; Elder, G.C.B.; Tan, M.H. Hindlimb suspension increases insulin binding and glucose metabolism. J. Appl. Physiol. 65:1833-1839, 1988.

9. Bonen, A.; Hood, D.A.; Tan, M.H.; Sopper, M.M.; Begin-Heick, N. Insulin binding in human skeletal muscle. Biochim. Biophys. Acta 801:171-176; 1984.

10. Bonen, A.; Malcolm, S.A.; Kilgour, R.D.; MacIntyre, K.P.; Belcastro, A.N. Glucose ingestion before and during intense exercise. J. Appl. Physiol. 50:766-771; 1981.

11. Bonen, A.; Tan, M.H. Dissociation between insulin binding and glucose utilization after intense exercise in mouse skeletal muscles. Horm. Metab. Res. (in press).

12. Bonen, A.; Tan, M.H.; Clune, P.; Kirby, R.L. Effects of exercise on insulin binding to human muscle. Am. J. Physiol. 248:E403-E408; 1985.

13. Bonen, A.; Tan, M.H.; Watson-Wright, W.M. Insulin binding and glucose uptake differences in rodent skeletal muscles. Diabetes 30:702-704; 1981.

14. Bonen, A.; Tan, M.H.; Watson-Wright, W.M. Effects of exercise on insulin binding and glucose metabolism in muscle. Can. J. Physiol. Pharmacol. 62:1500-1504; 1984.

15. Burant, C.F.; Treutelaar, M.K.; Landreth, G.E.; Buse, M.G. Phosphorylation of insulin receptors solubilized from rat skeletal muscle. Diabetes 33:704-708; 1984.

16. Burdett, E.; Beeler, T.; Klip, A. Distribution of glucose transporters and insulin receptors in the plasma membrane and transverse tubules of skeletal muscle. Arch. Biochem. Biophys. 253:279-286; 1987.

17. Challiss, R.A.J.; Hayes, D.J.; Radda, G.K. An investigation of arterial insufficiency in the rat hindlimb. Correlation of skeletal muscle bloodflow and glucose utilization in vivo. Biochem. J. 240:395-401; 1986.

18. Chou, C.K.; Dull, T.J.; Russell, D.S.; Gherzi, R.; Lebwohl, D.; Ullrich, A.; Rosen, O.M. Human insulin receptors mutated at the ATP-binding site

lack protein tyrosine kinase activity and fail to moderate post-receptor effects of insulin. J. Biol. Chem. 262:1842-1847; 1987.

19. Costill, D.L.; Coyle, E.; Dalsky, G.; Evans, W.; Fink, W.; Hoopes, D. Effects of elevated plasma FFA and insulin on muscle glycogen usage during exercise. J. Appl. Physiol. 43:695-699; 1977.

20. Cushman, S.W.; Wardzala, L.J. Potential mechanism of insulin action on glucose transport in the isolated rat adipose cell. Apparent translocation of intracellular transport systems to the plasma membrane. J. Biol. Chem. 255:4758-4762; 1980.

21. Czech, M. The nature and the regulation of the insulin receptor: structure and function. Annu. Rev. Physiol. 47:357-381; 1985.

22. Davis, T.A.; Klahr, S.; Tegtmyer, E.D.; Osborne, D.F.; Howard, T.L.; Karl, I.E. Glucose metabolism in epitrochlearis muscle of acutely exercised and trained rats. Am. J. Physiol. 250:E137-E143; 1986.

23. Dohm, G.L.; Sinha, M.K.; Caro, J.F. Insulin receptor binding and protein kinase activity in muscles of trained rats. Am. J. Physiol. 252:E170-E175; 1987.

24. Ebina, Y.; Araki, E.; Taira, M.; Shimada, F.; Mori, M.; Craik, C.S.; Siddle, K.; Pierce, S.B.; Roth, R.A.; Butler, W.J. Replacement of lysine residue 1030 in the putative ATP binding region of the insulin receptor abolishes insulin- and antibody-stimulated glucose uptake and receptor kinase activity. Proc. Nat. Acad. Sci. USA 84:704-708; 1987.

25. Flier, J.S.; Mueckler, M.; McCall, A.L.; Lodish, H.F. Distribution of glucose transporter messenger RNA transcripts in tissues of rat and man. J. Clin. Invest. 79:657-661; 1987.

26. Forsayeth, J.R.; Caro, J.F.; Sinha, M.K.; Maddox, B.A.; Goldfine, I.D. Monoclonal antibodies to the human insulin receptor that activate glucose transport but not insulin receptor kinase activity. Proc. Natl. Acad. Sci. USA 84:3448-3451; 1987.

27. Garretto, L.P.; Richter, E.A.; Goodman, M.N.; Ruderman, N.B. Enhanced muscle glucose metabolism after exercise in the rat: the two phases. Am. J. Physiol. 246:E471-E475; 1984.

28. Gherzi, R.; Russell, D.S.; Taylor, S.I.; Rosen, O.M. Reevaluation of the evidence that an antibody to the insulin receptor is insulinmimetic without activating the protein tyrosine kinase activity of the receptor. J. Biol. Chem. 262:16900-16905; 1987.

29. Gottesman, I.; Mandarino, L.; Nordink, G.; Rizza, R,; Gerich, J. Insulin increases the maximum velocity for glucose uptake without altering the Michaelis constant in man. Evidence that insulin increases glucose uptake merely by providing additional transport sites. J. Clin. Invest. 70:1310-1314; 1982.

30. Greco-Perotto, R.; Assimacopoulos-Jeannet, F.; Jeanrenaud, B. Insulin modifies the properties of glucose transporters in rat brown adipose tissue. Biochem. J. 247:63-68; 1987.

31. Greco-Perotto, R.; Zaninetti, D.; Assimacopoulos-Jeannet, F.; Bobbioni, E.; Jeanrenaud, B. Stimulatory effect of cold adaptation on glucose utilization by

brown adipose tissue. Relationship with changes in the glucose transporter system. J. Biol. Chem. 262:7732-7736; 1987.

32. Häring, H.U.; Machicao, F.; Kirsch, D.; Rinninger, F.; Holzl, J.; Eckel, J.; Bachmann, W. Protein kinase activity of the insulin receptor from muscle. FEBS Lett. 175:229-234; 1984.

33. Henriksen, E.J.; Tischler, M.E.; Johnson, D.G. Increased response to insulin of glucose metabolism in the 6-day unloaded rat soleus muscle. J. Biol. Chem. 261:10707-10712; 1986.

34. Hom, F.G.; Goodner, C.J. Insulin dose response characteristics among individual muscle and adipose tissues measured in the rat in vivo with ^{3}(H)2-deoxyglucose. Diabetes 33:153-159; 1984.

35. Horuk, R.; Matthaei, S.; Olefsky, J.M.; Baly, D.L.; Cushman, S.W. Simpson, I.A. Biochemical and functional heterogeneity of rat adipocyte glucose transporters. J. Biol. Chem. 261:1823-1828; 1986.

36. Jacobs, D.B.; Yung, C.Y. Sulfonylurea potentiates insulin-induced recruitment of glucose transport carrier in rat adipocytes. J. Biol. Chem. 260:2593-2596; 1985.

37. James, D.E.; Jenkins, A.B.; Kraegen, E.W. Heterogeneity of insulin action in muscle: influence of blood flow. Am. J. Physiol. 248:E422-E430; 1986.

38. James, D.E.; Kraegen, E.W.; Chisholm, D.J. Muscle glucose metabolism in exercising rats: comparison with insulin stimulation. Am. J. Physiol. 248:E575-E580; 1985.

39. Jandrain, B.; Krzentowski, G.; Pinney, F.; Masora, F.; Lacroix, M.; Luyckx, A.; Lefebvre, P. Metabolic availability of glucose ingestion 3h before prolonged exercise in humans. J. Appl. Physiol.: Respir. Environ. Exerc. Physiol. 56:1314-1319; 1984.

40. Joost, H.G.; Weber, T.M.; Cushman, S.W.; Simpson, I.A. Insulin-stimulated glucose transport in rat adipose cells. Modulation of transporter intrinsic activity by isoproterenol and adenosine. J. Biol. Chem. 261:10033-10036; 1986.

41. Joost, H.G.; Weber, T.M.; Cushman, S.W.; Simpson, I.A. Activity and phosphorylation state of glucose transporters in plasma membranes from insulin-, isoproterenol-, and phorbol-ester treated rat adipose cells. J. Biol. Chem. 262:11261-11267; 1987.

42. Kahn, R.C.; Crettaz, M. Insulin receptors and the molecular mechanisms of insulin action. Diabetes Metab. Rev. 1:203-227; 1985.

43. Karnieli, E.; Zarnowski, J.; Hissin, P.J.; Simpson, I.A.; Salans, L.B.; Cushman, S.W. Insulin-stimulated translocation of glucose transport systems in the isolated rat adipose cell. Time course, reversal, insulin concentration dependency, and relationship to glucose transport activity. J. Biol. Chem. 256:4772-4777; 1981.

44. Kasahara, M.; Hinckle, P.C. Reconstitution and purification of the D-glucose transporter from human erythrocytes. J. Biol. Chem. 252:7384-7390; 1977.

45. Katz, A.; Broberg, S.; Sahlin, K.; Wahren, J. Leg glucose uptake during maximal dynamic exercise in humans. Am. J. Physiol. 251:E65-E70; 1986.

46. Klip, A.; Ramlal, T.; Young, A.; Holloszy, J.O. Insulin-induced transloca-
    tion of glucose transporters in rat hindlimb muscles. FEBS Lett. 224:224-230;
    1987.

47. Klip, A.; Walker, D. The glucose transport system of muscle plasma mem-
    branes: characterization by means of [3H]Cytochalasin B binding. Arch. Bi-
    ochem. Biophys. 221:175-187; 1983.

48. Klip, A.; Walker, D.; Ransome, K.J.; Schroer, D.W.; Lienhard, G.E. Iden-
    tification of the glucose transporter in rat skeletal muscle. Arch. Biochem.
    Biophys. 226:198-205; 1983.

49. Kono, T.; Robinson, F.W.; Blevins, T.L.; Ezaki, O. Evidence that translo-
    cation of the glucose transport activity is the major mechanism of insulin ac-
    tion on glucose transport in fat cells. J. Biol. Chem. 257:10942-10947; 1982.

50. Kono, T.; Suzuki, K.; Damsey, L.E.; Robinson, F.W.; Blevins, T.L. Energy-
    dependent and protein synthesis-independent recyling of the insulin-sensitive
    glucose transport mechanism in fat cells. J. Biol. Chem. 256:6400-6407; 1981.

51. Krzentowski, G.; Jandrain, B.; Pinney, F.; Mosora, F.; Lacroix, M.; Luyckx,
    A.S.; Lefebvre, P.J. Availability of glucose given orally during exercise. J.
    Appl. Physiol.: Respir. Environ. Exerc. Physiol. 56:315-320; 1984.

52. Kubo, K.; Foley, J.E. Rate-limiting steps for insulin-mediated glucose uptake
    into perfused rat hindlimb. Am. J. Physiol. 250:E100-E102; 1986.

53. Leblanc, J.; Nadeau, A.; Boulay, M.; Rousseau-Mignerom, S. Effects of physi-
    cal training and adiposity on glucose metabolism and 125^I-insulin binding to
    red blood cells. J. Appl. Physiol. 46:235-239; 1979.

54. LeMarchand-Brustel, Y.; Grimeaux, T.; Ballott, R.; van Obberghen, E. Insulin
    receptor tyrosine kinase is defective in skeletal muscle of insulin-resistant obese
    mice. Nature 315:676-679; 1985.

55. LeMarchand-Brustel, Y.; Jeanrenaud, B.; Freychet, P. Insulin binding and
    effects in isolated soleus muscle of lean and obese mice. Am. J. Physiol.
    234:E348-E358; 1978.

56. Martz, A.; Mookerjee, B.K.; Jung, C.Y. Insulin and phorbol esters affect the
    maximum velocity rather than the half-saturation constant of 3-O-methylglucose
    transport in rat adipocytes. J. Biol. Chem. 261:13606-13609; 1986.

57. Marunaka, Y.; Murayama, K.; Kitasato, H. Diverse effects of insulin-induced
    hyperpolarization on 3-O-methyl-d-glucose (3-O-MG) transport in frog skele-
    tal muscles. Horm. Metab. Res. 19:139-142; 1987.

58. Matthaei, S.; Garvey, W.T.; Horuk, R.; Hueschstaedt, T.P.; Olefsky, J.M.
    Human adipocyte glucose transport system: biochemical and functional heter-
    ogeniety of glucose carriers. J. Clin. Invest. 79:703-709; 1987.

59. Matthaei, S.; Olefsky, J.M.; Horuk, R. Biochemical characterization and sub-
    cellular distribution of the glucose transporter from rat brain microvessels.
    Biochim. Biophys. Acta 905:417-425; 1987.

60. Michel, G.; Vocke, T.; Fiehn, W.; Weicker, H.; Schwartz, W.; Bieger, P.
    Bidirectional alteration on insulin receptor affinity by different forms of physical
    exercise. Am. J. Physiol. 246:E153-E159; 1984.

61. Morgan, D.O.; Roth, R.A. Acute insulin action requires insulin receptor kinase activity: introduction of an inhibitory monoclonal antibody into mammalian cells blocks the rapid effects of insulin. Proc. Natl. Acad. Sci. USA 89:41-45; 1987.

62. Morrison, B.D.; Pessin, J.E. Insulin stimulation of the insulin receptor kinase can occur in the complete absence of B subunit autophosphorylation. J. Biol. Chem. 262:2861-2868; 1987.

63. Mueckler, M.M.; Caruso, C.; Baldwin, S.A.; Panico, M.; Blench, I.; Morris, H.R.; Allard, J.W.; Lienhard, G.E.; Lodish, H.F. Sequence and structure of a human glucose transporter. Science 229:941-945; 1985.

64. Narahara, H.T.; Ozand, P. Studies of tissue permeability: IX. The effect of insulin on the penetration of 3-methylglucose-^{3}H in frog muscle. J. Biol. Chem. 238:40-49; 1963.

65. Nesher, R.; Karl, I.E.; Kipnis, D.M. Dissociation of effects of insulin and contraction on glucose transport in rat epitrochlearis muscle. Am. J. Physiol. 249:C226-C232; 1985.

66. Nicholson, W.F.; Watson, P.A.; Booth, F.W. Glucose uptake and glycogenesis in muscles from immobilized limbs. J. Appl. Physiol. 56:431-435; 1984.

67. Penicaud, L.; Ferre, P.; Kande, J.; Leturque, A.; Issad, T.; Girard, J. Effect of anesthesia on glucose production and utilization in rats. Am. J. Physiol. 252:E365-E369; 1987.

68. Pirnay, F.; Criellard, J.M.; Pallikarakis, N.; Lacroix, M.; Mosora, F.; Krzentowski, G.; Luyckx, A.S.; Lefebvre, P.J. Fate of exogenous glucose during exercise of different intensities in man. J. Appl. Physiol. 53:1620-1624; 1982.

69. Ploug, T.; Galbo, H.; Richter, E.A. Increased muscle glucose uptake during contractions: no need for insulin. Am. J. Physiol. 247:E726-E731; 1984.

70. Ploug, T., Galbo, H.; Vinten, J.; Jorgensen, M.; Richter, E.A. Kinetics of glucose transport in rat muscle: effects of insulin and contractions. Am. J. Physiol. 253:E12-E20; 1987.

71. Richter, E.A.; Garretto, L.P.; Goodman, M.N.; Ruderman, N.B. Muscle glucose metabolism following exercise in the rat: increased sensitivity to insulin. J. Clin. Invest. 69:785-793; 1982.

72. Richter, E.A.; Garretto, L.P.; Goodman, M.N.; Ruderman, N.B. Enhanced muscle glucose metabolism after exercise: modulation by local factors. Am. J. Physiol. 246:E476-E482; 1984.

73. Richter, E.A.; Ploug, T.; Galbo, H. Increased muscle glucose uptake after exercise: no need for insulin during exercise. Diabetes 34:1041-1048; 1985.

74. Rosen, O. After insulin binds. Science 237:1452-1458; 1987.

75. Sasson, S.; Cerasi, E. Substrate regulation of the glucose transport system in rat skeletal muscle. Characterization and kinetic analysis in isolated soleus muscle and skeletal muscle cells in culture. J. Biol. Chem. 261:16827-16833; 1986.

76. Schultz, T.A.; Lewis, S.B.; Westbie, D.K.; Gerich, J.E.; Rushakoff, R.J.;

Wallin, J.D. Glucose delivery—a clarification of its role in regulating glucose uptake in rat skeletal muscle. Life Sci. 20:733-736; 1977.

77. Shoji, S. Effect of denervation on glucose uptake in rat soleus and extensor digitorum longus muscles. Muscle Nerve 9:69-72; 1986.

78. Shoji, S. Effects of stretch and starvation on glucose uptake of rat soleus and extensor digitorum longus muscles. Muscle Nerve 9:144-147; 1986.

79. Simpson, I.A.; Hedo, J.A. Insulin phosphorylation may not be a prerequisite for acute insulin action. Science 223:1301-1304; 1984.

80. Simpson, I.A.; Smith, U.; Cushman, S.W. Counterregulation of insulin-stimulated glucose transport by isoproterenol in rat adipose cells: modulation of intrinsic glucose transporter activity. Diabetes 66:1334-1338; 1983.

81. Simpson, I.A.; Yver, D.R.; Hissin, P.J.; Wardzala, L.J.; Karnieli, E.; Salans, L.B.; Cushman, S.W. Insulin-stimulated translocation of glucose transporters in the isolated rat adipose cells: characterization of subcellular fractions. Biochim. Biophys. Acta 763:343-407; 1983.

82. Smith, R.L.; Lawrence, J.C., Jr. Insulin action in denervated skeletal muscle. Evidence that the reduced stimulation of glycogen synthesis does not involve decreased insulin binding. J. Biol. Chem. 260:273-278; 1985.

83. Suzuki, K.; Kono, T. Evidence that insulin causes translocation of glucose transport activity to the plasma membrane from an intracellular storage site. Proc. Natl. Acad. Sci. USA 77:2542-2545; 1980.

84. Tan, M.H.; Bonen, A. The in vitro effects of corticosterone on insulin binding and glucose metabolism in mouse skeletal muscles. Can. J. Physiol. Pharmacol. 62:1460-1465; 1985.

85. Tan, M.H.; Bonen, A. Effect of exercise training on insulin binding and glucose metabolism in mouse soleus muscle. Can. J. Physiol. Pharmacol. 65:2231-2234; 1987.

86. Toyoda, N.; Flanagan, J.; Kono, T. Reassessment of insulin effects on the Vmax and Km values of hexose transport in isolated rat epididymal adipocytes. J. Biol. Chem. 262:2737-2745; 1987.

87. Turinsky, J. Dynamics of insulin resistance in denervated slow and fast muscles in vivo. Am. J. Physiol. 252:531-537; 1987.

88. Vranic, M.; Kawamori, R.; Pek, S.; Kovacevic, N.; Wrenshall, G.A. The essentiality of insulin and the role of glucagon in regulating glucose utilization and production during strenuous exercise in dogs. J. Clin. Invest. 57:245-255; 1976.

89. Walker, P.M.; Mickle, D.A.G.; Tanner, W.R.; Harding, R.; Romaschin, A.D. Decreased uptake of exogenous substrates following graded muscle stimulation. Am. J. Physiol. 246:H690-H695; 1984.

90. Wallberg-Henriksson, H. Repeated exercise regulates glucose transport capacity in skeletal muscle. Acta Physiol. Scand. 127:39-43; 1986.

91. Wallberg-Henriksson, H. Glucose transport in skeletal muscle. Influence of contractile activity, insulin, catecholamines and diabetes mellitus. Acta Physiol. Scand. (Supplementum 564); 1987.

92. Wallberg-Henriksson, H.; Holloszy, J.D. Contractile activity increases glucose uptake by muscle in severely diabetic rats. J. Appl. Physiol.: Respir. Environ. Exerc. Physiol. 57:1045-1049; 1984.

93. Wang, C. The D-glucose transporter is tissue-specific. Skeletal muscle and adipose tissue have a unique form of glucose transporter. J. Biol. Chem. 272:15689-15695; 1987.

94. Wardzala, L.J.; Jeanrenaud, B. Potential mechanism of insulin action on glucose transport in the isolated rat diaphragm. Apparent translocation of intracellular transport units to the plasma membrane. J. Biol. Chem. 256:7090-7093; 1981.

95. Wheeler, T.J.; Hauck, M.A. Reconstitution of the glucose transporter from rat skeletal muscle. Life Sci. 40:2309-2316; 1987.

96. Whitesell, R.R.; Abumrad, N.A. Increased affinity predominates in insulin stimulation of glucose transport in the adipocyte. J. Biol. Chem. 260:2894-2899; 1985.

97. Yki-Jarvinon, H.; Young, A.A.; Lamkin, C.; Foley, J.E. Kinetics of glucose disposal in whole body and across the forearm in man. J. Clin. Invest. 79:1013-1719; 1987.

98. Young, D.A.; Uhl, J.J.; Cartee, G.D.; Holloszy, J.O. Activation of glucose transport in muscle by prolonged exposure to insulin. J. Biol. Chem. 261:16049-16053; 1986.

99. Young, D.A.; Wallberg-Henriksson, H.; Sleeper, M.D.; and Holloszy, J.O. Reversal of the exercise-induced increase in muscle permeability to glucose. Am. J. Physiol. 253: E331-E335, 1987.

100. Young, J.C.; Garthwaite, S.M.; Bryan, J.E.; Cartier, L.J.; Holloszy, J.O. Carbohydrate feeding speeds reversal of enhanced glucose uptake in muscle after exercise. Am. J. Physiol. 245:R684-R688; 1983.

101. Zierler, K.; Rogus, E.M. Hyperpolarization as a mediator of insulin action: increased muscle glucose uptake induced electrically. Am. J. Physiol. 239:E21-E29; 1980.

102. Zierler, K.; Rogus, E.M. Rapid hyperpolarization of rat skeletal muscle induced by insulin. Biochim. Biophys. Acta 640:687-692; 1981.

Utilization of Fatty Acids During Exercise

John O. Holloszy

Washington University School of Medicine, St. Louis, Missouri, U.S.A.

Fatty acids stored as triglycerides and glucose stored as glycogen are the only quantitatively important energy sources during exercise. Of these, glycogen is the more important fuel for strenuous exercise that requires in the range of about 65% to 100% of $\dot{V}O_2$max. Liver glycogen is important because it is the major source of blood glucose, which is the primary substrate for the central nervous system. The reason for the importance of muscle glycogen for strenuous exercise is less well understood, but it has been shown empirically that strenuous exercise cannot be continued after muscle glycogen is depleted (2, 15). Glycogen cannot, however, serve as a major energy reservoir in animals. The energy yield from complete oxidation of carbohydrate is only about 4 kcal/g; furthermore, a gram of dry glycogen binds about 2 g of water. In contrast, oxidation of 1 g of fat yields 9 kcal; furthermore, triglycerides are nonpolar and are stored in nearly anhydrous form. As a result, a gram of fat stores more than 6 times as much energy as a gram of hydrated glycogen. Thus, it is not surprising that triglycerides rather than glycogen were selected as the major energy store during evolution.

Whereas glycogen stores can readily be depleted during a single bout of exercise, the amount of energy stored as triglycerides in the great majority of people greatly exceeds the possible caloric expenditure during a bout of exercise. For example, a 70-kg person with a body fat content of 7 kg has a fuel reserve of about 60,000 kcal in triglycerides. Fatty acids derived from lipolysis of triglycerides have two major roles as substrate during exercise. During prolonged strenuous exercise, for which muscle glycogen is essential, fatty acids serve as an important secondary fuel, which, by sparing glycogen, prolongs the exercise time before glycogen depletion and exhaustion occur. During mild exercise, fatty acids can serve as the primary fuel (24), making possible very prolonged activity, such as walking, even in the fasting state.

The major site of triglyceride storage is the cytoplasm of adipose cells. Small amounts of triglycerides are also present in the blood and in the cytoplasm of other cells, including muscle. The triglycerides stored in adipose tissue and muscle provide most of the FFA oxidized during exercise. Under physiological conditions, plasma triglycerides provide only a minor portion of the FFA oxidized during exercise (14).

Plasma FFA

Lipolysis of triglycerides stored in adipocytes is accelerated during exercise as the result of an increase in the activity of adipose-cell lipase. Adipose-cell lipase activity is regulated by hormones, the two most important of which are catechol-amines and insulin (10). Catecholamines stimulate adenylate cyclase, and the cyclic AMP formed serves as a second messenger in the activation of lipolysis. In con-trast, insulin inhibits lipolysis, which helps to explain why plasma FFA are higher in the fasted state, when insulin levels are low, than in the fed state.

During prolonged exercise there is usually an initial small decrease in plasma FFA concentration as the result of increased utilization; this is followed by a progressive increase, as lipolysis and FFA release accelerate (Figure 1). This rise in FFA is mediated in large part by the increasing β-adrenergic stimulus to the adipocytes during prolonged exercise. The decline in plasma insulin during exercise contributes fur-ther to the increase in lipolysis (10). In an individual studied under a given set of physiological conditions, the rate of plasma FFA turnover varies linearly with plasma concentration over the physiological range (12). The turnover rate is, of course, greater during exercise than at rest at a given plasma FFA concentration because

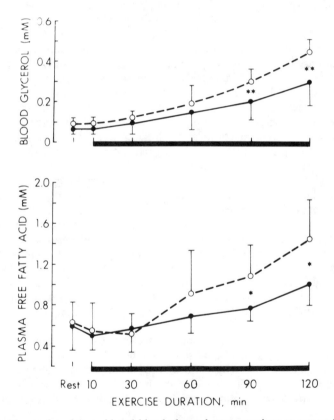

Figure 1.   Plasma free fatty acid and blood glycerol concentrations at rest and during cycle ergometer exercise before (open circles) and after (closed circles) a strenuous, 12-week program of training that resulted in a 30% increase in peak $\dot{V}O_2$. Values are means $\pm$ SD for 9 subjects at all time points, except for 120-min values, which are means $\pm$ SD for 6 subjects. (From ref. 20.)

of the greater rate of FFA oxidation; that is, both push, as determined by concentration, and pull, as determined by rate of oxidative metabolism, determine the rate of FFA utilization.

Little is known regarding the process by which FFAs are taken up by skeletal muscle. Evidence is accumulating that in hepatocytes and cardiac myocytes, a major portion of FFA influx occurs via a saturable process in which fatty acid transport is mediated by a specific carrier protein in the cell membrane (29). It is currently not known whether a similar transport system exists in skeletal muscle, nor is it known whether transport of FFAs can limit the rate of their utilization during exercise.

Fatty Acid Binding Proteins

Fatty acids are strongly hydrophobic and must therefore be bound to protein in order to be transported in aqueous medium. In plasma, this fatty acid binding and transport function is served by albumin. Most tissues, including skeletal muscle, contain fatty acid binding proteins (FABPs) that are thought to serve as intracellular carriers of fatty acids (11). On entering the muscle cell, fatty acids can either be stored as triglycerides or become part of the FABP-bound pool of FFA in the cytoplasm, where they are available for conversion to fatty acyl-CoA, transport into the mitochondria, and oxidation.

Intramuscular Triglycerides

Early studies of FFA turnover during exercise using [14C]-labeled fatty acids showed that during 60-120 min of exercise, plasma FFA accounted for only about 50% of the fat oxidized (13, 14). This finding provided the first good evidence suggesting that intramuscular triglycerides provide a significant amount of the fatty acids oxidized during prolonged exercise. Subsequent muscle biopsy studies have supported this interpretation (3, 7-9, 20, 22). Some of these studies are summarized in Table 1.

The triglyceride content of human skeletal muscle averages about 12 g/kg wet weight, although a wide range of higher and lower values occur (3, 7-9, 20), probably as the result of interindividual differences in the proportions of the different muscle fiber types, nutritional states, physical activity levels, and so on. Some of the large differences in muscle triglyceride concentration between studies may also be due to technical problems, including contamination of muscle biopsies with adipose tissue, resulting in erroneously high values, or hydrolysis of intramuscular triglycerides during handling of the biopsy sample, resulting in low values.

It appears that skeletal muscle triglyceride stores can be only partially depleted during exercise. Studies of the time course of the decrease in muscle triglycerides have not (to my knowledge) been performed, probably because of the technical difficulties involved. However, it appears from comparison of studies involving exercise of different durations that the decrease in muscle triglycerides that occurs during exercise is probably completed within 2-3 hours, leaving a residual of 6-8 g/kg wet

Table 1   Intramuscular Triglyceride Utilization During Exercise: A Summary of 4 Studies

Study	Subjects	Exercise	Duration (min)	Decrease in muscle[a] TG concentration (g/kg wet wt.)
Carlson et al. (3)	Untrained	Treadmill, 67% $\dot{V}O_2$max	99	2.2 ± 0.6
Essen et al. (7)	Trained	Cycle, 55% $\dot{V}O_2$max	60	3.0 ± 0.7
Hurley et al. (20)	Untrained	Cycle, 64% $\dot{V}O_2$max	110[b]	2.6 ± 1.1
	Trained[c]	Cycle, same[c]	110[b]	5.3 ± 1.9
Fröberg et al. (9)	Elite skiers	Ski race	447	7.4 ± 1.5

[a]In all of the studies, the biopsies were of the vastus lateralis muscle. [b] 6 men exercised 120 min, and 3 exercised 90 min. [c]The same men were re-studied after 12 weeks of intense exercise/training. The exercise test was of the same absolute intensity before and after training.

weight; thus, a similar amount of triglyceride remains in the muscles after many hours of exercise (3, 7-9, 20). A portion of this residual triglyceride could perhaps be nonavailable, structural lipid; however, most still appears to be in sarcoplasmic lipid droplets that are markedly reduced in size (22). The finding that the lipid droplets are not completely depleted suggests that after prolonged exercise, when plasma FFA levels are high, the rate of FFA influx into the intramuscular triglyceride pool balances their rate of efflux (i.e., synthesis and lipolysis are in equilibrium).

In the majority of studies, the decrease in muscle triglyceride concentration has been in the range of 2-6 g/kg wet weight (3, 7-9, 20). The largest decrease in muscle triglyceride concentration that has been reported occurred during a 7-hour–long ski race (Table 1; ref. 9). This very large decrease was made possible by very high initial muscle triglyceride stores; apparently, these elite endurance athletes develop very high muscle triglyceride stores as part of their adaptive response (9, 22). Interestingly, the residual muscle triglyceride level was very similar to that reported in most other studies, about 7 g/kg wet weight (9). It seems probable that by the time the muscle triglyceride stores stop decreasing, plasma FFA concentration has increased sufficiently to supply all of the muscles' FFA requirements. The factors involved in the regulation of lipolysis of muscle triglycerides during exercise are poorly understood. This is a fertile area for future research.

The Glucose–Fatty Acid Cycle

As first shown by Randle et al. (25, 26), oxidation of fatty acids inhibits glucose uptake, glycolysis, glycogenolysis, and pyruvate oxidation in cardiac muscle. These effects appear to be mediated in part by (a) the accumulation of citrate, which inhibits phosphofructokinase activity, resulting in accumulation of glucose-6-P, which inhibits hexokinase; and (b) inhibition of pyruvate dehydrogenase by the products of fatty acid oxidation, acetyl CoA and NADH. Randle and co-workers (25, 26) proposed that this phenomenon, which they termed the "glucose-fatty acid cycle," also occurred in other tissues, such as skeletal muscle, and played an important role in regulation of whole-body substrate metabolism. However, subsequent studies by a number of other investigators failed to show an inhibitory effect of fatty acids on glucose metabolism in skeletal muscle, leading them to conclude that the glucose–fatty acid cycle is limited to heart muscle (cf. 27, 28). This conclusion did not seem compatible with the extensive evidence that elevation of plasma FFA reduces carbohydrate utilization. This provided the stimulus to further research to determine whether or not glucose–fatty acid cycle activity occurs in skeletal muscle.

One approach that was used involved feeding a fat meal to raise plasma triglycerides, followed by a heparin injection to release lipoprotein lipase. This procedure results in a marked elevation of plasma FFA. It was found that raising FFA levels slows muscle glycogen depletion during exercise in humans (5) and rats (17, 28). Studies on rats further showed that elevation of plasma FFA slows liver glycogen depletion (17, 28) and markedly increases endurance (17). The increase in endurance appears to be due to the glycogen-sparing effect of increased FFA utilization. Studies on well-oxygenated perfused rat hindlimb muscles have further shown that fatty acids partially inhibit glucose uptake and glycogen depletion in muscle during contractile activity (27). It now seems clear, from the results of these and similar studies, that the glucose–fatty acid cycle functions in skeletal as well as heart muscle.

Effects of Endurance Exercise Training

One of the most important metabolic adaptations to endurance exercise training is an increased reliance on fat oxidation for energy during exercise. The glycogen-sparing effect of this adaptation undoubtedly plays a major role in the increase in endurance for prolonged exercise that occurs with training. As reviewed above, one mechanism for increasing the rate of fat oxidation is to raise plasma FFA levels. However, plasma FFA concentration is generally lower in the trained than in the untrained state during submaximal exercise of the same absolute intensity (Figure 1; refs. 20, 21, 30).

The lower plasma FFA concentration in the trained state appears to be due to slower lipolysis, probably as a result of the marked blunting of the catecholamine response, that is, a decreased beta-adrenergic stimulus (10, 30). The evidence that lipolysis is decreased includes the finding that blood glycerol concentration during exercise of the same intensity is lower after training (20, 30). Changes in plasma glycerol level usually reflect changes in the rate of lipolysis in adipose tissues (16). Measurements of ^{13}C-palmitate turnover during prolonged exercise of the same intensity, in a study of the effect of an intense, 12-week–long program of endurance training, showed approximately a 40% lower rate of palmitate appearance (i.e., release) in the trained state (6). The ^{13}C-palmitate oxidation data from this study provided evidence that the rate of oxidation of plasma FFA was reduced about 35%. This is not surprising in view of the reduced availability of plasma FFA to the skeletal muscles and the linear relationship between plasma FFA concentration and the rate of plasma FFA oxidation (12).

Despite the decreased availability and oxidation of plasma FFA, the rate of fat oxidation, estimated from the respiratory exchange ratio, was markedly higher in subjects performing the same exercise after, as compared to before, training (Figure 2). The source of the additional fatty acids used in the trained state appears to be the intramuscular triglyceride stores. As shown in Table 1, cycle ergometer exercise of the same duration and intensity resulted in roughly twice as great a decrease in muscle triglyceride concentration in the trained, as compared to the untrained, state (20). It is not clear whether the increased utilization of muscle triglyceride in the trained state confers any physiological advantage or is only a compensatory mechanism for the decreased β-adrenergic stimulation of lipolysis in adipose tissue. It is also not known how the greater rate of intramuscular triglyceride lipolysis is mediated in the trained state.

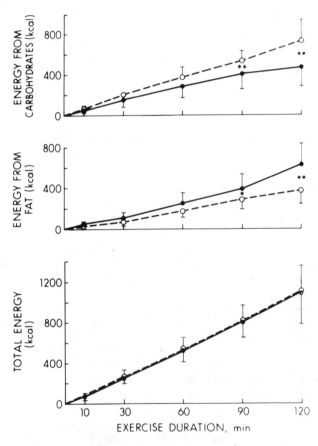

Figure 2. Cumulative total energy used, calculated from $\dot{V}O_2$; energy from fat oxidation; and energy from carbohydrate oxidation, calculated from R, during prolonged exercise before (open circles) and after (closed circles) training. See Figure 1 for details. (From ref. 20.)

Mechanism for Increased Oxidation of Fat in the Trained State

The rate of plasma FFA oxidation at a given work rate is a function of concentration (12). In view of the lower plasma FFA level during exercise of a given absolute submaximal intensity in the trained state (20), one mechanism that seems to be clearly ruled out as an explanation for the increased oxidation of fat is a greater availability of plasma FFA. However, plasma FFA concentration is only one of the factors that determines the concentration of fatty acids in the cytoplasm, and it is the concentration of fatty acids to which the mitochondria are exposed in the cytoplasm, not the plasma FFA concentration, that directly determines the rate of fat oxidation. In this context, another mechanism that might play a role in explaining the higher rate of fat oxidation in the trained state could be a higher cytoplasmic fatty acid concentration. Although this seems a reasonable possibility in view of the increased rate of lipolysis of intramuscular triglycerides, preliminary studies, in which fatty acids were measured in muscles of trained and sedentary rats at rest and after a bout of exercise, showed no difference in fatty acid concentration between trained and untrained muscle (Holloszy, unpublished results).

Endurance training results in an increase in muscle mitochondrial content and oxidative capacity (1, 4, 18, 19, 23). This adaptation includes an increase in the levels of activity of the enzymes involved in the activation of fatty acids, in their transport into the mitochondria, and in β-oxidation (23). As a consequence, when the mitochondrial fraction of muscles or whole homogenates of muscle are exposed to a given fatty acid concentration, the rate of fatty acid oxidation is higher in trained than in untrained muscle, roughly in proportion to the increased oxidative capacity (1, 23). If the preliminary finding that the cytoplasmic concentration of fatty acids is similar in trained and untrained muscle is confirmed, the increase in the enzymes responsible for fatty acid oxidation probably plays the primary role in accounting for the increased oxidation of fatty acids in the trained state. An additional factor may be a decreased availability of competing substrate as the result of slower rates of glycogenolysis and glycolysis.

This adaptation, by sparing glycogen by means of the glucose–fatty acid cycle, plays a major role in the increased ability to perform prolonged, strenuous exercise (i.e., increased endurance) in the trained state.

Acknowledgments

The author's research is supported by N.I.H. grants AG00425, DK 18986, and AG00078.

References

1. Baldwin, K.M.; Klinkerfuss, G.H.; Terjung, R.L.; Mole, P.A.; Holloszy, J.O. Respiratory capacity of white, red and intermediate muscle: adaptive response to exercise. Am. J. Physiol. 222:373-378; 1972.

2. Bergstrom, J.; Hermansen, L.; Hultman, E.; Saltin, B. Diet, muscle glycogen and physical performance. Acta Physiol. Scand. 71:140-150; 1967.

3. Carlson, L.A.; Ekelund, L.-G.; Fröberg, S.O. Concentration of triglycerides, phospholipids and glycogen in skeletal muscle and of free fatty acids and β-hydroxybutyric acid in blood in man in response to exercise. Eur. J. Clin. Invest. 1:248-254; 1971.

4. Chi, M.M.-Y.; Hintz, C.S.; Coyle, E.F.; Martin, W.H., III; Ivy, J.L.; Nemeth, P.M.; Holloszy, J.O.; Lowry, O.H. Effects of detraining on enzymes of energy metabolism in individual human muscle fibers. Am. J. Physiol. 244:C276-C287; 1983.

5. Costill, D.L.; Coyle, E.; Dalsky, G.; Evans, W.; Fink, W.; Hoopes, D. Effects of elevated plasma FFA and insulin on muscle glycogen usage during exercise. J. Appl. Physiol.: Respir. Environ. Exerc. Physiol. 43:695-699; 1977.

6. Dalsky, G.P.; Martin, W.H.; Hurley, B.; Matthews, D.; Bier, D.; Hagberg, J.; Holloszy, J.O. Oxidation of plasma FFA during endurance exercise. Med. Sci. Sports Exerc. 16:202; 1984.

7. Essen, B. Intramuscular substrate utilization during prolonged exercise. Ann. N.Y. Acad. Sci. 301:30-44; 1977.

8. Essen, B.; Hagenfeldt, L.; Kaijser, L. Utilization of blood-borne and intramuscular substrates during continuous and intermittent exercise in man. J. Physiol. (Lond.) 265:489-506; 1977.

9. Fröberg, S.O.; Mossfeldt, F. Effect of prolonged strenuous exercise on the concentration of triglycerides, phospholipids, and glycogen in muscles of man. Acta Physiol. Scand. 82:167-171; 1971.

10. Galbo, H. Hormonal and metabolic adaptations to exercise. New York: Thieme-Stratton; 1983:64-67.

11. Glatz, J.F.C.; Vandervusse, G.J.; Veerkamp, J.H. Fatty acid-binding proteins and their physiological significance. NIPS 3:41-43; 1988.

12. Hagenfeldt, L. Turnover of individual free fatty acids in man. Fed. Proc. 34:2236-2240; 1975.

13. Hagenfeldt, L.; Wahren, J. Human forearm muscle metabolism during exercise: II. Uptake, release and oxidation of FFA and glycerol. Scand. J. Clin. Lab. Invest. 21:263-276; 1968.

14. Havel, R.J.; Pernow, B.; Jones, N.L. Uptake and release of fatty acids and other metabolites in legs of exercising men. J. Appl. Physiol. 23:90-99; 1967.

15. Hermansen, L.; Hultman, E.; Saltin, B. Muscle glycogen during prolonged severe exercise. Acta Physiol. Scand. 71:129-139; 1967.

16. Hetenyi, G., Jr.; Perez, G.; Vranic, M. Turnover and precursor-product relationships of non-lipid metabolites. Physiol. Rev. 63:606-667; 1983.

17. Hickson, R.C.; Rennie, M.J.; Conlee, R.K.; Winder, W.W.; Holloszy, J.O. Effects of increased plasma fatty acids on glycogen utilization and endurance. J. Appl. Physiol. 43:829-833; 1977.

18. Holloszy, J.O. Biochemical adaptations in muscle. Effects of exercise on mitochondrial oxygen uptake and respiratory enzyme activity in skeletal muscle. J. Biol. Chem. 242:2278-2282; 1967.

19. Holloszy, J.O.; Coyle, E.F. Adaptations of skeletal muscle to endurance exercise and their metabolic consequences. J. Appl. Physiol. 56:831-838; 1984.

20. Hurley, B.F.; Nemeth, P.M.; Martin, W.H., III; Hagberg, J.M.; Dalsky, G.P.; Holloszy, J.O. Muscle triglyceride utilization during exercise: effect of training. J. Appl. Physiol. 60:562-567; 1986.

21. Koivisto, V.; Hendler, R.; Nadel, E.; Felig, P. Influence of physical training on the fuel-hormone response to prolonged low intensity exercise. Metabolism 31:192-197; 1982.

22. Lithell, H.; Örlander, J.; Schéle, R.; Sjödin, B.; Karlsson, J. Changes in lipoprotein-lipase activity and lipid stores in human skeletal muscle with prolonged heavy exercise. Acta Physiol. Scand. 107:257-261; 1979.

23. Molé, P.A.; Oscai, L.B.; Holloszy, J.O. Adaptation of muscle to exercise. Increase in levels of palmityl CoA synthetase, carnitine palmityltransferase, and palmityl CoA dehydrogenase and in the capacity to oxidize fatty acids. J. Clin. Invest. 50:2323-2330; 1971.

24. Phinney, S.D.; Bistrian, B.R.; Evans, W.J.; Gervino, E.; Blackburn, G.L. The human metabolic response to chronic ketosis: preservation of submaximal exercise capacity with reduced carbohydrate oxidation. Metabolism 32:769-776; 1984.

25. Randle, P.J.; Garland, P.B.; Hales, C.N.; Newsholme, E.A. The glucose fatty-acid cycle. Its role in insulin sensitivity and the metabolic disturbances of diabetes mellitus. Lancet 1:785-789; 1963.

26. Randle, P.J.; Newsholme, E.A.; Garland, P.B. Regulation of glucose uptake by muscle: 8. Effects of fatty acids, ketone bodies and pyruvate, and of alloxan diabetes and starvation, on the uptake and metabolic rate of glucose in rat heart and diaphragm muscles. Biochem. J. 93:652-665; 1964.

27. Rennie, M.J.; Holloszy, J.O. Inhibition of glucose uptake and glycogenolysis by availability of oleate in well-oxygenated perfused skeletal muscle. Biochem. J. 168:161-170; 1977.

28. Rennie, M.J.; Winder, W.W.; Holloszy, J.O. A sparing effect of increased plasma fatty acids on muscle and liver glycogen content in the exercising rat. Biochem. J. 156:647-655; 1976.

29. Stremmel, W. Fatty acid uptake by isolated rat heart myocytes represents a carrier-mediated transport process. J. Clin. Invest. 81:844-852; 1988.

30. Winder, W.W.; Hickson, R.C.; Hagberg, J.M.; Ehsani, A.A.; Mclane, J.A. Training-induced changes in hormonal and metabolic responses to submaximal exercise. J. Appl. Physiol. 46:766-771; 1979.

PART VII

Ion Regulation in Exercise

Acid-Base Regulation and Peter Stewart

John R. Sutton
McMaster University, Hamilton, Ontario, Canada

It was originally intended that Dr. Peter Stewart would make these introductory remarks. His approach to the already well-accepted physicochemical principles of acid-base regulation is quantitative and, therefore, more rigorous than that usually taken. Using "strong ion difference" (SID), he has made us appreciate the need to examine individual electrolyte changes as they affect acid-base regulation, as well as changes in PCO_2 and weak acids (A_{tot}). Perhaps his greatest contribution has been to create an awareness that some variables such as $[H^+]$ and HCO_3^- do not cause, but are the net result of, changes in other variables and may therefore be considered "dependent," whereas others such as SID, A_{tot}, and PCO_2 effect changes and are thus independent variables. Because illness prevents his being with us, we have dedicated this acid-base session of the International Biochemistry of Exercise Symposium to Dr. Peter Stewart.

References

1. Stewart, P.A. How to understand acid-base: a quantitative acid-base primer for biology and medicine. New York: Elsevier–North Holland; 1981.
2. Stewart, P.A. Modern quantitative acid-base chemistry. Can. J. Physiol. Pharmacol. 61:1444-1461; 1983.

[H$^+$] Control in Exercise:
Concepts and Controversies

Norman L. Jones
McMaster University, Hamilton, Ontario, Canada

There is no need to justify a symposium on acid-base control in a meeting devoted to the biochemistry of exercise, for changes in H$^+$ concentration have wide-ranging effects on exercise metabolism, extending from hormonal changes to rate-limiting enzyme changes in muscle and other tissues. The approach taken by all the contributors to the symposium may need some explanation, which is the reason for these introductory remarks to be given by Dr. Peter Stewart, who, unfortunately, was unable to attend. The approach is quantitative and based on classical physicochemical concepts, universally accepted since they were first introduced in the early part of this century (1). Stated in these terms, the approach is noncontroversial, but it differs in several important respects from the approach taken by most acid-base physiologists at the present time and thus to some extent challenges the current ways in which acid-base disturbances are assessed. Because the principles and "laws" are no different now from when they were first discovered, changes in concepts, or in the way we view physiology, appear at first sight rather subtle and perhaps due to semantics. Neither of these suppositions is true, as will become evident. Because all the contributors to the symposium have changed from the conventional to the quantitative approach, following Stewart's precepts (9, 10), we hope to highlight the benefits and advantages of this change in our habits. Furthermore, the study of acid-base physiology is an exercise in integrative physiology; a return to the physicochemical bases allows acid-base concepts to be integrated with water and electrolyte balance, control of intravascular volume, cellular ion shifts, and the membrane potential.

Dr. Stewart (9) pointed out that by confusing dependent with independent variables in acid-base systems, many current concepts are flawed; second, he pointed out that we may now solve the mathematical (simultaneous) equations with little effort, whereas previously this was beyond our power. Although Dr. Stewart's analysis encompasses all aspects of acid-base physiology, the present summary will focus on the aspects that particularly interest exercise physiologists and biochemists.

Current Concepts

Without wishing to caricature the concepts involved in [H$^+$] control during exercise, we may list a number of the components.

1. The major perturbation in exercise is provided by increases in lactic acid concentration in muscle and blood.

2. Lactic acid is mainly buffered by bicarbonate in the following conceptual scheme: LaH + $NaHCO_3 \rightarrow$ NaLa + CO_2 + H_2O. Thus, increases in lactate ([La^-]) are associated with equimolar reductions in [HCO_3^-] and increases in CO_2 output by the lungs. Therefore, production of 1 mole of LaH is accompanied by 22.4 L of CO_2; this is the basis of the ventilatory "anaerobic threshold" (12).

3. [H^+] is "determined" by the balance between PCO_2 (the respiratory component) and [HCO_3^-] (the metabolic component), as described by the Henderson-Hasselbalch equation, or Henderson's equation, [H^+] = 24 (PCO_2/[HCO_3^-]). This suggests that control of [H^+] is achieved through changes in PCO_2 or bicarbonate.

4. Exercise imposes a "proton load" on the body that has to be buffered if acid-base stability is to be achieved.

5. Bicarbonate acts as a buffer, is consumed by protons, is exchanged with chloride in the red cell, and is actively reabsorbed or excreted in the urine.

The Alternative: A Systems Approach

We may take a systems approach to acid-base control in major body fluid compartments in general, and to plasma and muscle in particular, by identifying the independent variables and parameters that are not altered by changes outside a system, and identifying the dependent variables that are controlled by both the independent variable in a system and by changes in other systems. The systems may then be described as a series of equations (9); the independent variables are specified, and the simultaneous solution of the equations yields the dependent variables, of which the most important are [H^+] and [HCO_3^-].

Water

In dilute aqueous solutions, the relative concentrations of [H^+] and [OH^-] have to satisfy the ion product for water (Kw'); in body fluids at 37° C Kw' = 4.4 × 10^{-14}: [H^+] = (4.4 × 10^{-14})/[OH^-]. In this equation (Eq. 1), the parameter is Kw', but [H^+] and [OH^-] are both dependent variables if the solution contains other ionic constituents.

Strong Ions

Strong ions are fully dissociated in aqueous solutions. In body fluids the main strong ions are Na^+, K^+, and Cl^-; if these were the only ions present, [H^+] would be determined by Eq. 1 and the law of electrical neutrality (Eq. 2): [Na^+] + [K^+] + [H^+] − [Cl^-] − [OH^-] = 0. The effects of the strong ions may be lumped into a term that expresses the net negative or positive charge that they exert, the "strong ion difference" ([SID]), where [SID] is normally [Na^+] + [K^+] − [Cl^-]; other strong ions, such as lactate, will also contribute to [SID]. In this system the independent variable is [SID], the dependent variables [H^+] and [OH^-].

Buffers

Buffers are usually weak acids (HA) that exist in a partially dissociated state (H$^+$, A$^-$) in the body pH range. The extent to which they are dissociated is determined by the dissociation constant, KA. The most important buffers are the plasma proteins (5), proteins and phosphates in cells (3), and hemoglobin in red cells. The effect of buffers in any site is dependent on their total concentration ([A$_{tot}$]). Thus, in this system, for plasma at 37°C (Eq. 3 and 4), [H$^+$] × [A$^-$] = KA × [HA] and [HA] + [A$^-$] = [A$_{tot}$]. In this system, [A$_{tot}$] is the independent variable and KA the parameter; [H$^+$] and [A$^-$] are dependent variables.

Carbon Dioxide

The carbon dioxide system, when conventionally defined, is only a weak buffer. It gains considerable power, however, through control of PCO$_2$ by alveolar ventilation, bringing about changes in total plasma CO$_2$ content. The overall effect is expressed in Henderson's equation (Eq. 5): [H$^+$] = .24 PCO$_2$/[HCO$_3^-$] Eq/L, where PCO$_2$ is in mmHg. In this equation PCO$_2$ is independent, [H$^+$] and [HCO$_3^-$] both dependent. Bicarbonate itself dissociates into H$^+$ and carbonate (CO$_3^{2-}$), the KA for this reaction being 6 × 10^{-11} (Eq. 6): [H$^+$] = (6 × 10^{-11}) [HCO$_3^-$]/[CO$_3^{2-}$] Eq/L.

Interaction Between Systems

We return to the law of electrical neutrality, which must be satisfied when all systems are in equilibrium (Eq. 7): [SID] + [H$^+$] − [HCO$_3^-$] − [CO$_3^{2-}$] − [A$^-$] − [OH$^-$] = 0. The linkage between variables is shown schematically in Figure 1. The six equations may be solved simultaneously, given the parameters and the independent

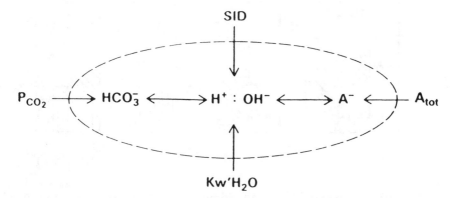

Figure 1. The acid-base systems. The arrows indicate the influence that variables may exert on each other; single-ended arrows indicate the effect of the independent variables [SID], PCO$_2$, and [A$_{tot}$] on the dependent variables [H$^+$], [OH$^-$], [HCO$_3^-$], [A$^-$], and (not shown) [CO$_3^{2-}$].

variables; notice that these variables appear only once in the series: [SID] (Eq. 7), [A$_{tot}$] (Eq. 4), and PCO$_2$ (Eq. 5). The dependent variables appear in more than one equation or more than one system: [H$^+$], [HCO$_3^-$], [A$^-$], [CO$_3^{2-}$], and [OH$^-$]. The equations are readily solved by a calculator program that may be modified through changes in parameters to define the acid-base state in any other tissue (interstitial fluid, red cells, muscle, etc.; see Figure 2). The equations clearly define the role and power of the independent variables in changing [H$^+$] and also identify that changes in [HCO$_3^-$] cannot occur independently.

[H$^+$] in Heavy Exercise

We may illustrate the application of these principles to studies carried out in heavy exercise (3); these data (Table 1) will be only briefly reviewed because they form

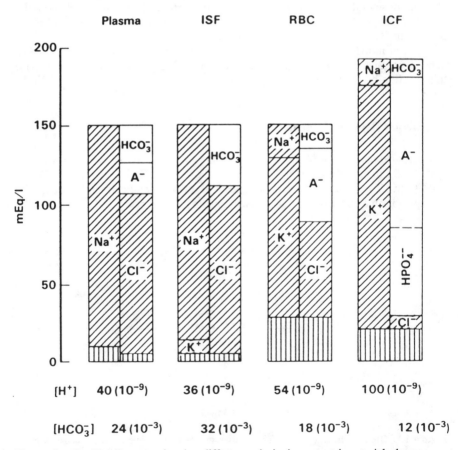

Figure 2. Gamble diagrams showing differences in ionic content in arterial plasma, interstitial fluid, red cells, and intracellular fluid of resting humans. Strong ions are cross-matched; SID has been left clear.

Table 1   Independent and Dependent Variables in Acid-Base Status at Rest and Following 30 s of Maximal Dynamic Cycling Exercise

Variable	Arterial plasma			Active muscle		
		Postexercise (min)			Postexercise (min)	
	Rest	0.5	3.5	Rest	0.5	3.5
K$^+$	5	7	5	142	138	123
La$^-$	1	10	14	6	47	30
SID	37	34	31	154	106	101
PCO$_2$	40	37	30	46	106	48
A$_{tot}$	17	18	19	180	155	160
H$^+$	38	47	54	132	328	417
HCO$_3^-$	25	19	14	9	7	3
A$^-$	14	16	17	145	98	98

Note. Adapted from 3.

part of other presentations by Heigenhauser and Lindinger. In arterial plasma rapid changes in all the variables may occur. In addition to increases in [La$^-$], increases in [K$^+$] and [Cl$^-$] contribute to changes in [SID] (4); in the first 2-3 min following exercise, [K$^+$] and [Cl$^-$] fall to resting levels, but [La$^-$] may continue to increase. PCO$_2$ usually falls by about 10 Torr. Thus, in terms of independent variables, at 3 min postexercise, [SID] and PCO$_2$ are reduced, and A$_{tot}$ is increased due to hemoconcentration (2, 8). The dependent variables show an increase in [H$^+$], a fall in [HCO$_3^-$] (2), and a decrease in [A$^-$]. The fall in [HCO$_3^-$], roughly equimolecular to the increase in [La$^-$], is seen to be the result of a series of changes in all the systems and not merely the "buffering" of LaH by HCO$_3^-$.

In muscle, not surprisingly, the changes at a comparable time postexercise are seen to be more extensive and more complex (6, 7, 8). In addition to the large increase in [La$^-$], there is a substantial fall in [K$^+$], which contributes to a large reduction in [SID]. A large increase in PCO$_2$ occurs immediately following exercise, but by 3 min postexercise, it has fallen to resting levels. The dependent variables show a very large increase in [H$^+$], a small absolute decrease in [HCO$_3^-$], and a large reduction in [A$^-$], representing the effect of buffering by the intracellular weak acid system. Thus, in contrast to plasma, decreases in [K$^+$] are able to contribute as much as increases in [La$^-$] to increases in [H$^+$], and reductions in [A$^-$] are far more important than reductions in [HCO$_3^-$] in minimizing increases in [H$^+$].

Current Concepts Reexamined

There is no denying that the relationships expressed in the equations have their roots in the classical acid-base work of 1920-1940 (1, 5, 11) and thus do not describe anything new. How then are the concepts changed, and what new information have we obtained?

1. We can examine the systems to quantify their individual contributions to the acid-base changes in any system. For example, we see that a reduction in intramuscular $[K^+]$ may contribute almost equally to increases in $[H^+]$ as the increase in $[La^-]$ in muscle after severe exercise.

2. The "reaction" between LaH and HCO_3^- is recognized as a naive shortcut that obscures understanding and that does not actually occur.

3. The Henderson-Hasselbalch equation is seen to express the relationship between $[H^+]$, the independent variable PCO_2, and the dependent variable $[HCO_3^-]$; although clearly a valid mathematical description, its use in any extended way to imply that $[H^+]$ is *controlled* by $[HCO_3^-]$ is invalid.

4. Bicarbonate, being dependent on all the acid-base systems, cannot be assigned an active role in acid-base control. The relationships identify its true role in buffering, establish that $[HCO_3^-]$ cannot change without changes in PCO_2 or [SID], and show that it cannot be consumed or diluted unless the independent variables change. Additionally, we may state that HCO_3^- need not "exchange with" Cl^- (a movement of Cl^- has to be followed by a change in $[HCO_3^-]$, even if PCO_2 is constant). Also, plasma $[HCO_3^-]$ is modified by the kidneys only through their regulated handling of Na^+, K^+, and Cl^-, and through the renal PCO_2.

5. A proton (H^+) load has no meaning quantitatively in acid-base terms, although its expression in terms of the balance between strong ions, acting as conjugate acids or bases, allows an effect to be calculated through changes in [SID] using the quantitative approach.

Probably the most important feature of Stewart's approach is the clear identification of which variables are capable of independent action and which are dependent on the result of more than one reaction. The illogicality of assigning an active role to a dependent variable becomes immediately apparent. The only impediments to the approach are the accuracy of the analyses required and a debate regarding the specific values for the constants used in equations. However, analytical improvements and continuing research should solve these problems and establish its validity in the next few years.

References

1. Henderson, L.J. Blood. New Haven, CT: Yale University Press; 1928.

2. Hermansen, L.; Orheim, A.; Sejersted, O.M. Metabolic acidosis and changes in water and electrolyte balance in relation to fatigue during maximal exercise of short duration. Int. J. Sports Med. 5:110-115; 1984.

3. Kowalchuk, J.M.; Heigenhauser, G.J.F.; Lindinger, M.I.; Sutton, J.R.; Jones, N.L. Factors influencing hydrogen ion concentration in muscle after intense exercise. J. Appl. Physiol. 65:2080-2089; 1988.

4. Medbo, J.I.; Sejersted, O.M. Acid-base and electrolyte balance after exhausting exercise in endurance-trained and sprint-trained subjects. Acta Physiol. Scand. 125:97-109; 1985.

5. Peters, J.P.; Van Slyke, D.D. Hemoglobin and oxygen: carbon dioxide and acid-base balance. Baltimore: Williams & Wilkins; 1931.

6. Sahlin, K.; Alvestrand, A.; Brandt, R.; Hultman, E. Intracellular pH and bicarbonate concentration in human muscle during recovery from exercise. J. Appl. Physiol.: Respir. Environ. Exerc. Physiol. 45:474-480; 1978.

7. Sjögaard, G. Electrolytes in slow and fast muscle fibers of humans at rest and with dynamic exercise. Am. J. Physiol. 245:R25-R31; 1983.

8. Sjögaard, G.; Adams, R.P.; Saltin, B. Water and ion shifts in skeletal muscle of humans with intense dynamic knee extension. Am. J. Physiol. 248: R190-R196; 1985.

9. Stewart, P.A. How to understand acid-base: a quantitative acid-base primer for biology and medicine. New York: Elsevier North Holland; 1981.

10. Stewart, P.A. Modern quantitative acid-base chemistry. Can. J. Physiol. Pharmacol. 61:1444-1461; 1983.

11. Van Slyke, D.D.; Hastings, A.B.; Hiller, A.; Sendroy, J. Studies of gas and electrolyte equilibria in blood: IV. The amounts of alkali bound by serum albumin and globulin. J. Biol. Chem. 79:769-780; 1928.

12. Wasserman, K. Anaerobiosis, lactate, and gas exchange during exercise: the issues. Fed. Proc. 45:2904-2909; 1986.

Acid-Base Systems in Skeletal Muscle and Their Response to Exercise

Michael I. Lindinger and George J.F. Heigenhauser
McMaster University Medical Center, Hamilton
and University of Guelph, Guelph, Ontario, Canada

The purpose of this paper is to describe a physicochemical model of acid-base balance in skeletal muscle. The model consists of skeletal muscle cells with uniform intracellular compartments, bounded by the sarcolemma, where the total ionic status of the intracellular fluid is determined by the independent variables: PCO_2, the concentrations of strong ions as represented by the strong ion difference ($[SID]$), and total concentration of weak acids and bases ($[A_{tot}]$). The relationships between these variables and the dependent variables $[H^+]$, $[OH^-]$, $[HCO_3^-]$, $[CO_3^{2-}]$, $[A^-]$, and $[HA]$ have been described by Stewart (28, 29), as summarized in the preceding chapter by Jones (13).

The physiological and biochemical characteristics of resting and fatigued skeletal muscle, such as metabolism, contractile properties, and membrane properties, are highly dependent upon the ionic composition of the extra- and intracellular fluids. The skeletal muscle intracellular fluid compartment, as all body fluid compartments, may be analyzed as a physicochemical system within which the fundamental laws of physical chemistry must be followed. Stewart (28, 29) has formalized the physicochemical theories of Henderson (9), Van Slyke (31, 32), Singer and Hastings (26), Harned and Owen (8), and Edsall and Wyman (4) into a concept of body fluid acid-base homeostasis that recognizes that $[H^+]$, $[OH^-]$, $[HCO_3^-]$, $[CO_3^{2-}]$, $[A^-]$, and $[HA]$ are dependent on the concentrations of strong and weak ions and on the PCO_2.

Presently, the major limitation of this analysis of skeletal muscle is that all the different intracellular fluid compartments are considered to be one large compartment with homogenous distribution of intracellular constituents. The major advantage of the method is that it allows the researcher to achieve a good indication of the changes in muscle physicochemical status that accompany the fatigue and recovery processes. This paper will attempt to demonstrate how these physicochemical changes are intimately related to the biochemistry and physiology of exercising muscle.

Fatigue

Skeletal muscle fatigue has been defined as an inability to maintain an expected force or power output due to a reduction in the number of simultaneously attached actin-myosin cross-bridges in the force-generating state (5, 12). It is highly unlikely that of the many changes occurring in skeletal muscle or in the blood perfusing the muscle during exercise, any one is in itself causative of fatigue. Rather, there is likely to be a host of closely associated events that occur simultaneously, or nearly so, that lead to the observed decrements in muscle force production.

The biochemical factors associated with skeletal muscle fatigue may be divided into three fundamental events: (a) impairment of metabolism and reduction of energy production; (b) alteration of sarcolemmal, transverse tubular, and sarcoplasmic reticulum membrane properties; and (c) impaired function of the contractile proteins. Ultimately, maintained muscle function and force output is dependent on a *required* energy production by the muscle cell to regulate intracellular organellar environments by maintaining transmembrane ionic and chemical gradients and osmotic equilibria. In the event of energy demands exceeding immediately available energy production, homeostasis of the intracellular environment cannot be maintained, and changes that are now well known to be associated with muscle fatigue occur (Table 1). With the exception of glycogen, all of the substances listed in Table 1 are ionic in nature and thus directly influence the physicochemical status of the intracellular compartment.

Table 1   Biochemical Factors Contributing to Fatigue in Exercising Skeletal Muscle

Glycogen depletion	Decrease in $[Ca^{2+}]$
Phosphocreatine depletion	Decrease in $[Mg^{2+}]$
ATP depletion	Decrease in $[K^+]$
Increase in lactate	Increase in $[Na^+]$
Increase in inorganic phosphate	Increase in $[Cl^-]$
Increase in inosine monophosphate	Increase in $[H^+]$

Physical Chemistry of Skeletal Muscle

This section describes the relationships between independent and dependent ionic variables in skeletal muscle and discusses briefly how changes in one or more of the independent variables, such as occurs with exercise, differentially affect the dependent variables. The equations describing the mass action and chemical equilibria for weak acids, carbon dioxide, and strong ions in aqueous solutions (described by Jones, ref. 13) may be combined to yield a single equation that may be solved for $[H^+]$ when [SID], $[A_{tot}]$, and PCO_2 are known (equation 7A.1.2 from ref. 28):

$$[H^+]^4 + \{K_A + [SID]\}[H^+]^3 + \{K_A([SID] - [A_{tot}]) -$$
$$(K_C \times PCO_2 + K'_w)\}[H^+]^2 - \{K_A(K_C \times PCO_2 + K'_w) +$$
$$K_3 \times K_2 \times PCO_2\}[H^+] - K_A \times K_3 \times K_c \times PCO_2 = 0$$

The values for the constants in muscle intracellular fluid are given in Table 2. These equations and constants can be used to generate the curves shown in Figure 1.

Table 2   Values and Sources of the Constants Used in the Calculations

Constant	Value	Source (ref. no.)
K'_W	4.40×10^{-14} (Eq/L)^2	8
$K_c{}^a$	2.34×10^{-11} (Eq/L)^2/mmHg	25
K_3	6.0×10^{-11} Eq/L	4
K_A	1.64×10^{-7} Eq/L (Rest)	This study
K_A	1.98×10^{-7} Eq/L (Exercise)	This study

^{a}Calculated from $K_C = K \times S$, where K is the apparent dissociation constant for CO_2 and S is the CO_2 solubility coefficient. $K = 7.41 \times 10^{-7}$ Eq/L and $S = 0.0351$ Eq/L • mmHg^{-1} at 37° C at intracellular ionic strength of 300 mOsm (25). All values for 37° C and ionic strength of 300 mOsm.

Figure 1 shows how the dependent variables, presented on the ordinate axes, are affected by a change in only one of the independent variables while the other independent variables are held constant. The range of PCO_2, [A_{tot}], and [SID] values are representative of the expected physiological ranges in skeletal muscle. A brief

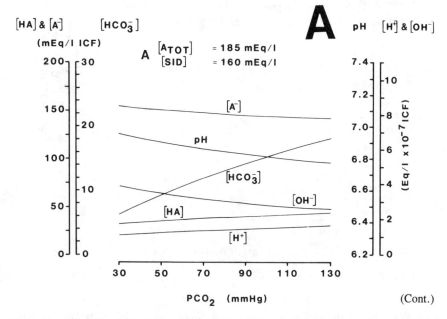

(Cont.)

Figure 1. The effects of changes in the independent variables PCO_2, [A_{tot}], and [SID] on the concentrations of the dependent variables. Changes in PCO_2 (upper panel) exert the least effect on the dependent variables, whereas changes in [SID] (lower panel) exert the greatest effects.

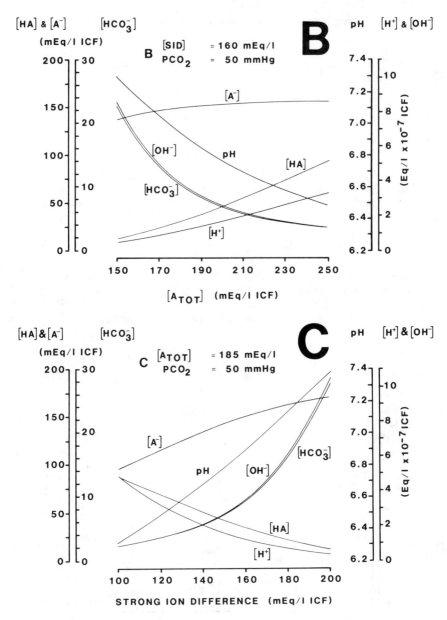

Figure 1. Continued

study of the figure shows that in skeletal muscle, changes in PCO_2 exert a markedly smaller effect on the dependent variables (Figure 1A) than do changes in $[A_{tot}]$ or [SID].

The value for the intracellular weak acid dissociation constant K_A for $[A_{tot}]$ in skeletal muscle is derived from the relative abundance of the major weak electrolytes and their individual apparent dissociation constants in muscle as listed in Table 3. With the exception of creatine, all of these compounds are ionized within the pH range of 6.0-7.0, and their degree of protonation changes as dictated by changes in the independent variables. Changes in the protonated state of weak acids and bases as related to the associated pH change may be demonstrated as follows: (a) the valency of histidine changes from -0.9 at pH 7.0 to -0.74 at pH 6.5, and to -0.46 at pH 6.0; (b) for inorganic phosphate (P_i), the valencies are -1.39, -1.2, and -1.03 at pH of 7.0, 6.5, and 6.0; (c) over this pH range, the valency of MgATP is considered as -2, those of MgADP and the glycolytic phosphates as -1. These valency changes are important in understanding how the values of [AH] and [A⁻] change with changes in the independent variable.

From Table 3 it is apparent that the relative abundance of the intracellular weak acids changes with exercise, and this will cause a corresponding change in K_A. Creatine and P_i increase in direct proportion to the amount of phosphocreatine (PCr^{2-}) that becomes hydrolyzed. PCr^{2-}, a strong acid anion, is 99.7% in the divalent form at pH 7.0 and 97% in the divalent form at pH 6.0; its pK' is 4.5. Thus, PCr^{2-}

Table 3   Acidic Dissociation Constants (@ 25° C) of Intramuscular Weak Acids and Bases and Their Relative Abundance in Muscle at Rest and After Intense Exercise

Substance	pK	Ka (Eq/L×10⁻⁷)	mmol/kg dry wt.		% abundance	
			Rest	Exer	Rest	Exer
Histidine	$pK_2 = 6.04$					
	$pK_3 = 9.33$					
	pK' = 6.75	1.78	165 ± 10	165 ± 10	60	38
Creatine	$pK_1 = 2.63$					
	$pK_2 = 11.02$					
	pK' = 6.83	1.50	48 ± 3	120 ± 30	15	25
P_i	$pK_2 = 7.20$					
	$pK_3 = 12.38$					
	pK' = 6.78	1.66	26 ± 2	98 ± 10	8	20
ATP	pK' = 6.97	1.07	25 ± 3	13 ± 2	7	3
ADP	pK' = 6.75	1.78	3 ± 1	4 ± 1	1	1
Glyc-P[a]	pK' = 6.11	7.9	3 ± 2	22 ± 4	1	4
Other			?	?	8	9
Total			270 ± 21	422 ± 57	100	100
A_{tot}	pK_A		6.79	6.70		
	K_A (Eq/L×10⁻⁷)		1.64	1.98		

Note. Adapted from Hultman and Sahlin (11); dissociation constants from Robinson and Stokes (23) and Hultman and Sahlin (11). The model assumes that the in vivo pKs for weak acids at 35° C are similar to in vitro values at 25° C.

[a]Glycolytic phosphates.

hydrolysis has two direct effects on cell physicochemistry: It leads to an increase in the [SID], and it causes an increase in [A_{tot}]. ATP decreases with intense exercise, whereas the concentrations of ADP and the glycolytic phosphates increase. The result is a 20% increase in the K_A of exercised muscle, as shown at the bottom of Table 3.

The effects of changes in [A_{tot}] on the dependent variables are shown in Figure 1B. As explained above on theoretical grounds and as can be shown experimentally (see below), there is a tendency for [A_{tot}] to increase by 5-10% with intense exercise. With increases in [A_{tot}], there is very little increase in the dissociated form [A^-] but a more marked increase in its protonated form [AH]. There are pronounced changes in the concentrations of the other dependent variables as [A_{tot}] changes; however, because [A_{tot}] changes little with exercise, the effect on the dependent variables is less than that of changes in [SID].

Physiological changes in [SID] with exercise exert the largest effect of the independent variables on the dependent variables (Figure 1C). With intense short-term exercise, as described below, muscle intracellular [SID] may decrease by 30 mEq/L or more and may account for about 80% of the increase in [H^+]. Within the operative [SID] range in skeletal muscle, changes in the dependent variables are nearly linearly related to the change in [SID]. Intracellular [SID] is calculated as follows: [SID] = [Na^+] + [K^+] + [$Mg^{2+}/2$] − [Cl^-] − [Lac^-] − [PCr^{2-}]. Note that the [Mg^{2+}] is halved because about 50% is strongly bound to ATP and ADP (Table 3) inside the cell. Lactate (Lac^-) and phosphocreatine (PCr^{2-}) are strong acid anions with pKs of 3.8 and 4.5, respectively.

With exercise the effects of increases in [Na^+], [Mg^{2+}], and [Cl^-] are relatively small and tend to cancel each other, whereas the decrease in [PCr^{2-}] raises [SID], and decreases in [K^+] and increases in [Lac^-] lower [SID]. Following intense exercise, PCr^{2-} is rapidly regenerated (16) and, together with Lac^- removal and K^+ repletion, is important in restoring intracellular ionic status during the recovery process.

A criticism of the approach we have used is that the analysis uses ion concentrations rather than ion activities. It can be shown, by using literature values for ion activity coefficients, that whereas quantitatively different results for [SID] may be obtained, estimated changes in [SID] ''activity'' with exercise lead to a similar quantitative interpretation. Because of the curvilinear relationship between [SID] and [H^+] in muscle (Figure 1), for a given fall in [SID] the [H^+] increases more when the initial [SID] is low than when the initial [SID] is high. Therefore, a high [SID] in resting muscle may have a protective effect against large changes in the dependent ionic variables caused by strong ion disturbances.

Decreases in [SID] cause large decreases in [A^-] and increases in [AH] (Figure 1C). These changes, in combination with increased [AH] resulting from increases in [A_{tot}] (Figure 1B, Figure 2A), are indicative of a general increase in the protonated state of intracellular proteins. Therefore, changes in the two independent variables [SID] and [A_{tot}] may alter the catalytic activity of enzymes that are classically considered ''pH sensitive'' (3). Such ''pH effects'' have been proposed both for the regulation of glycolysis at the level of phosphorylase (1, 12) and phosphofructokinase (12, 30), and also for the impairment of contraction at the level of the sarcoplasmic reticulum (6, 21) and at the myofilaments (2, 10).

The regulation of the glycolytic enzyme phosphofructokinase (PFK) is known to display pH sensitivity in vitro (30). The catalytic conversion of fructose-6-phosphate to fructose-1,6-bisphosphate by PFK is inhibited by conditions that result in low physiological pH, resulting in the accumulation of fructose-6-phosphate and its precursor, glucose-6-phosphate. PFK may exert a regulatory influence via glucose-6-phosphate inhibition of the flux-generating step from glycogen catalyzed by phosphorylase b.

The effects of changes in the ionic state of intracellular weak acids due to changes in the independent variables are very pronounced, and the case of P_i provides a good example. There is evidence that suggests that a large increase in the diprotonated form of P_i ($H_2PO_4^-$) over that of the monoprotonated form (HPO_4^{2-}) with exercise-induced increases in P_i leads to fatigue by at least two different mechanisms: inhibition of energy production at the level of phosphorylase at the beginning of the glycogenolytic pathway (15) and inhibition of actomyosin kinetics (2). With intense exercise, free $[P_i]$ may increase by 20 mM or more (2, 11). Assuming an increase of 20 mM from the degradation of PCr^{2-} and a fall in pH to 6.5 during intense exercise, the $[H_2PO_4^-]$ will increase to 23 mEq/L from 2.5 mEq/L, whereas the proportion of HPO_4^{2-} to total P_i decreases from 37% to 20% (Table 4). The diprotonated form is believed to be inhibitory to force production (22) and phosphorylase activity (15) in muscle.

Table 4   Effects of Phosphocreatine (PCr^{2-}) Hydrolysis and Increased [H^+] on Inorganic Phosphate (HPO_4^{2-} and $H_2PO_4^-$)

	Rest pH = 7.0		Exercise pH = 6.5		pH = 6.0
	mmol/L	mEq/L	mmol/L	mEq/L	mEq/L
$[PCr^{2-}]$	25	50	7	14	14
Total $[P_i]$	4	5.5	24	28.8	24
$[H_2PO_4^-]$	2.5	2.5	19.4	23.0	22.5
$[HPO_4^{2-}]$[a]	1.5	3.0	4.6	5.8	1.5
(% of $[P_i]$)	37	53	19	20	6.2

[a]Believed to be the biologically active species (22). With very intense exercise, the effective intracellular $[HPO_4^{2-}]$ may decrease from 6.6 to 1.6 mEq/L despite a 2-fold increase in $[P_i]$.

It is useful to know how much of a change in one of the independent variables is required to cause a 5% change in one of the dependent variables; these data are presented in Table 5. Changes in the dependent variables are highly sensitive to small changes in [SID] and [A_{tot}], but because the changes in [SID] with exercise tend to be quantitatively larger, they exert the greater influence on muscle total ionic status. The value of K_A, which represents the degree of dissociation between H^+ and AH, is also of quantitative importance because its value will change with exercise-induced changes in intracellular weak acid composition. With the exception of HCO_3^- and carbonate (CO_3^{2-}, not shown), the concentrations of the dependent variables are relatively insensitive to PCO_2.

Table 5 also shows that small errors in the measurement and calculation of [SID] and [A_{tot}] may lead to significant errors in calculated values of the dependent variables. Here it is important to stress that we are not so much interested in the absolute values for [H^+] but in understanding the relative contributions of the changes in the variables seen with exercise, and their association with muscle fatigue and recovery mechanisms.

Table 5   Change in the Independent Variables Required to Cause 5% Change in the Dependent Variables in Skeletal Muscle

Independent variables		Dependent variables				
		[H^+] (Eq/L $\times$ 10^{-7})	[OH^-]	[AH] (mEq/L)	[A^-] (mEq/L)	[HCO_3^-] (mEq/L)
Initial values		0.887	4.96	63.2	116.8	13.2
PCO_2	Increase by	11 (22)	11	18 (36)	32 (64)	4 (8)
50 mmHg	Decrease by	10 (20)	10	17 (34)	26 (52)	4
[A_{tot}]	Increase by	4 (2.2)	4	4	60 (33)	4
180 mEq/L	Decrease by	4	4	4	30 (17)	5 (3)
[SID]	Increase by	3 (2.3)	3	4 (3.1)	8 (6.2)	3
130 mEq/L	Decrease by	2.5 (1.9)	2.5	4	8	2.5
K_A	Increase by	0.11 (6.7)	0.11	0.67 (41)	1.75 (107)	0.12 (7)
1.64 $\times$ 10^{-7}	Decrease by	0.11	0.11	0.42 (26)	0.65 (40)	0.11

Note. Change in independent variable as a percentage of initial value of independent variable is indicated in parentheses.

Experiment

Male Sprague-Dawley rats ($n = 21$) weighing 430-530 g (478 $\pm$ 11 g mean $\pm$ SEM) were randomly assigned to two groups: resting nonexercised controls ($n = 13$) and rats exercised to exhaustion by swimming with tail weights ($n = 8$). Muscle pH was measured using the distribution of DMO 2.5-3.5 hours following injection of 0.50 ml of 5.7 μCi ^{14}C-DMO and 20.0 μCi ^{3}H-mannitol (New England Nuclear) via a tail vein.

Resting controls ($n = 13$) were quickly killed by cervical dislocation, and 2-3 ml of blood was immediately collected in a heparinized syringe from the abdominal aorta of each. The blood was immediately analyzed for pH, blood gases, and plasma ions and metabolites. The entire soleus and plantaris muscles, the medial (red) gastrocnemius, and a large (0.3- to 0.5-g) portion of the superficial (white) gastrocnemius were removed from both legs. Muscles were immediately freeze-clamped with aluminum tongs cooled in liquid nitrogen, wrapped in aluminum foil, and stored in liquid nitrogen until analyzed.

The exercise group rats were fitted with tail weights (amounting to about 5% of body mass) and individually swum to exhaustion in a 35° C water bath (19). The exhausted animal was removed from the water and immediately killed by cervical dislocation. Blood and muscles were immediately sampled as described above and analyzed as described elsewhere (17-19).

For each muscle, two 30- to 40-mg dry weight samples were used for measurement of muscle homogenate pH during CO_2 and strong ion titrations. Both samples were initially treated as follows. The muscle was weighed, then homogenized with a glass rod in 1.00 ml of solution (145 mM KCl, 10 mM NaCl, and 5 mM sodium iodoacetate [ref. 27]) within a 10-by-75-mm polyethylene test tube. The tube was placed in a 37° C water bath for equilibration to temperature; 20 μl of 2-octanol (an antifoam agent) and 20 ul of a rabbit muscle carbonic anhydrase solution (100,000 Units/ml homogenizing solution) were added. The carbonic anhydrase increased the rate of equilibration from 15-20 min to about 5 min during titrations; the carbonic anhydrase contributed less than 3% to the muscle homogenate $[A_{tot}]$ and was neglected. Equilibration of the homogenate to the gas mixtures was performed by passing a fine stream of bubbles from PE-50 tubing through the homogenate. Homogenate pH was monitored with a pH electrode (Radiometer model #GK2421C, for microsamples) connected to a Radiometer PHM 72 digital acid-base analyzer. The homogenate was equilibrated to 0.1% CO_2 by bubbling with air for 5 min; the pH was recorded when a stable reading was obtained.

For the first muscle sample, the homogenate was titrated with 5%, 10%, and 15% CO_2 in air, and each end point in homogenate pH was recorded. Upon completion of the CO_2 titration, the homogenate was reequilibrated to air, and the pH of the homogenate was reduced to about 6.0 by the addition of 0.2 N HCl. During continuous air bubbling, the homogenate was then titrated with strong ion (0.2 N NaOH) dispensed from a Gilson microburette in 5- to 20-μl aliquots. The end point homogenate pH was recorded about 5 min after each addition.

The second muscle sample was titrated with increasing CO_2 (as before). Samples of resting control muscle were then equilibrated with 5% CO_2 for titration with strong ion (0.2 N NaOH), whereas samples of exercised muscles were equilibrated to 15% CO_2 for titration with 0.2 N NaOH.

Homogenate $[A_{tot}]$ was calculated from the equation $[A_{tot}] = \{([SID] - [HCO_3^-]) \times (K_A + [H^+])\}/K_A$, where bicarbonate $[HCO_3^-]$ was calculated from homogenate PCO_2, pH and K_3 and K_c from Table 2. Homogenate [SID] was calculated from the known ionic composition of the homogenate solution and the known muscle sample [SID] (excluding the contribution from $[PCr^{2-}]$, because PCr is rapidly degraded in the homogenate at 37° C [ref. 27]). The homogenate K_A used for each titration was one that gave identical $[A_{tot}]$ values for each end point pH/[SID]/PCO_2 relationship for each given muscle sample. These K_As were different from the intracellular K_A (Table 3) because of the somewhat different composition of each muscle homogenate. The calculated value of homogenate $[A_{tot}]$ also contained the contributions of creatine and P_i liberated from the hydrolysis of PCr^{2-}. In resting muscle with $[PCr^{2-}]$ averaging 35, 48, 55, and 58 mEq/L (19), the creatine and P_i contributions to homogenate $[A_{tot}]$ averaged 30, 40, 45, and 50 mEq/L in SL, RG, PL, and WG, respectively. In exercised samples the creatine and P_i contributions to subtract from homogenate $[A_{tot}]$ were 25, 10, 10, and 10 mEq/L, based on $[PCr^{2-}]$ at the end of exercise. These calculations have been detailed by Lindinger et al. (17).

The dependent acid-base variables $[H^+]$, $[OH^-]$, dissociated weak acid $[A^-]$, undissociated weak acid $[AH]$, and bicarbonate $[HCO_3^-]$ were calculated for each muscle sample using the intracellular [SID], an intramuscular PCO_2 of 50 mmHg (resting muscle) or 82 mmHg (exercised muscle), and the $[A_{tot}]$ derived from muscle homogenate titrations. The equations used for the calculations are outlined in the preceding chapter (13) and by Lindinger et al. (17). Results are expressed as mean $\pm$ SE. Statistical differences between muscles and treatments were assessed by analysis of variance. The Student's t test was used to compare means when a significant F ratio was obtained. Statistical significance was accepted at $p \leqslant 0.05$.

Results and Discussion

The mean time to fatigue of swimming rats was 4.4 ± 0.5 min. The composition of abdominal aortic blood in fatigued rats was pH 6.89 ± 0.02, $[Lac^-]$ 20 ± 1 mEq/L, and PCO_2 82 ± 12 mmHg. The changes in the intracellular independent variables $[A_{tot}]$ and [SID] with intense swimming exercise are shown in Figure 2; intramuscular PCO_2 is considered to have increased from 50 to 82 mmHg. $[A_{tot}]$ increased signifi-

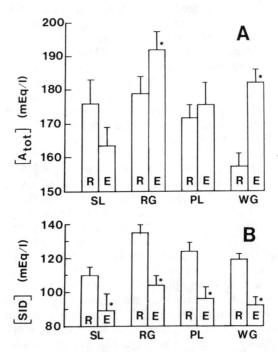

Figure 2. The $[A_{tot}]$ and [SID] values in soleus (SL), red gastrocnemius (RG), plantaris (PL), and white gastrocnemius (WG) muscles at rest (R, $n = 13$) and at the end of intense swimming exercise (E, $n = 8$). Asterisks indicate exercise means significantly different ($p < 0.05$) from rest means.

cantly in RG and WG, and [SID] was significantly reduced to about 80% of resting values in all muscles.

The major contributors to the reduction in [SID] in all muscles were the increase in [Lac⁻] and the decrease in [K⁺] (Table 6). The increase in [Lac⁻] was approximately equal to the decrease in [PCr²⁻] at the end of exercise (19), and the reduction in [SID] was largely equal to the loss of intracellular K⁺ (Table 6). These ionic changes increased progressively with increasing proportion of fast-twitch fibers within the muscle, such that the WG showed the largest increase in [Lac⁻] and the largest decreases in [K⁺] and [SID]. The increase in [Lac⁻] contributed 50% and 67% to the fall in [SID] in SL and WG, respectively. In all muscles the fall in [SID] was the major contributor to the increase in [H⁺]; therefore, increased [Lac⁻] was the most important factor directly responsible for the ionic disturbances at the *end* of intense exercise.

The changes in the independent variables resulted in increases in [AH] (Figure 3A); decreases in [A⁻] (Figure 3B), [OH⁻] (Figure 4A), and [HCO₃⁻] (Figure 4B); and increases in [H⁺] in all muscles. Decreases in intracellular [HCO₃⁻] at the end of

Table 6 Intramuscular Fluid Volumes and Intracellular Ion Concentrations in Rat Hindlimb Muscles at Rest (R) and at the End of Intense Exercise (E)

Variable	Soleus		Red gastroc.		Plantaris		White gastroc.	
	R	E	R	E	R	E	R	E
TTW	766	776	760	778	761	778	758	777
	±7	±6	±3	±5	±2	±3	±3	±3
ECFV	79	80	58	63	57	73	64	78
	±14	±14	±10	±10	±8	±12	±10	±18
ICFV	688	698	703	717	702	707	701	714
	±13	±14	±11	±14	±8	±10	±13	±14
[Na⁺]	7.2	9.0	9.6	13.3	10.6	14.0	5.9	14.6
	±1.5	±3.7	±0.7	±2.8	±1.3	±2.6	±0.9	±2.6
[K⁺]	117	112	144	128	136	123	143	128
	±6	±10	±6	±6	±7	±6	±6	±6
[Mg²⁺]	24	21	31	29	29	28	31	26
	±1	±1	±1	±2	±2	±2	±2	±3
[Cl⁻]	8.5	12.8	5.1	9.3	5.9	9.1	8.7	11.2
	±3.2	±2.9	±1.4	±2.2	±1.2	±1.9	±1.1	±7.0
[Lac⁻]	1.9	17.7	4.9	32.9	7.0	35.7	7.2	43.3
	±0.2	±2.0	±0.4	±4.0	±0.7	±3.5	±1.1	±3.7
[PCr²⁻]	34.6	11.4	55.4	11.0	53.8	12.6	60.6	11.0
	±3.4	±3.0	±4.4	±3.4	±2.8	±6.2	±3.6	±5.2

Note. TTW, total tissue water; ECFV, extracellular fluid volume; ICFV, intracellular fluid volume. Units: fluid volumes, ml/kg wet wt.; strong ions, mEq/L intracellular fluid.

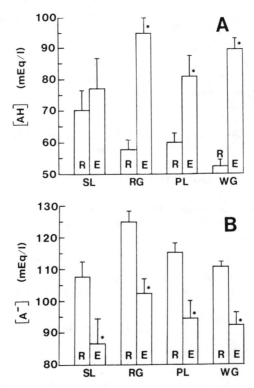

Figure 3. The concentrations of undissociated ([AH]) and dissociated ([A⁻]) weak acid in the intracellular compartment of rat hindlimb muscles at rest and after intense exercise. Abbreviations as in Figure 2.

intense exercise are not as large as may be expected, due to the large generation and accumulation of CO_2 in the body fluids. Based on these results, $[HCO_3^-]$ may be expected to fall to much lower values during the initial minutes of the postexercise recovery period as CO_2 is rapidly washed out. The combined effects of increased [AH] and decreased [A⁻] with exercise (Figure 3) greatly reduces the proportion of weak acids in the ionized form, the form that is considered to be biologically active (15, 22). This effect appears to be important in the slowing of glycogenolysis and actomyosin kinetics described in the preceding section.

The differences in the ionic status of skeletal muscle at rest and following exercise are related to muscle fiber-type composition and muscle function. The [SID] at rest and following exercise (Figure 2B) reflects the intracellular concentrations of strong ions (Table 6). Compared to fast-twitch muscles (WG and PL), the low [SID] in resting SL (Figure 2B) results from the significantly lower $[K^+]$ and higher $[Cl^-]$ (Table 6), in turn resulting in a higher resting $[H^+]$ (Figure 5). In all muscles following exercise, the final [SID] was similar (Figure 2B) and resulted in similar $[H^+]$ values for all muscles (Figure 5). However, the decrease in [SID] was greater in fast-twitch muscles (−27 mEq/L) than in SL (−20 mEq/L); therefore, the increase in $[H^+]$ (Figure 5) was greater in fast-twitch WG (+117 nEq/L) than in SL

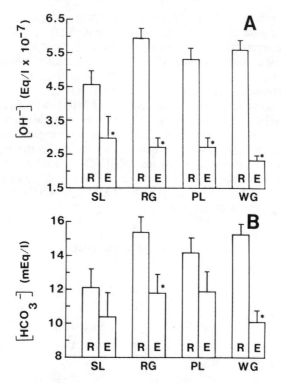

Figure 4. The concentrations of hydroxyl ion ([OH⁻]) and bicarbonate ([HCO₃⁻]) in the intracellular compartment of rat hindlimb muscles at rest and after intense exercise. Abbreviations as in Figure 2.

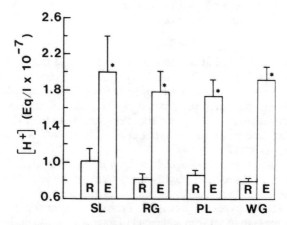

Figure 5. The concentration of hydrogen ion ([LH⁺]) in the intracellular compartment of rat hindlimb muscles at rest and after intense exercise. Abbreviations as in Figure 2.

(+93 nEq/L), reflecting the larger increase in [A_{tot}] and decreases in [SID] seen in WG with exercise (Figure 2). The high resting [SID] in WG may effectively prolong continued muscle function during exercise by preventing even larger changes in protein ionization state and [H^+]. The significant decreases in [OH^-] (Figure 4A) and in [H^+] (Figure 5) in all muscles also reflect the general increase in protonated state of the intracellular environment with intense exercise.

Muscle pH values determined by the DMO and [SID] methods are compared in Table 7. Intracellular pH measured by DMO distribution yielded values consistently lower than the [SID] method by about 0.1 unit in both resting and exercised muscle. There was no significant difference between techniques in the magnitude of the exercise-induced decreases in pH. At rest, pH-[SID] showed a significant decrease as the percentage of fast-twitch fibers decreased (WG 100% fast-twitch; SL 13% fast-twitch); this trend was not evident with pH-DMO, which showed no differences between resting muscle pH (Table 7).

Table 7   Intramuscular pH as Determined by the DMO and SID Methods

Muscle	Condition	pH-DMO	pH-SID
Soleus	Rest	7.03 ± .03	7.00 ± .04
	Exercise	6.66 ± .04	6.76 ± .07
Red gastroc.	Rest	6.98 ± .02	7.09 ± .03
	Exercise	6.62 ± .05	6.77 ± .05
Plantaris	Rest	6.99 ± .03	7.07 ± .03
	Exercise	6.65 ± .05	6.78 ± .05
Wh. gastroc.	Rest	6.98 ± .03	7.08 ± .02
	Exercise	6.64 ± .03	6.72 ± .03

Note. Values are means ± SE (n = 13 at rest; n = 8 with exercise). All exercise values are significantly lower than resting values.

The values for muscle pH at rest and exercise calculated from [SID] and the distribution of the weak acid DMO (Table 7) are within the range of values tabulated by Roos and Boron (24) from a variety of mouse and rat skeletal muscles in which intracellular pH was measured in vitro and in vivo using microelectrodes and weak acid distribution techniques. They are also very similar to the pH values obtained using the homogenate technique of Spriet et al. (27) on both wet and freeze-dried rat hindlimb muscles (17).

There is evidence that physiological changes in the intracellular concentrations of Na^+ and K^+ may substantially modify the activity of the key glycolytic enzyme, pyruvate kinase (14). Pyruvate kinase catalyzes the conversion of phosphoenolpyruvate plus ADP to pyruvate plus ATP. From the magnitude of the decrease in [K^+] and the increase in [Na^+] seen at the end of intense exercise (Table 6), it appears from the available data (14) that the velocity of the pyruvate kinase reaction could be inhibited by at least 20%. Substantial inhibition of pyruvate kinase activity during muscle contraction could result in the accumulation of metabolic intermediates between fructose-1,6-bisphosphate and phosphoenolpyruvate, and in reduced pyruvate and lactate production, as well as in a fall in glycolytic ATP production. The mechanism of the allosteric regulatory effects of monovalent cations on enzyme activity appears to be mediated through structural and conformational changes in the protein's active site (20).

The use of fundamental physicochemical concepts to understand muscle biochemistry and physiology is not new. In his review on muscle electrolytes, Fenn (7) attempted to explain his results on "the basis of the physicochemical organization of the muscle," and he realized that changes in muscle electrolytes were related to acid-base changes in the blood. He referred to a "diffusion of acid" as "the chloride shift" and "a diffusion of base into the muscles" as "the potassium shift." The present study has provided quantitative evidence that the total ionic status of the intracellular fluids of skeletal muscle is determined by the concentrations of strong ions, weak acids and bases, and CO_2 in the intracellular fluids. Changes in acid-base status cannot occur without a concomitant change in at least one of these three independent physicochemical variables, which in turn cause changes in the concentrations of the dependent variables.

Summary

Intracellular acid-base status at rest and following exercise in muscles of differing fiber-type composition can be estimated with reasonable accuracy from measurements of the three independent quantities PCO_2, $[A_{tot}]$, and [SID]. In resting hindlimb muscles, average [SID] was about 125 mEq/L, and $[A_{tot}]$ was about 176 mEq/L. At rest, SL had a significantly higher $[H^+]$ (107 ± 11 nEq/L) than PL, RG, and WG (86 ± 6 nEq/L). With exercise, a significantly greater rise in $[H^+]$ in WG ($+117$ nEq/L) than in soleus ($+93$ nEq/L) was due primarily to a greater fall in [SID] in WG (-27 mEq/L) than in SL (-20 mEq/L) and secondarily to a 25-mEq/L increase in WG $[A_{tot}]$ while soleus $[A_{tot}]$ remained unchanged. The effect of increasing PCO_2 from 50 mmHg to 82 ± 7 mmHg was similar for all muscles. Compared to SL, the greater fall in WG [SID] with exercise was due to higher $[Lac^-]$ (43 ± 4 vs. 18 ± 2 mEq/L) and to greater depletion of K^+ (-15 vs. -5 mEq/L). We conclude that of the changes in the independent variables that occur during intense exercise, those of [SID] exert the greatest effects on intracellular ionic status. Large changes in muscle [SID] with exercise contribute to muscle fatigue by altering (a) intracellular ion concentrations, (b) membrane resting potential, and (c) protonated states and activities of intracellular proteins involved in the contractile apparatus, metabolism, and ion transport.

Acknowledgments

The authors gratefully acknowledge Dr. M. Ganagarajah and Sandra Peters for their excellent technical assistance, and Drs. Lawrence Spriet and Norman Jones for their critical reading of the manuscript. This study was supported by MRC and NSERC of Canada.

References

1. Chasiotis, D.; Hultman, E.; Sahlin, K. Acidotic depression of cyclic AMP accumulation and phosphorylase *b* to *a* transformation in skeletal muscle of man. J. Physiol. (Lond.) 335:197-204; 1982.

2. Cooke, R.; Franks, K.; Luciani, G.B.; Pate, E. The inhibition of rabbit skeletal muscle contraction by hydrogen ions and phosphate. J. Physiol. (Lond.) 395:77-97; 1988.

3. Dixon, M.; Webb, E.C. Enzymes. 3d ed. New York: Academic Press; 1979:138-164.

4. Edsall, J.T.; Wymann, J. Biophysical chemistry. New York: Academic Press; 1958:578-587. (Vol. 1).

5. Edwards, R.H.T. Human muscle function and fatigue. In: Porter, R.; Whelan, J., eds. Human muscle fatigue: physiological mechanisms. London: Pitman Medical; 1981:1-18. (CIBA Foundation Symposium 82).

6. Fabiato, A.; Fabiato, F. Effects of pH on the myofilaments and the sarcoplasmic reticulum of skinned cells from cardiac and skeletal muscles. J. Physiol. (Lond.) 276:233-255; 1978.

7. Fenn, W.O. Electrolytes in muscle. Physiol. Rev. 16:450-487; 1936.

8. Harned, H.S.; Owen, B.B. The physical chemistry of electrolyte solutions. 3d ed. New York: Van Nostrand-Reinhold; 1958.

9. Henderson, L.J. The theory of neutrality regulation in the animal organism. J. Biol. Chem. 21:427-448; 1908.

10. Hibberd, M.G.; Dantzig, J.A.; Trentham, D.R.; Goldman, Y.E. Phosphate release and force generation in skeletal muscle fibers. Science 228:1317-1319; 1985.

11. Hultman, E.; Sahlin, K. Acid-base balance during exercise. Exerc. Sport Sci. Rev. 8:41-128; 1980.

12. Hultman, E.; Sjoholm, H. Biochemical causes of fatigue. In: Jones, N.L.; McCartney, N.; McComas, A.J., eds. Human muscle power. Champaign, IL: Human Kinetics; 1986:215-238.

13. Jones, N.L. [H⁺] control in exercise—concepts and controversies (this volume).

14. Kachmar, J.F.; Boyer, P.D. Kinetic analysis of enzyme reactions: II. The potassium activation and calcium inhibition of pyruvic phosphopherase. J. Biol. Chem. 200:669-682; 1953.

15. Kasvinsky, P.J.; Meyer, W.L. The effect of pH and temperature on the kinetics of native and altered glycogen phosphorylase. Arch. Biochem. Biophys. 181:616-631; 1977.

16. Kowalchuk, J.M.; Heigenhauser, G.J.F.; Lindinger, M.I.; Sutton, J.R.; Jones, N.L. Factors influencing hydrogen ion concentration in muscle after intense exercise. J. Appl. Physiol. 65:2080-2089; 1988.

17. Lindinger, M.I.; Ganagarajah, M.; Heigenhauser, G.J.F. Relationships between ionic composition and pH in mammalian skeletal muscle. J. Appl. Physiol. (submitted).

18. Lindinger, M.I.; Heigenhauser, G.J.F. Intracellular ion content of skeletal muscle measured by instrumental neutron activation analysis. J. Appl. Physiol. 63:426-433; 1987.

19. Lindinger, M.I.; Heigenhauser, G.J.F.; Spriet, L.L. Effects of intense swimming exercise and tetanic electrical stimulation on skeletal muscle ions and metabolites. J. Appl. Physiol. 63:2331-2339; 1987.

20. Mildvan, A.S. Mechanism of enzyme action. Annu. Rev. Biochem. 43:357-399; 1974.

21. Nakamura, Y.; Schwartz, A. The influence of hydrogen ion concentration on calcium binding and release by skeletal muscle sarcoplasmic reticulum. J. Gen. Physiol. 59:22-32; 1972.

22. Nosek, T.M.; Fender, K.Y.; Godt, R.E. It is diprotonated inorganic phosphate that depresses force in skinned skeletal muscle fibers. Science 236:191-193; 1987.

23. Robinson, R.A.; Stokes, R.H. Electrolyte solutions. 2d rev. ed. London: Butterworth; 1970.

24. Roos, A.; Boron, W.F. Intracellular pH. Physiol. Rev. 61:296-433; 1981.

25. Siesjo, B.K.; Thews, G. Ein verfahren zur Bestimmung der CO_2-Leitfaigkeit der CO_2-Diffusionskoeffizienten und des scheinbaren CO_2-Loslichkeitoeffizienten in Gehirngeweben. Pflügers Arch. 276:192-210; 1962.

26. Singer, R.B.; Hastings, A.B. Improved clinical method for estimation of disturbances of acid-base balance of human blood. Medicine 27:223-242; 1948.

27. Spriet, L.L.; Soderlund, K.; Thompson, J.A.; Hultman, E. pH measurement in human skeletal muscle samples: effect of phosphagen hydrolysis. J. Appl. Physiol. 61:1949-1954; 1986.

28. Stewart, P.A. How to understand acid-base: a quantitative acid-base primer for biology and medicine. New York: Elsevier; 1981.

29. Stewart, P.A. Modern quantitative acid-base chemistry. Can. J. Physiol. Pharmacol. 61:1444-1461; 1983.

30. Trivedi, B.; Danforth, W.H. Effect of pH on the kinetics of frog muscle phosphofructokinase. J. Biol. Chem. 241:4110-4112; 1966.

31. Van Slyke, D.D. On the measurement of buffer values and on the relationship of buffer value to the dissociation constant of the buffer and the concentration and reaction of the buffer solution. J. Biol. Chem. 52:525-570; 1922.

32. Van Slyke, D.D.; Hastings, A.B.; Hiller, A.; Sendroy, J. Studies of gas and electrolyte equilibria in blood: XIV. The amounts of alkali bound by serum albumin and globulin. J. Biol. Chem. 79:769-780; 1928.

The Role of the Physicochemical Systems in Plasma in Acid–Base Control in Exercise

George J.F. Heigenhauser, Norman L. Jones, John M. Kowalchuk, and Michael I. Lindinger

McMaster University, Hamilton, University of Waterloo, Waterloo, and University of Guelph, Guelph, Ontario, Canada

During intense exercise, the high turnover rate of ATP is largely dependent on glycolytic metabolism. In muscle at these high glycolytic rates, intracellular hydrogen ion concentration ($[H^+]_i$) has been shown to increase from approximately 100 nEq/L at rest to approximately 300 nEq/L following heavy exercise of short duration (14). The large increases in $[H^+]_i$ have been implicated in the fatigue that is found in this type of exercise. A number of loci for fatigue have been suggested: excitation-contraction coupling (6), the interaction between actin and myosin (25), the inhibition of glycolytic flux at the level of phosphorylase (3) and phosphofructokinase (38), and the impairment of ionic pumps in the sarcoplasmic reticulum and sarcolemma (24). Changes in $[H^+]_i$ may be minimized by intracellular physicochemical buffering or by exchange of CO_2 and strong electrolytes between the intramuscular fluid compartment and the extracellular fluid compartment.

In most studies that have investigated the changes occurring in $[H^+]_i$, the approach has been to relate changes that occur in PCO_2 and $[H^+]$ between arterial and venous blood flowing through the muscle capillaries to changes in $[H^+]_i$. An assumption is made that changes in $[H^+]$ of arterial and venous blood reflect transmembrane fluxes of H^+ between muscle and the capillary blood flowing through the muscle. However, as emphasized by Stewart (36, 37), three fundamental laws govern the $[H^+]$ in aqueous solutions: the conservation of mass, the maintenance of electrical neutrality, and the dissociation equilibrium of weak electrolytes (A_{tot}) and water. Strong electrolytes, including lactate, which are completely or almost completely dissociated in solution influence $[H^+]$ through a strong ion difference [SID] (the difference between the sum of all strong base cations and strong acid anions), and CO_2 also contributes to the acid-base status. In solutions such as muscle cytosol and blood, $[H^+]$ is a dependent variable, and its concentration is determined by the independent variables of PCO_2, $[A_{tot}]$, and [SID]. Because weak electrolytes, generated intramuscularly by glycolytic metabolism, are generally impermeable to the muscle membrane, the regulation of $[H^+]_i$ occurs primarily through the exchange of strong ions between the muscle and extracellular fluid and through the regulation of intramuscular PCO_2 by the movement of CO_2 down its diffusion gradient.

In this context the apparent flux of H^+ must be considered in relation to the effects of transmembrane movements of strong ions, water, and PCO_2. Any changes in $[H^+]_i$ and blood arteriovenous $[H^+]$ differences cannot occur unless in association with a change in the [SID] in each of the fluid compartments, that is, changes in either the strong base cations (Na^+, K^+, Ca^{2+}, Mg^{2+}) or the strong acid anions (Cl^-, or lactate [Lac^-]). Regulation of $[H^+]_i$ occurs by the translocation of strong base cations or strong acid ions and not necessarily by translocation of H^+ per se. In muscle, there is some evidence (1) that a "regulatory" process may translocate H^+ across the muscle membrane; however, this is always associated with appropriate movement of strong ions such as Na^+ and Cl^- with [SID] influencing the $[H^+]$ in the blood or muscle.

Carbon dioxide is soluble in both water and fat and diffuses rapidly into capillary blood. Intracellular PCO_2 is dependent on the interaction between the intracellular CO_2 production, the muscle-capillary PCO_2 gradient, and the capillary blood flow, which removes the CO_2 from the muscle and transports it to the lungs. In most exercise studies, base excess is calculated to assess the change in $[H^+]$ in plasma or blood due to an increase of a "metabolic acid"; usually, metabolic acid is assumed to be lactic acid. Using this approach, studies in humans (22) and animals (2, 4) have reported that Lac^- does not always appear in the plasma or blood in stoichiometric equivalents with H^+. Even though Lac^- is well recognized as an important contributor to the increases in plasma $[H^+]$, it should also be recognized that changes in other strong ions and $[A_{tot}]$ are also important. Additionally, when an exchange of ions, CO_2, or H_2O occurs between muscle and plasma, the magnitude of the change in $[H^+]$ is quite different in each of the fluid compartments, and in some instances, in the opposite direction.

The purposes of this paper are to discuss the physicochemical changes that occur in the femoral venous and arterial plasma during short-duration, high-intensity exercise and to relate these changes to $[H^+]$. The series of human studies to be reported were carried out in our laboratory over the past few years (14, 16, 17). In these studies, each subject exercised maximally for 30 s on an isokinetic cycle ergometer. Blood was sampled simultaneously from the radial artery and the femoral vein; muscle biopsies were taken from the vastus lateralis. Blood samples and muscle biopsy samples were taken while the subject was seated on the cycle prior to exercise and during the recovery period. A detailed description of the exercise protocol and methods used in these studies has been published (14, 16-21).

Changes in Muscle Metabolites

Compared with resting muscle, large changes in intramuscular metabolites were observed immediately following 30 s exercise (Table 1). Little change occurred in $[ATP]_i$, whereas $[PCr^{2-}]_i$ decreased approximately 80% from resting values. During the 30 s of exercise, glycogen utilization was 18 mmol/kg wet weight of muscle and resulted in a large accumulation of the Lac^- intramuscularly. During the 10 min of recovery, $[PCr^{2-}]_i$ returned to resting values, whereas $[Lac^-]_i$ decreased but remained considerably elevated throughout recovery, compared with resting values.

Changes in Fluid and Electrolytes in Muscle

Increases in total muscle H_2O were observed during the 30 s of exercise and during the 10-min recovery period (Table 2). A 6% increase in total muscle water was

Table 1 Muscle Metabolite Concentrations at Rest and Following 30 s Maximal Exercise

		Time postexercise (min)		
	Rest	0.5	3.5	9.5
Adenosine triphosphate	7.9	3.7	6.0	7.8
Creatine phosphate	21.6	4.8	13.4	21.3
Lactate	5.5	47.0	29.9	26.4

Note. Values expressed in mEq/L of intracellular water.

Table 2 Muscle Total Tissue Water (TTW), Extra- (ECFV) and Intracellular (ICFV) Fluid Volumes, and Intracellular Strong Ion Concentrations at Rest and Following 30 s Maximal Exercise

		Recovery (min)		
	Rest	0.5	3.5	9.5
TTW (ml/g dw)	3.20	3.30	3.43*	3.41*
ECFV (ml/d dw)[a]	0.40	0.50*	0.50*	0.46*
ICFV (ml/g dw)[a]	2.78	2.80	2.93	2.96
[Lac$^-$] (mEq/L ICF)	5.5	47.0*	29.9*	26.4*
[K$^+$] (mEq/L ICF)	142	138	123	128
[Na$^+$] (mEq/L ICF)	9.3	11.4	11.5	9.7
[Cl$^-$] (mEq/L ICF)	8.8	9.1	13.0	9.6
[Mg^{2+}] (mEq/L ICF)	21	24	19	22
[Ca^{2+}] (mEq/L ICF)	2.5	2.6	2.3	2.7

[a]Calculated from data of Sjögaard and Saltin (33).
*Significantly different from rest value ($p < .05$).

observed at 0.5 min postexercise; this persisted for the remainder of the recovery period. Immediately following exercise there were small increases in [Na$^+$]$_i$ and [Cl$^-$]$_i$ and a small decrease in [K$^+$]$_i$, compared to resting values. These changes approached resting values by the end of the 10-min recovery period.

The [H$^+$]$_i$ at rest and during the recovery period was calculated from the independent variables, [SID]$_i$, PCO$_2$, and [A$_{tot}$]$_i$. The physicochemical systems and the equations necessary to calculate [H$^+$]$_i$ from the independent variables are described in the two preceding papers. The equilibrium constants for the equations are listed in Table 2 of Lindinger and Heigenhauser's paper (20). PCO$_2$ was assumed to be equal to the femoral venous PCO$_2$, and [SID]$_i$ was calculated from strong ions tabulated in Table 2. At the present time, we have not titrated human muscle with NaOH and

CO_2 to determine $[A_{tot}]_i$; $[A_{tot}]_i$ and K_A of human muscle were assumed to be similar to those obtained for rat plantaris.

The $[H^+]_i$ increased from 118 nEq/L at rest to peak at 281 nEq/L at 3.5 min postexercise (Table 3). Immediately postexercise, the increase in $[H^+]_i$ could be accounted for equally by decreases in $[SID]_i$ and increases in K_A and PCO_2. By the end of 10 min recovery, the increases in $[H^+]_i$ were accounted for solely by decreases in $[SID]_i$. The changes in $[SID]_i$ were due to both a decrease in $[K^+]_i$ and an increase in $[Lac^-]_i$ during the recovery period. The values of $[H^+]_i$ at any given $[Lac^-]_i$, calculated from the physicochemical variables, are similar to those obtained by the homogenate technique applied to human muscle (12, 29, 34). However, as emphasized previously (20), the increases in $[H^+]_i$ were due not only to increases in $[Lac^-]_i$ but also to decreases in $[K^+]_i$ and to an increase in K_A.

Table 3 Calculation of the Effects of Changes of PCO_2, [SID], [A_{tot}], and K_A on Muscle [H⁺]

		Time postexercise (min)		
	Rest	0.5	3.5	9.5
[SID] (mEq/L)	111	96 (39%)	74 (91%)	72 (100%)
PCO_2 (mmHg)	46	106 (32%)	48 (1%)	40 (3%)
[A_{tot}] (mEq/L)*	175	175	175	175
K_A (10^{-7}Eq/L)*	1.64	1.97 (29%)	1.80 (8%)	1.64
H⁺ (nEq/L)	118	212	281	256
pH	6.93	6.67	6.55	6.59

Note. Values expressed per liter intramuscular water. The change in the total increase of [H⁺] from rest, expressed as a percentage, is indicated in parentheses.

*Assumed to be equal to those obtained by NaOH and CO_2 titration of rat plantaris (19).

Changes in Arterial and Femoral Venous Plasma

Compared with resting values, a decrease in plasma volume was observed in both the arterial and the femoral venous blood (Tables 4 and 5). A 13.5% and a 9.8% decrease were observed in the femoral venous and arterial blood, respectively, immediately following exercise. In plasma the weak electrolytes are primarily the plasma proteins. Following exercise there was an increase in plasma protein concentration

Table 4   Plasma Strong Ion Concentrations in Femoral Vein at Rest and During Recovery From 30 s Maximal Exercise

| | | | | Time postexercise (min) | | | | |
	Rest	0	0.5	1.0	1.5	2.5	3.5	5.5	9.5
[Na⁺]	138	150	149	147	145	143	141	139	138
[K⁺]	5.4	7.8*	6.9*	6.1	5.7	5.3	5.2	5.2	5.3
[Ca²⁺]	1.1	1.4*	1.3*	1.3*	1.2*	1.2*	1.2	1.2	1.2
[Lac⁻]	1.0	9.7*	13.1*	14.8*	15.7*	16.9*	17.6*	15.5*	15.2*
[Cl⁻]	102	108	105	102	104	101	101	100	99
[Hb]	13.5	15.6	14.8*	14.9*	14.6*	14.8*	14.7	14.0*	14.5
[Plasma proteins]	7.3	8.4	8.0	8.1	7.9	8.0	7.9	7.6	7.8

Note. All concentrations but Hb (g/100 ml) and plasma proteins (g/dl) are measured in mEq/L. Values are means.

*Significantly different ($p < .05$) from resting value.

Table 5   Plasma Strong Ion Concentrations in Radial Artery at Rest and During Recovery From 30 s Maximal Exercise

| | | | | Time postexercise (min) | | | | |
	Rest	0	0.5	1.0	1.5	2.5	3.5	5.5	9.5
[Na⁺]	137	144*	145*	144*	143*	141*	141*	139*	138
[K⁺]	4.5	6.9*	6.3*	5.6*	5.2*	4.8	4.6	4.5	4.6
[Ca²⁺]	1.1	1.2*	1.2*	1.2*	1.2*	1.2*	1.2*	1.2	1.1
[Lac⁻]	0.9	6.3	9.6*	12.2*	13.5*	13.9*	13.8*	13.8*	12.3*
[Cl⁻]	105	112	111	109	108	104	102	102	101
[Hb]	12.9	14.3*	14.3*	14.1*	14.1*	14.1*	14.0*	14.3*	13.8*
[Plasma proteins]	7.0	7.7	7.7	7.6	7.6	7.6	7.5	7.7	7.5

Note. All concentrations but Hb (g/100 ml) and plasma proteins (g/dl) are measured in mEq/L. Values are means.

*Significantly different ($p < .05$) from resting value.

in both the femoral venous and the arterial blood, which paralleled the decrease in plasma fluid volume (Tables 4 and 5). These decreases in blood volume persisted for the remainder of the recovery period.

All the plasma concentrations of strong inorganic ions were increased in both the arterial and the venous femoral plasma immediately following exercise and gradually returned to resting values during the first 5 min of recovery (Figure 1, Tables 4 and 5). Except for [K$^+$], all the concentration changes of the inorganic ions could be accounted for by changes in plasma fluid volume. Immediately following exercise, plasma [Lac$^-$] increased to 9.7 and 6.3 mEq/L in venous and arterial samples, respectively (Figure 1, Tables 4 and 5). In both arterial and venous plasma, [Lac$^-$]

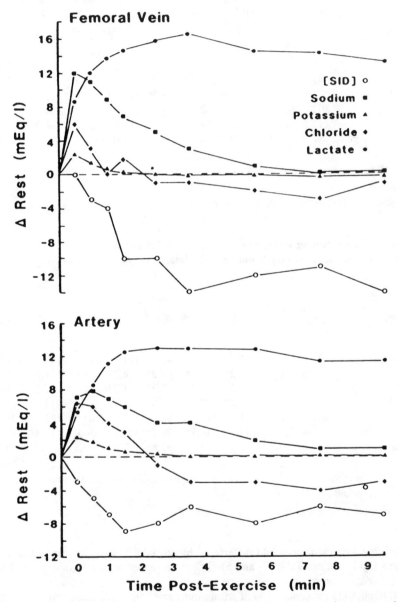

Figure 1. Mean changes in plasma strong ion concentrations postexercise compared with preexercise values in femoral venous and arterial plasma. Reprinted with permission of the American Physiological Society.

peaked at 4 min postexercise and decreased throughout the recovery period, but remained elevated compared to rest.

During the first minute of recovery, femoral venous [SID] remained similar to resting values (42 mEq/L), but it decreased to 33 mEq/L by 1.5 min of recovery (Figure 1). Thereafter, [SID] in femoral venous plasma remained stable throughout the recovery period. In contrast, arterial plasma [SID] decreased to 37 mEq/L immediately after exercise and reached stable levels at 1 min of recovery (Figure 1). Femoral venous PCO_2 was 100 mmHg immediately following exercise and peaked at 106 mmHg at 1 min of recovery; thereafter, it decreased rapidly during the early part of recovery (Figure 2). By the end of the recovery period, PCO_2 was below resting values. Within 2 min postexercise, arterial PCO_2 fell to 30 mmHg and remained at that level throughout the remaining 8 min of recovery.

Femoral venous [H$^+$] increased from 42 nEq/L at rest to 95 nEq/L at 30 s postexercise and decreased throughout the recovery period (Figure 2). Arterial [H$^+$] followed the same pattern as the femoral venous [H$^+$], but the magnitude of the increase was less (11 nEq/L compared with 53 nEq/L). The femoral venous and arterial [H$^+$] did not return to preexercise values by the end of the 10-min recovery period.

In order to account for the changes in [H$^+$] that occurred in the femoral venous and arterial plasma, the physicochemical approach of Stewart was used. The description of this approach to ''acid-base'' regulation was outlined in the initial presentation of this symposium by Dr. N.L. Jones (13). This approach to acid-base regulation in plasma is not new; it was used in the classical research in acid-base chemistry of blood (9, 27, 39, 40). Although it is controversial, is has helped clarify the interrelationships that occur in the independent variables ([SID], [A$_{tot}$], and PCO_2) that determine [H$^+$] in the plasma. The contributions of the independent variables to changes in plasma [H$^+$] were determined at rest and 0.5, 3.5, and 9.5 min of the recovery period, using the physicochemical equations of Stewart (36, 37). The equilibrium constants for the system equations are listed in Table 6.

At 0.5 min postexercise, 90% of the increase in [H$^+$] in the femoral venous plasma can be accounted for by the increased PCO_2, but by 3.5 min into the recovery period, the effect of PCO_2 was small (Table 7). By the end of the recovery period, femoral venous PCO_2 fell below resting values and had an alkalinizing effect. The small decrease in [SID] observed immediately following exercise increased [H$^+$] by 6%, but by the end of the recovery period, it accounted for 94% of the increase in [H$^+$]. The small increase in [A$_{tot}$] accounted for only 4-6% of the increase in [H$^+$] throughout the recovery period. Throughout recovery, in arterial plasma (Table 8) the decreased [SID] and increased [A$_{tot}$] accounted for 77-85% and 15-23%, respectively, of the increased [H$^+$]. Immediately following exercise, the increase in [H$^+$] (resulting from the decreased [SID] and increased [A$_{tot}$]) was reduced by 29% through a decrease in PCO_2, and this alkalinizing influence was increased throughout the remainder of the recovery period.

In order to validate the physicochemical approach in plasma, we have compared the directly measured values for plasma [H$^+$] in the femoral venous and the arterial plasma with those calculated by the physicochemical approach. The calculated values for [H$^+$] are similar to the measured [H$^+$], except for the resting arterial [H$^+$] (Tables 7 and 8). We have also examined the effect of experimental error of each of the independent variables on the calculated [H$^+$] in the femoral venous plasma at 0.5 min postexercise. The standard deviation of measurement for [SID] is 1.4 mEq/L; this would lead to a potential error of $\pm$ 2 nEq/L (4%). Measurement of PCO_2 in plasma

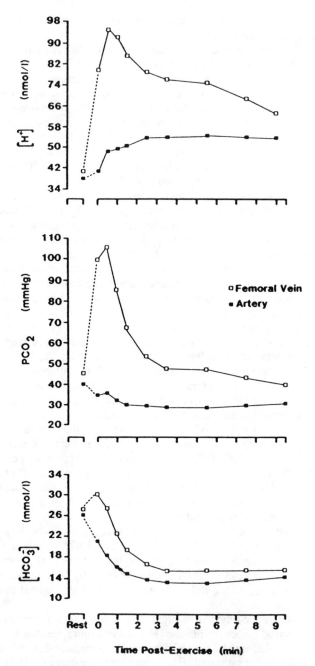

Figure 2. Hydrogen ion concentration ($[H^+]$), PCO_2, and $[HCO_3^-]$ in femoral venous and arterial plasma postexercise. Reprinted with permission of the American Physiological Society.

**Table 6 Constants Used in Calculations of Plasma [H⁺]
Using the Physicochemical Equations**

Equation	Constant	Reference #
$[H^+] \times [A^-] = K_A[HA]$	$K_A = 3.0 \times 10^{-7}$	36
$[H^+] \times [HCO_3^-] = K_c PCO_2$	$K_c = 2.46 \times 10^{-11}$	36
$[H^+] \times [CO_3^-] = K_3[HCO_3^-]$	$K_3 = 6.0 \times 10^{-11}$	5
$[H^+] \times [OH^-] = K_W$	$K_W = 4.4 \times 10^{-14}$	8

**Table 7 Calculation of the Effects of Changes of PCO_2, [SID], and $[A_{tot}]$
on Femoral Venous [H⁺]**

| | Rest | Time postexercise (min) | | |
		0.5	3.5	9.5
[SID] (mEq/L)	42	39 (6%)	29 (86%)	30 (94%)
PCO_2 (mmHg)	46	106 (90%)	48 (10%)	40 (15%)
$[A_{tot}]$ (mEq/L)	17	19 (4%)	18.5 (4%)	18.5 (6%)
[H⁺] (nEq/L)[a]	42	99	76	62
[H⁺] (nEq/L)[b]	41	95	76	64

Note. The change in total increase of [H⁺] from rest, expressed as a percentage, is indicated in parentheses.

[a]Calculated using physicochemical equations.

[b]Measured using pH electrode.

is accurate to ± 1 mmHg, which is equivalent to ± 1 nEq/L (2%) error. A measurement error of ± 10% for plasma proteins would lead to a ± 2 nEq/L (4%) error in [H⁺].

The total "acid load" in plasma traditionally has been analyzed in terms of a respiratory (CO_2) component and a metabolic (non-CO_2) component (30, 31). The contribution of plasma metabolic [H⁺] is estimated by titrating plasma with strong ions and is termed *base excess*. Using this approach, the components that contribute to the non-CO_2 or metabolic component of the acid load cannot be determined and are generally accepted to result from increases in plasma [Lac⁻]. Using this approach, Stainsby and colleagues (2, 4) reported that the efflux of H⁺ exceeded that of Lac⁻

**Table 8 Calculation of the Effects of Changes of PCO₂, [SID], and [A_tot]
on Arterial Plasma [H⁺]**

	Rest	Time postexercise (min)		
		0.5	3.5	9.5
[SID] (mEq/L)	37	32 (77%)	31 (85%)	31 (85%)
PCO₂ (mmHg)	41	37 (29%)	30 (79%)	32 (74%)
[A_tot] (mEq/L)	17	19 (23%)	18.5 (15%)	18.5 (15%)
[H⁺] (nEq/L)^a	38	47	53	55
[H⁺] (nEq/L)^b	45	51	54	54

Note. The change in total increase of [H⁺] from rest, expressed as a percentage, is indicated in parentheses.
^{a}Calculated using physicochemical equations.
^{b}Measured using pH electrode.

in an electrically stimulated in situ dog preparation by factors of 5 and 11 during steady state and non–steady state contractions, respectively.

Similar results have been reported in human studies. Medbo and Sejersted reported that following exercise the metabolic H⁺ accumulation in the extracellular space exceeded Lac⁻ accumulation by 30-45% (22). If we used base excess to determine the metabolic [H⁺], the metabolic [H⁺] in femoral venous plasma at 0.5 min postexercise would be 5 times less than the [Lac⁻]. Using base excess to account for [H⁺] in plasma in our studies and that of Medbo and Sejersted (22), it may be considered that H⁺ and Lac⁻ move independently from muscle to the plasma. However, the discrepancy between the [H⁺] and [Lac⁻] can be accounted for if the physicochemical approach is used. In the present study, the increase in metabolic acid resulted from an increase in [A_tot] and a small decrease in [SID]. The decrease in [SID] was 3 mEq/L, whereas the [Lac⁻] increased by 9 mEq/L. The increase in the acidic anion [Lac⁻] was almost totally offset by increases in the basic cations, [Na⁺] and [K⁺], accounting for the appearance of [H⁺] and [Lac⁻] in nonstoichiometric equivalents. When the data of Medbo and Sejersted (22) are analyzed using the physicochemical approach, the discrepancy between H⁺ and Lac⁻ accumulation in the extracellular space is also resolved.

In plasma, the primary weak electrolytes are proteins (28). Even though there are many species of plasma proteins, they can be considered to behave as a single weak electrolyte with a single K_A. The total concentration of weak electrolytes is obtained from the plasma protein concentration, which is considered to have a 2.42 anion equivalent for every gram of plasma protein. The "average" K_A of the plasma proteins is 3.0×10^{-7}. These values have recently been validated by Rossing and colleagues (28). In our studies, plasma $[A_{tot}]$ changed in parallel with the fluid shift from plasma to the interstitial and intracellular spaces (Tables 4 and 5). An increase in plasma proteins of 1.0 g/dl ($[A_{tot}]$ of 2.42 mEq/L), which is similar to the magnitude found in our studies, will result in a 3.6 nEq/L increase in plasma $[H^+]$ without concomitant changes in PCO_2 and [SID]. It is clear that the changes that occur in plasma volume with exercise will influence plasma $[H^+]$, but they are not considered when using the concept of base excess (30, 31).

For PCO_2 to be an independent variable, the body must be an "open system" for CO_2, and the circulatory and respiratory systems must function so that CO_2 is eliminated from the lungs as fast as it is produced in the tissues. A rapid efflux of CO_2 occurred during the first 3 min postexercise. Femoral venous PCO_2, which had increased to 106 mmHg by 0.5 min postexercise, fell to 50 mmHg by 3 min postexercise. This was associated with large increases in total body CO_2 production, respiratory exchange ratio, and ventilation (Figure 3). For the remainder of the recovery period, ventilation remained elevated in relation to the CO_2 efflux from muscle, resulting in a decreased PCO_2 (respiratory alkalosis) in both the femoral venous and arterial plasma.

The resting physicochemical properties of the individual fluid compartments determine the magnitude of the influence of the independent variables on $[H^+]$ changes that occur from rest to exercise. In muscle the [SID] and $[A_{tot}]$ are 2.5 and 10 times greater, respectively, than in plasma (Tables 3 and 7). At 0.05 min postexercise, $[H^+]_i$ increased by 94 nEq/L from rest, whereas the femoral venous plasma $[H^+]_i$ increased by 57 nEq/L. The increase in PCO_2 from 46 to 106 mmHg increased $[H^+]$ by 30 nEq/L and 51 nEq/L in muscle and femoral venous plasma, respectively. In

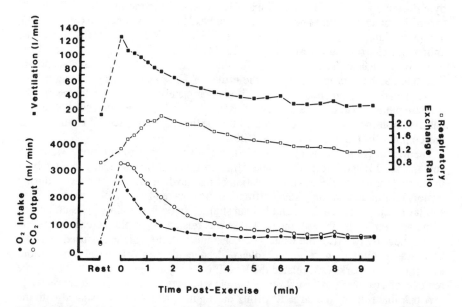

Figure 3. Oxygen uptake, carbon dioxide output, respiratory exchange ratio, and ventilation during 10 min of recovery. Reprinted with permission of the American Physiological Society.

muscle a decrease in [SID] of 15 mEq/L observed 0.5 min postexercise resulted in an increase in [H^+] of 37 nEq/L; if a similar change in [SID] had been observed in femoral venous plasma, it would have resulted in an increase of 44 nEq/L in [H^+]. Thus, the higher [SID] and [A_{tot}] of muscle attenuated the changes in [H^+] resulting from changes in the independent physicochemical variables that occurred during exercise.

The time course of the effects of independent variables on [H^+] is different in muscle and femoral venous plasma (Tables 3 and 7). In plasma the [H^+] increase is initially due primarily to a large increase in PCO_2. The influence of PCO_2 is quickly resolved by 3.5 minutes into the recovery period; thereafter, the increase in [H^+] is due primarily to a decrease in [SID]. In muscle at 0.5 min postexercise, a decreased [SID] and increased PCO_2 and K_A contribute equally to the increase in [H^+]. By 3.5 min postexercise, K_A of the weak electrolytes returns toward resting values, and the influence of PCO_2 is reduced. For the remainder of the recovery period, the major contributor to the increase in [H^+]$_i$ is a decrease in [SID].

The Role of K^+ in Heavy, Intense Exercise

A small net influx of Na^+ and Cl^- into muscle and a large net efflux of K^+ were observed immediately following exercise. These fluxes were reflected in both the femoral arteriovenous difference and the intramuscular ion concentration. At 3.5 min postexercise, approximately 45% of the increase in [H^+]$_i$ could be accounted for by a decrease in [K^+]$_i$. The net efflux of K^+ from contracting muscle has been observed by other investigators. In human studies, there was a net flux of K^+ from the intracellular to the extracellular space (22, 32, 33). With electrically stimulated animal muscle, several investigators (7, 10, 11, 15, 21, 23) have shown a net efflux of K^+ from muscle. The mechanism for the increase in K^+ release is not known. One that has been proposed is that the efflux of K^+ is electrogenic in origin; that is, during an action potential, K^+ efflux is not completely counteracted by the Na^+/K^+ ATPase pump, resulting in a net loss of [K^+]$_i$ (10, 11, 15). The increase in K^+ efflux has also been postulated to be mediated by special Ca^{2+}-activated K^+ channels that are common in the T tubule system (26).

The loss of [K^+]$_i$ via the electrogenic mechanism is open to question. Mohrman and Sparks (23) and Streter (35) found large transient K^+ fluxes related to glycolysis in the first minute of electrical stimulation of mammalian muscle. However, during prolonged stimulation, only small effluxes or an uptake of K^+ are observed. We had similar results in both animal and human studies. In both swimming rats and in the stimulated rat hindlimb (21), the [K^+]$_i$ loss was related to a rapid increase in muscle glycolytic activity. Also, the white gastrocnemius [K^+]$_i$ loss in the perfused rat hindlimb was greater than from the soleus, despite identical electrical stimulation. Mohrman and Sparks (23) related the K^+ efflux to regulation of [H^+]$_i$; however, the removal of a cation from the cytosol of muscle will increase rather than decrease [H^+]$_i$.

A possible role for the large K^+ efflux during muscle activity associated with the rapid increase in glycolytic activity may be in osmoregulation. The increases in [Lac^-], inorganic phosphate, and hexose phosphate concentrations represent an increase of approximately 70 mOsm intramuscularly during the 30 s of exercise (14). Because water will move quickly into muscle in response to these osmotic pressure gradients, an immediate 25% increase in muscle water would be expected. However, only a 6% increase in total muscle water was observed in our studies. The rapid and large flux of K^+ from muscle would be an efficient mechanism to reduce the large osmotic load generated by the accumulation of metabolites during sudden intense muscle contractions. From a teleological viewpoint, the decreased $[K^+]_i$ would further increase $[H^+]_i$, tending to inhibit glycolytic flux and thus prevent further accumulation of osmotically active metabolites. Further investigation is necessary to characterize the mechanism for these large K^+ fluxes.

Conclusions

Our studies illustrate the use of a physicochemical approach to quantify the major factors that influence $[H^+]$ in plasma. Although this approach is controversial, the series of equations used to quantify the effects of the independent variables are based on classical physicochemical principles. Using this approach, plasma $[H^+]$ and, more important, the effect of each of the independent variables on plasma $[H^+]$ may be calculated.

Acknowledgments

The authors gratefully acknowledge the excellent technical assistance of Tanya Chypchar, Dr. M. Ganagarajah, George Obminski, Sandra Peters, and Dr. John R. Sutton. We also wish to thank Dr. Peter Stewart, who spent 3 months with us, introducing us to the "classical physicochemical approach" to acid-base regulation. This study was supported by a grant to Drs. Heigenhauser and Jones from the Medical Research Council of Canada. Dr. Heigenhauser is a Career Investigator of the Heart and Stroke Foundation of Ontario.

References

1. Aickin, C.C.; Thomas, R.C. An investigation of the ionic mechanism of intracellular pH regulation in mouse soleus fibres. J. Physiol. (Lond.) 273:295-316; 1977.

2. Barbee, R.W.; Stainsby, W.N.; Chirtel, S.J. Dynamics of O_2, CO_2, lactate and acid exchange during contractions and recovery. J. Appl. Physiol. 54:1687-1692; 1983.

3. Chasiotis, D.; Hultman, E.; Sahlin, K. Acidotic depression of cyclic AMP accumulation and phosphorylase b to a transformation in skeletal muscle of man. J. Physiol. (Lond.) 335:197-204; 1982.

4. Chirtel, S.J.; Barbee, R.W.; Stainsby, W.N. Net O_2, CO_2, lactate and acid exchange by muscle during progressive working contractions. J. Appl. Physiol. 56:161-165; 1984.

5. Edsall, J.T.; Wymann, J. Biophysical chemistry. New York: Academic Press; 1958:578-587. (Vol. 1).

6. Fabiato, A.; Fabiato, F. Effects of pH on the myofilaments and the sarcoplasmic reticulum of skinned cells from cardiac and skeletal muscles. J. Physiol. (Lond.) 276:233-255; 1978.

7. Fenn, W.O. Factors affecting the loss of potassium from stimulated muscles. Am. J. Physiol. 124:213-229; 1938.

8. Harned, H.S.; Owen, B.O. The physical chemistry of electrolyte solutions. 3d ed. New York: Van Nostrand-Reinhold; 1958.

9. Hastings, A.B.; Van Slyke, D.D.; Neill, J.M.; Heidelberger, M.; Harington, C.R. Studies of gas and electrolyte equilibria in blood: VI. The acid properties of reduced and oxygenated hemoglobin. J. Biol. Chem. 59:89-153; 1924.

10. Hirche, H.; Schumacher, E.; Hagemann, H. Extracellular K^+ concentration and K^+ balance of the gastrocnemius muscle of the dog during exercise. Pflügers Arch. 387:231-237; 1980.

11. Hnik, P.; Holas, M.; Krekule, I.; Kriz, N.; Mejsnar, J.; Smiesko, V.; Ujec, E.; Vyskocil, F. Work-induced potassium changes in skeletal muscle and effluent venous blood assessed by liquid ion-exchanger microelectrodes. Pflügers Arch. 362:85-94; 1976.

12. Hultman, E.; Sahlin, K. Acid-base balance during exercise. Exerc. Sport Sci. Rev. 8:41-128; 1980.

13. Jones, N.L. [H^+] control in exercise—concepts and controversies (this volume).

14. Jones, N.L.; McCartney, N.; Graham, T.; Spriet, L.L.; Kowalchuk, J.M.; Heigenhauser, G.J.F.; Sutton, J.R. Muscle performance and metabolism in maximal isokinetic cycling at slow and fast speeds. J. Appl. Physiol. 59:132-136; 1985.

15. Juel, C. Potassium and sodium shifts during in vitro muscle contraction and the time course of the ion-gradient recovery. Pflügers Arch. 406:458-463; 1986.

16. Kowalchuk, J.M.; Heigenhauser, G.J.F.; Lindinger, M.I.; Sutton, J.R.; Jones, N.L. Factors influencing hydrogen ion concentration in muscle following intense exercise. J. Appl. Physiol. 65:2080-2089; 1988.

17. Kowalchuk, J.M.; Heigenhauser, G.J.F.; Lindinger, M.I.; Sutton, J.R.; Obminski, G.; Jones, N.L. Role of lungs and inactive muscle in acid-base control after maximal exercise. J. Appl. Physiol. 65:2090-2096; 1988.

18. Lindinger, M.I.; Heigenhauser, G.J.F. Intracellular ion content of skeletal muscle measured by instrumental neutron activation analysis. J. Appl. Physiol. 63:426-433; 1987.

19. Lindinger, M.I.; Ganagarajah, M.; Heigenhauser, G.J.F. Relationships between ionic composition and pH in mammalian skeletal muscle. J. Appl. Physiol. (submitted for publication).

20. Lindinger, M.I.; Heigenhauser, G.J.F. Acid–base systems in skeletal muscle and their response to exercise (this volume).

21. Lindinger, M.I.; Heigenhauser, G.J.F.; Spriet, L.L. Effects of intense swimming exercise and tetanic electrical stimulation on skeletal muscle ions and metabolites. J. Appl. Physiol. 63:2331-2339; 1987.

22. Medbo, J.I.; Sejersted, O.M. Acid-base and electrolyte balance after exhausting exercise in endurance-trained and sprint-trained subjects. Acta Physiol. Scand. 125:97-109; 1985.

23. Mohrman, D.E.; Sparks, H.V. Role of potassium ions in the vascular response to a brief tetanus. Circ. Res. 35:384-390; 1974.

24. Nakamura, Y.; Schwartz, A. The influence of hydrogen ion concentration on calcium binding and release by skeletal muscle sarcoplasmic reticulum. J. Gen. Physiol. 59:22-32; 1972.

25. Nosek, T.M.; Fender, K.Y.; Godt, R.E. It is diprotonated inorganic phosphate that depresses force in skinned skeletal muscle fibers. Science 236:191-193; 1987.

26. Pallotta, B.S.; Magleby, K.L.; Barrett, J.N. Single channel recordings of Ca^{2+}-activated K^+ currents in rat muscle cell culture. Nature 293:471-474; 1981.

27. Peter, J.P.; Van Slyke, D.D. Quantitative clinical chemistry: I. Interpretations. Baltimore: Williams and Wilkins; 1932.

28. Rossing, T.H.; Maffeo, N.; Fencl, V. Acid-base effects of altering plasma protein concentration in human blood in vitro. J. Appl. Physiol. 61:2260-2265; 1986.

29. Sahlin, K.; Harris, R.C.; Nylind, B.; Hultman, E. Lactate content and pH in muscle samples obtained after dynamic exercise. Pflügers Arch. 367:143-149; 1976.

30. Siggaard-Andersen, O. Blood acid-base alignment nomogram. Scand. J. Clin. Invest. 15:211-217; 1963.

31. Singer, R.B.; Hastings, A.B. Improved clinical method for estimation of disturbances of acid-base balance of human blood. Medicine 27:223-242; 1948.

32. Sjögaard, G.; Adams, R.P.; Saltin, B. Water and ion shifts in skeletal muscle of humans with intense dynamic knee extension. Am. J. Physiol. 248: R190-R196; 1985.

33. Sjögaard, G.; Saltin, B. Extra- and intracellular water spaces in muscle of man at rest and with dynamic exercise. Am. J. Physiol. 243:R271-R280; 1982.

34. Spriet, L.L.; Söderlund, K.; Thompson, J.A.; Hultman, E. pH measurement in human skeletal muscle samples: effect of phosphagen hydrolysis. J. Appl. Physiol. 61:1949-1954; 1986.

35. Sreter, F.A. Cell water, sodium and potassium in stimulated red and white mammalian muscles. Am. J. Physiol. 205:1295-1298; 1963.

36. Stewart, P.A. How to understand acid-base: a quantitative acid-base primer for biology and medicine. New York: Elsevier/North Holland; 1981.

37. Stewart, P.A. Modern quantitative acid-base chemistry. Can. J. Physiol. Pharmacol. 61:1444-1461; 1983.

38. Trivedi, B.; Danforth, W.H. Effect of pH on the kinetics of frog muscle phospho-fructokinase. J. Biol. Chem. 241:4110-4112; 1966.

39. Van Slyke, D.D. On the measurement of buffer values and on the relationship of buffer value to the dissociation constant of the buffer and the concentration and reaction of the buffer solution. J. Biol. Chem. 52:525-570; 1922.

40. Van Slyke, D.D.; Hastings, A.B.; Miller, A.; Sendroy, J. Studies of gas and electrolyte equilibria in blood: XIV. The amounts of alkali bound by serum albumin and globulin. J. Biol. Chem. 79:769-780; 1928.

Ion Regulation in Exercise:
Lessons From Comparative Physiology

Donald C. Jackson
Brown University, Providence, Rhode Island, U.S.A.

The rationale for considering comparative aspects of exercise or any other topic in physiology, in addition to satisfying our curiosity about how animals function, is that particular animals often illustrate physiological mechanisms in a clear or dramatic fashion or reveal novel mechanisms not present in higher forms. Either of these outcomes can sharpen understanding of our own response to exercise. In this paper I will first consider responses to exercise in selected lower animals, vertebrates and invertebrates, in which the acid-base responses to exertion display both clear similarities and divergences from the familiar human responses. Second, I will discuss examples from higher vertebrates, mammals and birds, of exercise in hostile environments made possible by physiological mechanisms that are still poorly understood.

Methods

A major challenge for the comparative physiologist is how to study exercise and its consequences in appropriate fashion in diverse organisms. The usual objectives are either to define the limits of an animal's exercise capacity or to describe the mechanisms that permit the normal activity carried on by the animal in nature. To achieve these objectives, a number of approaches have been used, each with advantages and limitations; they can be conveniently divided into three categories.

The most commonly employed approach utilizes the treadmill principle, in which the intensity of activity is controlled and constant and the animal is stationary relative to the measuring apparatus. The application of this approach has been readily made to walking, running, or crawling species using conventional treadmills and, with some ingenuity and patience, to swimming and flying species using circular water channels and wind tunnels, respectively. This method has the advantages of graded activity up to some maximum level, variable time duration, and repetitive or continuous measurements of physiological variables even during activity. However, it may oversimplify the normal exercise of some animals, which is rarely at a constant level for an extended period of time.

A second, less refined approach is to stimulate an animal to maximal activity until it becomes refractory, that is, exhausted. This may be accomplished by mechanical or electrical prodding or by inverting the animal and forcing repeated righting reactions. This method has the advantage of defining the limits of performance and response, as well as reproducing in some respects the burst activity characteristic of many species (1). In addition, many animals either do not perform adequately on a treadmill or cannot be induced to exercise to exhaustion in this fashion. An obvious negative aspect of the stimulation method is the stress imposed on the experimental animal, although it can be argued that this mirrors the stress of an animal responding to a life-threatening event in nature.

A final method is to study animals under natural conditions in the field. This has the advantage of being realistic in terms of normal behavior, but is uncontrolled and not always well defined. In some circumstances in which the particular activity is predictable and confined (17), it has been a useful approach. With the advent of highly sophisticated and miniaturized telemetry and microprocessor-controlled data acquisition and storage (14), it should find increased applications, although the retrieval of the animal and its data after the study may be a problem in some cases.

Principles of Acid-Base Change

Most comparative exercise studies have focused on the acid-base state of blood, and from observed changes have inferred effects derived from respiratory gas exchange and from ion fluxes into or out of blood. Except under conditions of mild activity in lower animals, oxygen delivery to active muscles is inadequate to sustain aerobic metabolism, so that some anaerobic production of lactic acid is a common feature of these studies. In many cases in which the activity level is severe or exhausting, anaerobic processes are the major suppliers of energy. Therefore, a key problem confronting animals, both during and after activity, is to deal with the lactate ions and associated protons generated within the active tissue. Likewise, the metabolic production of CO_2 and the additional, and often predominant, generation of this volatile acid from the titration of bicarbonate pose further challenges to the animal's acid-base homeostasis.

These effects may be assessed using the approach described by Stewart (27) in which the independent variables (SID, PCO_2, and A_{tot}) are identified that determine, on the basis on the fundamental equilibrium reactions of the system, the dependent variables (pH or $[H^+]$, $[HCO_3]$, etc.). It must be stressed at the outset, however, that the studies cited, without exception, have not used this approach in the analysis of data, so some reinterpretation is required.

During and after activity, CO_2 in excess of the resting rate is produced via either aerobic metabolism or acid titration. In humans and many other mammals, blood P_{CO_2} is regulated at or slightly below its resting value during mild exercise by closely matching alveolar ventilation with metabolic CO_2 production, whereas at activity levels exceeding the anaerobic threshold, relative hyperventilation causes P_{CO_2} to fall. In contrast, although most lower animals maintain or even lower P_{CO_2} during mild exercise, heavy exercise almost always results in a transient respiratory acidosis due to their less effective gas exchange capacities.

The contribution of SID to acid-base state during exercise is both a more complicated and a more controversial topic. By definition, SID is the difference in concentration between all the strong cations and all the strong anions in a solution (such as plasma). An accurate assessment of this important variable therefore requires measurement of all the quantitatively significant strong ions in the solution, a condition that makes identification of small changes extremely difficult to accomplish. The more commonly employed acid-base analysis, in which the so-called H^+ load on the extracellular fluid is calculated (31), is also technically difficult because it requires an accurate knowledge of the in vivo buffering capacity of the blood. Once the changes in acid-base state are documented, a further challenge is to define the ion transfer mechanisms that produced these changes. Here the SID approach, where successfully applied, has a distinct advantage over the more traditional acid-base analysis because the alterations in the individual ionic concentrations provide a clear indication of possible mechanisms involved. Although any net change in strong cation vis-à-vis strong anion represents a change in SID, the underlying global event in strenuous exercise is an increase in lactate anion. Lactate is produced within active muscle tissue in stoichiometrically equivalent amounts with proton (23), but formation of undissociated lactic acid is minimal because of the low dissociation constant ($K_a \cong 10^{-4}$).

Lactate may remain within muscle cells or leave as undissociated lactic acid or as lactate anion. If the latter, then another ion must move to preserve charge balance; if this is a strong ion, such as Cl entry into the cell, SID will be unaffected by the exchange. If, however, a weak ion balances the lactate, such as HCC_3 entry, then SID will rise in the cell and fall in the extracellular fluid as a result. Extracellular SID may be further affected by exchange of ions with either other body fluid compartments or with the environment. The net effect of these events on the plasma, the usual indicator of extracellular composition, is likely to be complex and not easy to interpret.

An indication of the mechanisms involved can be learned by comparing the change in plasma SID with the change in plasma lactate concentration, as in schematic diagram Figure 1. In the control or resting state, lactate is considered negligible and SID ($[B^+]-[A^-]$) is at some positive value for the particular animal. Three exercise-induced conditions associated with lactate production and exchange can occur. The increase in plasma lactate can be equal in concentration to the decrease in SID, the increase in plasma lactate may exceed the decrease in SID, or the increase in lactate may be less than the decrease in SID. In conventional terms these different states are interpreted as coupled (first case) or uncoupled (second and third cases) effluxes of H^+ and lactate from muscle cells to extracellular fluid and/or removal of these ions from extracellular fluid. When lactate increase exceeds SID decreases (or H^+ load), compensatory changes in other plasma strong ions have occurred to diminish the acidotic effect. But when the opposite is true and lactate increase is less, then additional strong ion changes exacerbating the acid effect must have occurred.

Sustainable Activity

Certain animals can remain active for long periods when the supply of oxygen matches utilization. Acid-base disturbances are minimal under these conditions. For example, many fish cruise for long periods powered by a small mass of well-perfused red muscle. Only during rapid escape or predatory maneuvers must they switch to their large mass of white, largely glycolytic fibers for locomotion. Similarly, marine

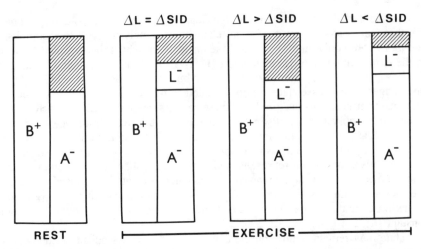

Figure 1. Possible relationships between the change in plasma lactate and the change in plasma SID as a result of exercise. See text for discussion.

turtles regularly swim for great distances to breeding and foraging areas; laboratory studies on juvenile green turtles *(Chelonia mydas)* reveal that speeds up to 0.7 m • sec^{-1}, which elevate metabolic rate 3-fold, are sustained with no acid-base disturbance (7). Adult green turtles have also been studied during their natural nesting period (17). This more strenuous activity of cumbersome terrestrial locomotion and nest-building may last for 2 to 3 hours at up to 10 times resting oxygen consumption, but it results in only mild increases in plasma lactate, with partial compensation by hyperventilation.

Varanid lizards, like marine turtles, are reptiles capable of sustained activity. Indeed, these lizards are considered to be nearly mammalian in certain of their metabolic qualities. A study of their acid-base response to treadmill running bears this out (10). Monitor lizards, *Varanus salvator*, ran on a treadmill for 45 minutes at 0.5 km • h^{-1}, a speed that demands 85% of their maximal aerobic capacity. Although an initial lactate surge and acidosis occurred in the blood, lactate values fell throughout the balance of the exercise period, and pH ([H$^+$]) was restored to normal by the end of exercise by hyperventilatory reduction in blood P$_{CO_2}$ (Figure 2). No SID values were provided in this study, but the relationship between lactate and HCO$_3$ suggests that the rise in lactate exceeded the fall in SID, indicative of modest compensatory changes in other strong ions.

In contrast to the extraordinary performance of the varanids and marine turtles, many other reptilian species lack both their aerobic scope and their sustainable aerobic capacity. Even routine activities require some reliance on anaerobiosis, and higher metabolic demands may be predominantly met by anaerobic glycolysis (1). The acid-base responses of reptiles and other animals relying on substantial anaerobic glycolysis during exercise will be considered in the next section.

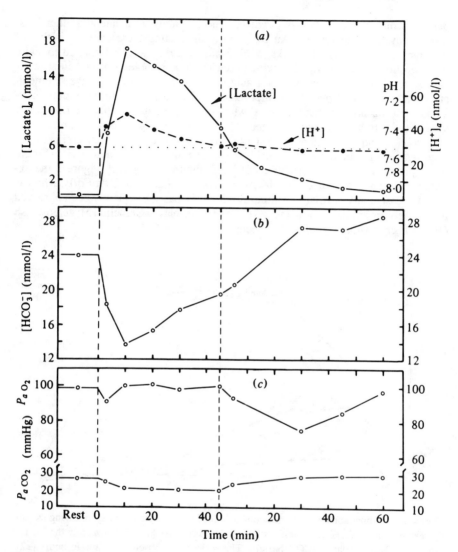

Figure 2. Blood gas and acid-base during and after moderate treadmill exercise in the monitor lizard, *Varanus salvator* (10).

Strenuous or Exhaustive Exercise

The typical acid-base state of ectothermic animals at the conclusion of a severe bout of experimentally induced exercise is a combined respiratory and metabolic acidosis. The respiratory disturbance is corrected rapidly, although not usually to below normal, while the metabolic disturbance, relating to lactate and other ions, takes many hours to restore. An early study illustrating these changes is that of Piiper et al. (22). Dogfish sharks, *Syliorhinus stellaris*, were stimulated to swim to exhaustion (10-25 min), after which arterial blood samples were taken at intervals up to 22 hours and analyzed for acid-base status. Blood P_{CO_2} peaked immediately but was normal by 1 hour after exercise. Blood pH fell to its minimum by 2 hours but was normal after 6-8 hours, whereas blood lactate continued to rise slowly after activity to a maximum after about 6 hours and was returned to control only after some 24 hours. Beginning soon after the onset of recovery, a discrepancy existed between the increase in [lactate] and what Piiper et al. called $\Delta[H^+]$ (Figure 3), in principle the same variable as SID (cf. Figure 1). Note in Figure 3 the extreme condition at 8 hours, when lactate was maximal at about 20 mEq/L, whereas SID was essentially normal. A similar discrepancy has subsequently been observed in a variety of animals following severe exercise: elasmobranch (15); teleost fish (16, 29); crocodilian reptile (25); decapod crustaceans (4, 20, 32).

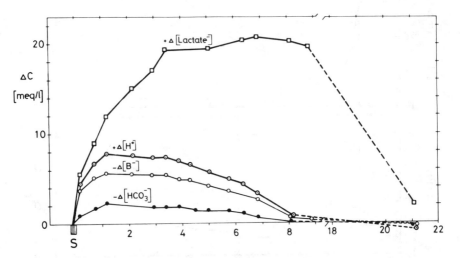

Figure 3. Comparison between metabolic acid load ($\Delta[H^+]$) and [lactate] following exhaustive exercise in the shark, *Syliorhinus stellaris*. The term [ΔH^+] is calculated from the changes in non-HCO$_3^-$ ([B$^-$]) and HCO$_3^-$ buffers. The scale of the abscissa is time in hours (22).

Piiper et al. (22) postulated that the discrepancy was due to retention of H$^+$ within the active muscles. Subsequently, Turner et al. (29) made similar observations on the rainbow trout *(Salmo gairdneri)*; based on blood data following both exercise and lactic acid or Nalactate infusion, they likewise concluded that H$^+$ was preferentially retained in the tissues. These authors also observed significant strong ion responses in blood (increased cations and decreased anions) that appear to account for the discrepancy in terms of SID. About the same time as this latter study, however, additional studies on the shark (15) and the trout (16), though confirming most of the other authors' observations on the same species, recorded a substantial excretion of acid into the water by both animals following exercise that was subsequently taken back up as lactate was remetabolized. They concluded that H^+ actually exits the muscle cells faster than lactate, but its apparent deficit in the blood is due to removal to the ambient water. In the trout study, additional evidence of strong ion exchanges between the animal and the surrounding water agrees with the blood ionic changes reported by Turner et al. (29). In terms of the SID formulation, the phenomenon that Holeton et al. (16) refer to as "excretion of acid equivalents to the water" can be explained by Na uptake or Cl excretion by the gills, the balancing ion in each case being an unidentified weak ion. What they describe as more rapid loss of H^+ than lactate from muscle cells must also have a strong ion component, due, for example, to H^+/Na^+ or HCO_3^-/Cl^- exchange.

Similar results, including the acid excretion to the water, have been reported for the marine crab, *Callinectes sapidus* (4). Researchers postulated gill ionic exchanges, but large background concentrations of Na and Cl in both water and hemolymph make detection of small changes in these ions technically difficult. The same detection problem exists as well for the ambient environment of marine fishes, as noted earlier by Piiper et al. (22). Certain terrestrial crabs and lower vertebrates show a similar plasma lactate/SID discrepancy, but exchange with the environment is not a likely explanation in these animals during the time course of the experiments. In the land crab, *Cardisoma carnifex*, the ionic exchange accounting for the discrepancy appears to be movement of Ca, probably accompanied by carbonate, from the exoskeleton to the extracellular fluid (32), as may also be the case in the coconut crab, *Birgus latro* (26).

A very different picture of lactate dynamics, in which the apparent change in plasma SID exceeds the change in lactate following strenuous activity (see Figure 1), has been observed in several species. A dramatic example is the flathead sole, *Hippoglossoides elassodon*, a sluggish benthic marine teleost studied by Turner et al. (30). In this animal, lactate remained almost entirely within the active muscles, and blood levels rose only slightly, whereas the metabolic acid load in the blood rose substantially more (Figure 4). The extracellular acid load, however, was less than that observed in the more active species discussed above, as was the increase in intracellular lactate level, indicating a lower intensity of exercise in the sole. A lactate/SID discrepancy of the same sort has also been observed in a related flatfish, *Platichthys stellatus* (31), and in two species of amphibians, *Bufo marinus* and *Cryptobranchus alleganiensis* (6). These latter species, like the sole, are generally inactive but may display short bursts of exertion.

Strategies of Lactate Efflux From Muscle

Similar changes in blood lactate and SID occur during exercise in humans (5), suggesting a coupled loss of lactate and H^+, perhaps occurring in part as undissociated lactic acid. Recent studies, however, have reported a modest excess of H^+ efflux (21, 24). In lower animals, lactate and SID changes generally differ, pointing to an uncoupling in the efflux process. Curiously, in some animals the uncoupling leads to greater change in lactate than in SID, whereas in others the opposite is true. What adaptive significance might these different outcomes have for the animals concerned?

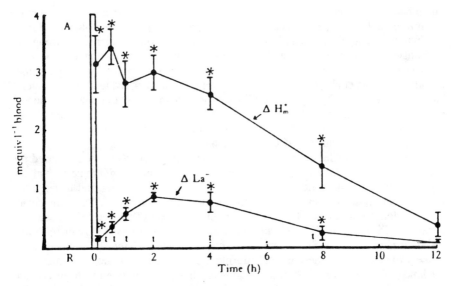

Figure 4. Comparison between metabolic acid load (ΔH^+_m) and lactate following exhaustive exercise in the flathead sole, *Hippoglossoides elassodon* (30).

In the case where Δlactate is greater than ΔSID, the advantage appears to be that the animal can neutralize much of the acid load extracellularly, either by acid excretion to the water (15, 16) or by enhancement of extracellular buffering capacity by release of $CaCO_3$ from bone (26, 32). By these mechanisms, muscle cell acidosis is relieved, facilitating recovery of muscle function, but without producing a severe extracellular acidosis. With respect to the animals in which Δlactate is less than ΔSID during recovery from exercise, the strategy may be based on retention of lactate within the muscle for subsequent reconversion to glycogen and preferential restoration of muscle cell pH to promote this end (30). The added load on the blood is nevertheless rather modest due to low overall lactate buildup in these sluggish animals. A similar strategy in a more energetic species, with its greater acid load, might overwhelm the capacity for extracellular pH regulation. It is not clear to what extent the sluggish Pleuronectes utilize branchial acid excretion in their regulatory strategy. Nor is it clear what the efflux mechanisms are that underlie these differences, although both lactate and H^+ efflux from muscle recovering from activity have been shown to be influenced by flow rate, pH, and buffer capacity of the perfusing fluid (13, 19).

Special Problems in Comparative Physiology of Exercise

The above examples illustrate the acid-base responses in lower animals that, relative to man and other mammals, are limited by their gas exchange and metabolic capacities. Other animals face different limitations, not due to less highly developed physiological systems but rather to the hostile environments in which they exercise.

Examples in this category are the marine mammals that spend most of their lives, active and otherwise, holding their breath beneath the water surface, and certain high-flying birds that can engage in demanding flapping flight at altitudes higher than the summit of Mt. Everest.

Apneic diving produces characteristic acid-base disturbances that begin with a pure respiratory acidosis due to CO_2 retention, which becomes a combined respiratory and metabolic acidosis (reduced SID) if the dive duration is long enough to lead to significant lactate accumulation. The classic work of Scholander (24) on restrained animals revealed that the severity of the acidosis is reduced by two mechanisms: first, peripheral vasoconstriction sequesters the lactic acid in the tissues apart from the circulating blood until reinitiation of breathing; second, metabolic depression occurring during forced diving conserves the oxygen supply and slows the development of acidosis. Subsequent work on voluntary diving animals, however, has emphasized the fact that in nature, animals are often quite active while beneath the surface—hunting, exploring, and so on. Active swimming during a dive tends to accelerate depletion of body oxygen stores and cause acidosis to develop more rapidly. Even more remarkable, then, is the observation that exploratory dives lasting up to 70 min have been recorded with Weddell seals in the Antarctic (18).

The gradual acidosis that occurs during prolonged diving may contribute to the diving ability of these animals in two ways, one obvious, the other less obvious. First, it is well known that the affinity of hemoglobin for oxygen is reduced by acidosis (the Bohr effect) and that this facilitates the unloading of O_2 from the blood in active tissues. For the seal and other diving animals, this response to acidosis enables effective exploitation of O_2 reserves without a drastic fall in blood or tissue P_{O_2}. This is a familiar adaptation of diving animals. The second effect is less substantiated and relates to a possible depressant effect on cellular metabolism. Recent results on Weddell seals (11) suggest that the surprisingly low apparent metabolism of these animals during active dives can be explained only by a low energetic requirement of swimming, coupled with arrested metabolism in inactive tissues. The latter effect may be due in part to the inhibitory effects of low pH on key metabolic enzymes (12).

Both anecdotal and experimental observations have documented the superior anoxic tolerance of birds compared to mammals (3). This is dramatically illustrated by the ability of birds to fly at high altitude under severely hypoxic conditions. A prime example is the bar-headed goose, which migrates from its wintering grounds in India to its northern breeding areas by flying across the Himalaya Mountains. The behavior is particularly remarkable because these birds fly directly from near sea level to these high elevations without the acclimation required by human climbers. Furthermore, geese continuously flap their wings and do not glide. Various hypotheses have been put forward to explain the performance of birds, including special features of their cardiovascular system (28), respiratory system (2), and blood gas transport system (3). How might birds' acid-base state during hypoxic exercise contribute to their extraordinary ability?

An immediate problem in attempting to answer this question is the uncertainty as to the nature of the acid-base changes under these conditions. Laboratory studies have shown that hypoxic exposure in resting birds elicits pronounced hyperventilation and respiratory alkalosis (9) but also that flight by a pigeon in a wind tunnel at 10 times the resting metabolic rate leads to compensated metabolic acidosis (8). No one yet has devised an experiment to measure metabolism and blood pH in a bar-headed goose flying over the Himalayas, but a reasonable guess is that its metabolism is exclusively aerobic and its blood is alkalotic. These are long flights, so a persistent deficit in O_2 delivery seems unlikely. The alkalosis, due to profound hypocapnia and in contrast to the situation in the diving seal, increases the affinity of hemoglobin for O_2 and facilitates the loading of O_2 into the blood at the low prevailing P_{O_2} levels. The bar-headed goose, at rest under sea level conditions, already has blood with higher affinity for O_2 than other waterfowl (3).

The extreme cases of the Weddell seal and the bar-headed goose serve to illustrate contrasting strategies by which acid-base state can promote adaptation to an otherwise hostile environment. They also reveal in clear fashion how acid-base state is closely linked with O_2 exchange. Shortage of O_2 in each case leads to the acid-base disturbance: in the seal, acidosis due to anaerobiosis; in the bird, alkalosis due to hyperventilation. These disturbances in turn ameliorate the chief problem confronting each animal: in the seal, the delivery of O_2 to the tissues; in the bird, the acquisition of O_2 from the environment.

Conclusion

All animals operate within the limitations imposed by their physiology and by their environments. For strenuous activity, a major limitation is the availability and exchange of oxygen. Acid-base state is generally regarded as an index of how well the uptake and delivery systems for O_2 are meeting these demands. Failure in this regard leads to acid-base disturbance (acidosis); a variety of mechanisms have evolved to deal with this secondary problem (hyperventilation, selective distribution of the acid load, acid excretion to the environment, mobilization of buffers from skeletal elements). In certain cases, however, the acid-base change is clearly an adaptive response to the problem of O_2 lack during exercise and not merely a consequence of system failure. As in other homeostatic systems, a unique value for a particular regulated variable may not be optimal under all conditions.

Acknowledgments

This paper was written while the author was a guest scientist at the Laboratoire d'Etude des Régulations Physiologiques of the CNRS in Strasbourg, France, supported by a Fogarty Senior International Fellowship (number 1 FO6 TW01356-01).

References

1. Bennett, A.F. Activity metabolism of the lower vertebrates. Annu. Rev. Physiol. 40:447-469; 1978.
2. Bernstein, M.H.; Schmidt-Nielsen, K. Ventilation and oxygen extraction in the crow. Respir. Physiol. 10:384-401; 1974.

3. Black, P.B.; Tenney, S.M. Oxygen transport during progressive hypoxia in high-altitude and sea-level waterfowl. Respir. Physiol. 39:217-239; 1980.

4. Booth, C.E.; McMahon, B.R.; DeFur, P.L.; Wilkes, P.R.H. Acid-base regulation during exercise and recovery in the blue crab, *Callinectes sapidus*. Respir. Physiol. 58:359-376; 1984.

5. Bouhuys, A.; Pool, J.; Binkhorst, R.A.; van Leeuwen, P. Metabolic acidosis of exercise in healthy males. J. Appl. Physiol. 21:1040-1046; 1966.

6. Boutilier, R.G.; McDonald, D.G.; Toews, D.P. The effects of enforced activity on ventilation, circulation and blood acid-base balance in the aquatic gill-less urodele, *Cryptobranchus alleganiensis*; a comparison with the semi-aquatic anuran, *Bufo marinus*. J. Exp. Biol. 84:289-302; 1980.

7. Butler, P.J.; Milsom, W.K.; Woakes, A.J. Respiratory, cardiovascular and metabolic adjustments during steady state swimming in the green turtle, *Chelonia mydas*. J. Comp. Physiol. [B] 154:167-174; 1984.

8. Butler, P.J.; West, N.H.; Jones, D.R. Respiratory and cardiovascular responses of the pigeon to sustained level flight in a wind tunnel. J. Exp. Biol. 71:7-26; 1977.

9. Colacino, J.M.; Hector, D.H.; Schmidt-Nielsen, K. Respiratory responses of ducks to simulated altitude. Respir. Physiol. 9:265-281; 1977.

10. Gleeson, T.T.; Bennett, A.F. Acid-base imbalance in lizards during activity and recovery. J. Exp. Biol. 98:439-453; 1982.

11. Guppy, M.; Hill, R.D.; Schneider, R.C.; Qvist, J.; Liggins, G.C.; Zapol, W.M.; Hochachka, P.W. Microcomputer-assisted metabolic studies of voluntary diving of Weddell seals. Am. J. Physiol. 250 (Regulatory Integrative Comp. Physiol. 19):R175-R187; 1986.

12. Hand, S.C.; Somero, G.N. Phosphofructokinase of the hibernator, *Citellus beecheyi*: temperature and pH regulation of activity via influences on the tetramer-dimer equilibrium. Physiol. Zool. 56:380-388; 1983.

13. Heisler, N. Lactic acid elimination from muscle cells. In: Grote, J., ed. Aktuelle probleme der atmungsphysiologie. Mainz, FRG: Akademic der Wissenshaften der Literatur; (in press).

14. Hill, R.D. Microcomputer monitor and blood sampler for free-diving Weddell seals. J. Appl. Physiol. 61:1570-1576; 1986.

15. Holeton, G.F.; Heilser, N. Contribution of net ion transfer mechanisms to acid-base regulation after exhausting activity in the larger spotted dogfish *(Scyliorhinus stellaris)* J. Exp. Biol. 103:31-46; 1983.

16. Holeton, G.F.; Neumann, P.; Heisler, N. Branchial ion exchange and acid-base regulation after strenuous exercise in rainbow trout *(Salmo gairdneri)*. Respir. Physiol. 51:303-318; 1983.

17. Jackson, D.C.; Prange, H.D. Ventilation and gas exchange during rest and exercise in adult green sea turtles. J. Comp. Physiol. 134:315-319; 1979.

18. Kooyman, G.L. Weddell seal: consummate diver. Cambridge, England: Cambridge Univ. Press; 1981.

386   Jackson

19. Mainwood, G.W.; Worsley-Brown, P. The effects of extracellular pH and buffer concentration on the efflux of lactate from frog sartorius muscle. J. Physiol. (Lond.) 250:1-22; 1975.

20. McDonald, D.G.; McMahon, B.R.; Wood, C.M. An analysis of acid-base disturbances in the haemolymph following strenuous activity in the dungeness crab, *Cancer magister*. J. Exp. Biol. 79:47-58; 1979.

21. Medbo, J.I.; Sejersted, O.M. Acid-base and electrolyte balance after exhausting exercise in endurance-trained and sprint-trained subjects. Acta Physiol. Scand. 125:97-109; 1985.

22. Piiper, J.; Meyer, M.; Drees, F. Hydrogen ion balance in the elasmobranch *Syliorhinus stellaris* after exhausting activity. Respir. Physiol. 16:290-303; 1972.

23. Portner, H.-O. Contributions of anaerobic metabolism to pH regulation in animal tissues: theory. J. Exp. Biol. 131:69-87; 1987.

24. Scholander, P.F. Physiological adaptations to diving in animals and man. Harvey Lect. 57:93-110; 1962.

25. Seymour, R.S.; Bennett, A.F.; Bradford, D.F. Blood gas tensions and acid-base regulation in the salt-water crocodile, *Crocodylus porosus*, at rest and after exhaustive exercise. J. Exp. Biol. 118:143-159; 1985.

26. Smatresk, N.J.; Cameron, J.N. Post-exercise acid-base balance and ventilatory control in *Birgus latro,* the coconut crab. J. Exp. Zool. 218:75-82; 1981.

27. Stewart, P.A. Modern quantitative acid-base chemistry. Can. J. Physiol. Pharmacol. 61:1442-1461; 1983.

28. Tucker, V.A. Respiratory physiology of house sparrows in relation to high altitude flight. J. Exp. Biol. 48:56-66; 1968.

29. Turner, J.D.; Wood, C.M.; Clark, D. Lactate and proton dynamics in the rainbow trout *(Salmo gairdneri)*. J. Exp. Biol. 104:247-268; 1983.

30. Turner, J.D.; Wood, C.M.; Hobe, H. Physiological consequences of severe exercise in the inactive benthic flathead sole *(Hippoglossoides elassodon):* a comparison with the active pelagic rainbow trout *(Salmo gairdneri)*. J. Exp. Biol. 104:269-288; 1983.

31. Wood, C.M.; McMahon, B.R.; McDonald, D.G. An analysis of changes in blood pH following exhausting activity in the starry flounder, *Platichthys stellatus*. J. Exp. Biol. 69:173-185; 1977.

32. Wood, C.M.; Randall, D.J. Haemolymph gas transport, acid-base regulation and anaerobic metabolism during exercise in the land crab *(Cardisoma carnifex)*. J. Exp. Zool. 218:23-35; 1981.

Anaerobic Capacity: Past, Present, and Prospective

Bengt Saltin

University of Copenhagen, Copenhagen, Denmark

Lars Hermansen had many research interests, but none was more important to him than the glycolytic energy release during exercise and the effects on muscle pH, and how this influences fatigue as well as the recovery from exercise. In evolution, the anaerobic capacity has been an essential component for survival, maybe more so for our ancestors as hunters than a high aerobic capacity. A remnant of this may be the extremely high potential for glycolysis that still persists in skeletal muscle of humans. This is shown by the high glycolytic enzyme levels, which need only to be minimally activated for a very pronounced ATP production to occur by glycolysis. Glycogen can also be stored in all skeletal muscle fiber types of humans to an extent that is above that found in most other species.

Today a high maximal anaerobic capacity has no practical significance other than in certain sport disciplines. What should be remembered, however, is the paramount role anaerobic energy release has in allowing for very quick alterations in muscle power output, which thereby does not depend on the gradual increase in aerobic ATP production. This presentation starts with an overview (past), followed by presenting some results from ongoing experiments at our institute (present). In closing, critical unsolved issues are identified and research strategies are discussed, as well as sites for possible adaptation (prospective).

Past

Oxygen Deficit (Debt) and Its Utilization

In 1919/1920 Krogh and Lindhard published a paper in the *Journal of Physiology* on "The Respiration at the Transition From Rest to Work" (48). The lag of oxygen uptake was quantified and defined as oxygen deficit (Figure 1). They also followed the oxygen uptake in recovery and made the observation that at light exercise intensities, the recovery oxygen uptake above basal (resting) metabolic rates (oxygen debt) matched the oxygen deficit, whereas more intense or exhaustive exercise led to larger debt than deficit (Figure 2). The reason was that recovery oxygen uptake was slow in returning to preexercise level. Indeed, it may not have returned to resting levels the same day as the exercise!

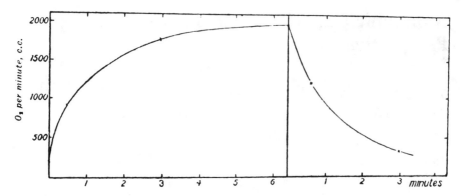

Figure 1. Original figure (No. 4) from the paper by Krogh and Linhard (48), where they measured the oxygen uptake in transition from rest to exercise and in recovery. The oxygen uptake after 5-6 min of exercise represents the energy demand at this intensity because the work was submaximal.

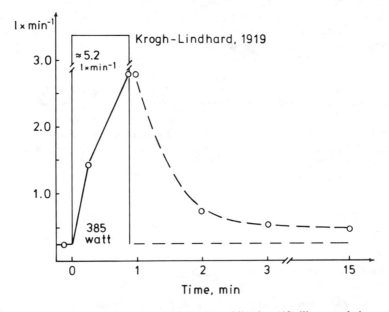

Figure 2. These data from Krogh and Linhard's publication (48) illustrate their results of very intense work performed to exhaustion. The same subject repeated the exercise at some interval (different days) to achieve complete measures of the oxygen uptake during the quite short exercise period ($\sim$ 50 s).

Long before measurements of oxygen deficit and debt were performed, lactic acid had been determined in blood and muscle and was associated with a lack or a limited supply of oxygen (3, 4, 49). Before these reports lactic acid had already been linked with intense physical exertion because a high level of lactic acid had been found in exhausted game (see 8). The literature an anaerobic energy metabolism flourished early in this century (for references, see 38) and culminated after Lundsgaard (54, 55) had demonstrated that muscle unable to produce lactic acid, due to iodoacetate poisoning, could still contract. This paved the way for understanding that CP and ATP are the energy-rich compounds that are the more immediate energy sources for muscle contraction (52, 53). Detailed studies followed on factors of importance for lactic acid formation in exercising humans (7, 65); how the lactacid and alactacid (ATP/CP) anaerobic energy yield contributed to the oxygen deficit (56); and how the repayment of the oxygen debt, as defined by Krogh and Linhard (48) and Meyerhof (61), occurred (13, 16, 45, 58). In essence, they could demonstrate a first, very fast component of repayment lasting some minutes and a second, quite slow component. Resynthesis of ATP and CP as well as reloading of hemoglobin and myoglobin were linked with the first phase, the metabolism of lactate with the second phase, although lactate clearance was not the only cause.

Early studies by A.V. Hill are also available on the utilization of the oxygen deficit in exercise. He found that an even pace was most economical in a race (31, 32). This concept has been challenged by Secher (79), who argues that in racing over a fixed distance, the intensity (speed) should be the highest at the onset of the exercise. This produces the fastest rate of acceleration of the oxygen uptake. A point that has support is the fact that the rate of rise in oxygen uptake at onset of exercise is a function of the relative exercise intensity (5, 50).

It is noteworthy that an oxygen deficit is a capacity; it is not a rate like maximal oxygen uptake, but it is utilized at a certain rate that may vary (see also Figures 1 and 2). The unloading of oxygen from hemoglobin and myoglobin is rapid, and the new, lower equilibrium concentrations for ATP and CP in the contracting muscles is also reached within 15-20 s (21, 40). The rate of the lactate production can be extremely high; 1-2 mmoles • kg^{-1} can be accumulated in the muscle over a few seconds (Figure 3), which demonstrates that, in contrast to earlier beliefs, an acceleration of the glycolysis starts at onset of dynamic exercise (35, 76). With this in mind, it could be anticipated that the entire oxygen deficit is utilized within 1 min or less. Data demonstrating complete usage in 1 min are available (39, 60). However, according to Medbø et al. (59), only 75% of the total oxygen deficit is utilized after 1 min of exercise, but after 2 min the whole capacity is exhausted. Special training may be critical and may be part of the explanation for differences in results.

Components of the Oxygen Deficit

The energy derived to cover the oxygen deficit is derived from glycolysis and also ATP and CP stores. At the start of the exercise, muscle ATP and CP concentrations are high ($\geq$ 30 mmoles • kg^{-1}); at exhaustion they are reduced up to 20% and 80-90%, respectively (47). Depending on the muscle mass involved in the exercise, the actual amount of this alactacid component of the oxygen deficit varies slightly. Moreover, aerobic processes are also included in a measure of the oxygen deficit because the oxygen bound to hemoglobin and myoglobin is reduced from the start to the end of an exercise period (12). The magnitude of these components

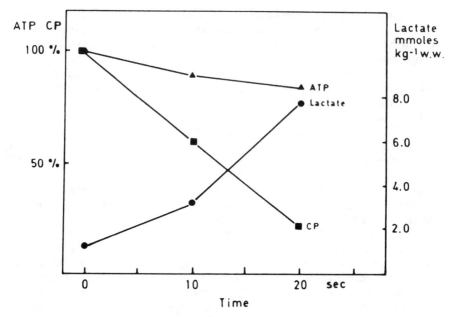

Figure 3.   The reduction of ATP and CP and the increase in lactate of contracting muscles are depicted after onset of exercise (76).

is smaller than the lactacid components, and at maximum they amount to 30-40% of the total oxygen deficit (Table 1).

More important is that training produces only minor alterations in the absolute values for the contributions of these variables to the oxygen deficit. ATP and CP concentrations in muscle are basically unaffected by any type of training (see 75), and the degree of depletion during exercise is more a function of the relative intensity than the training status (47). Endurance training increases the amount of hemoglobin (and myoglobin?) and thus the oxygen stored, but again the magnitude of this factor is small compared to the total oxygen deficit. Thus, an elevation in the maximal oxygen deficit is a function of greater lactate production.

How to Measure Anaerobic Work Capacity

An accepted method to measure a person's anaerobic capacity is not yet available. Several routes have been tried, but objections on theoretical grounds can be made against the various trials to quantify the anaerobic energy yield. Measurement of lactate in blood after exhaustive exercise has frequently been used, and Margaria and associates (57) have gone the furthest to use such a measure to estimate the anaerobic energy release (see also 34). There are, however, several difficulties with this method. One is in identifying when an equilibrium between muscle and blood lactate concentration exists. Other problems are the variability of dilution space for lactate and of lactate's turnover rate (25, 29). Before an equilibrium is reached between muscle and blood, the lactate evenly distributed in the various water spaces

Table 1   Components of the Oxygen Deficit

Components	O₂ equivalents (ml · kg⁻¹)		Percentage of total (%)	
	S^a	AT^b	S^a	AT^b
Oxygen stored to Hb and Mb	5	6	10	8
ATP and CP ("alactacid")	15	16	30	22
Glycolysis ("lactacid")	30	48	60	70
Total ml-O₂ Eq −kg⁻¹	50	70	100	100

Note. The exercise involves primarily the leg muscles (running or bicycling) (refs. 12, 21, 40, 47).

^{a}Sedentary subjects. ^{b}Anaerobically trained subjects.

of the body, a large fraction of the lactate has been metabolized. Thus, although everybody would agree that lactate in the blood is an indication of glycolysis, it is equally true that it cannot give a reasonable estimate of the anaerobic energy yield. Thus, it is not a quantitative measure of anaerobic capacity.

It was mentioned above that the oxygen deficit accumulated during exercise was repaid during recovery. A measure of the recovery oxygen uptake beyond preexercise or resting value (oxygen debt) has also been proposed and used as a measure of the anaerobic capacity after intense exhaustive exercise. The procedure has been used by, among others, Lars Hermansen in collaboration with Jan Karlsson (see 39). Several drawbacks with this method limit its value. More energy is needed to use lactate as substrate for the synthesis of glucose (glycogen) than is liberated when lactate is produced. Further, an unknown quantity of lactate is oxidized, which will then not appear as "extra" oxygen consumption. The largest problem is related to the fact that factors other than elevated lactate increase the oxygen consumption of the body (see 46). When oxygen uptake measurements in recovery are used to estimate anaerobic capacity, a factor (2 or more?) has been used to convert the oxygen debt into an anaerobic energy yield. This can hardly be a recommended procedure. The third route is to determine the oxygen deficit as was done in the "old days." In short-term submaximal exercise, the use of the oxygen deficit has been used extensively as a measure of the anaerobic energy release, which may be reasonable (40; see also Figure 1).

Problems arise with exhaustive exercise. If this work exhausts the subjects within a short time, we can assume that a maximal value for the oxygen deficit is reached. However, the energy cost of the exercise must be accurately known to calculate the oxygen deficit. This is not difficult at submaximal work loads, where the steady state oxygen uptake represents the energy costs. With exhaustive exercise, however, the validity of the estimate of the true energy cost is less certain. This uncertainty relates to both methods used to estimate the energy costs, which either assume a given mechanism efficiency or extrapolate from the submaximal relationship between work intensity and oxygen uptake. Such estimations are likely to underestimate the true energy expenditure during maximal work because mechanical efficiency may be lower in exhaustive than in submaximal exercise (73, 74). How much lower is unknown. In spite of some theoretical objections to using the maximal oxygen deficit (or accumulated oxygen deficit, as it is referred to by Medbø et al. [59]) as a measure of anaerobic capacity, it is the only method with the potential of being quantitative.

The most commonly used test to determine anaerobic capacity is probably the Wingate test. It has limited value. The work time is usually too short to exhaust the whole oxygen deficit. The shorter the work time, the more it is a measure of the components of oxygen deficit other than the contribution of glycolysis (see above and 9, 11). Further contractile factors and muscle strength may be more limiting than the energy delivery systems. Another limitation is that the test is performed on a bicycle. The basic limitation of a person's anaerobic work capacity is located in the contracting muscle (cells). Thus, a measure of the maximal anaerobic power is a reflection of the capacity of the specific muscles engaged in the test. Exercising on a bicycle is ideal for the cyclist, but it has less practical value for athletes in other sports.

Magnitude of the Anaerobic Capacity
(Maximal or "Accumulated" Oxygen Deficit)

Although the concept of oxygen deficit is old, it has not systematically been used to evaluate the range of anaerobic capacities of humans. It appears that the magnitude of the maximal oxygen deficit is a reproducible measurement. With time to exhaustion ranging from 2-17 min, the same peak values are observed (Figure 4). Further, acute changes in the barometric pressure does not affect the maximal oxygen deficit (Figure 4).

Some data on maximal oxygen deficit from the Scandinavian literature are summarized in Table 2. The subjects studied had anaerobic capacities of around 40-70 ml "O_2 eq" • kg^{-1}. The low and middle part of the range is rather well established. The high end contains only a few observations, and only a few subjects were national-class competitors. More important, the athletes were not in "peak" training at the time for the study. A value of close to 100 ml "O_2 eq" • kg^{-1} or more may be a likely estimate for a good miler or pursuit cyclist.

Young prepubescent children appear to have a much lower anaerobic capacity than adults, as judged by Eriksson et al.'s data (20). These 11- to 12-year-old boys had anaerobic capacities of only 35 ml "O_2 eq" • kg^{-1}, and endurance-type training had only a very minor influence on such capacity. Both muscle and blood lactate concentrations were also low in these boys. Based on these findings, it has frequently been concluded that anaerobic events are unsuitable for young kids. However, that is not a proper interpretation; it only means that they perform less well in sprint-type events. However, they probably have the advantage of recovering quickly

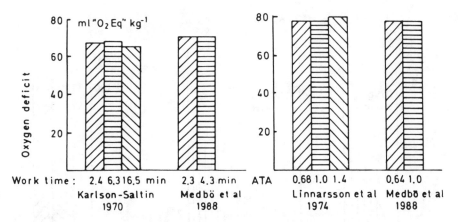

Figure 4. Summary of data in the literature on the maximal oxygen deficit in exhaustive exercise of different durations (left) and at different ambient pressures (right).

Table 2 Summary of Some Data in the Literature on Oxygen Deficit and Related Variables in Males

Reference	n	Age (years)	Training (status/test[a])	Weight (kg)	Oxygen deficit (L)	Work time (min)	Peak blood lactate (mM)
20	8	11.5	SED/B	44.7	1.48	~ 5	4.7
20	8	12.1	ET/B	45.4	1.64	~ 5	5.9
5	4	29	ET/B	77	6.25	~ 3	14.8
40	3	26	ET/B	74	4.95	~ 2.4	13.4
51	6	29	ET/B	75	5.75	~ 4	15.6
27	6	25	ET/R	70	3.15	~ 0.9	12.6
27	6	25	ST/R	75	4.06	~ 0.95	17.0
59	4	22	SED/R	74	4.72	~ 2	16.6
59	7	26	ST+ET/R	78	6.04	~ 2	16.6

Training status: sedentary, SED; endurance trained, ET; sprint trained, ST. Type of exercise used in the test: bicycling, B; running, R.

because less lactate has to be removed. After puberty, adolescent children have glycolytic enzyme activities similar to adults, and they then also exhibit "normal" blood lactate concentrations after exhaustive work.

Of importance is the fact that when more than the leg muscles are intensely involved in the exercise, as in whole-body exercise, the maximal oxygen deficit is much larger (Figure 5). This could be anticipated because the magnitude of the maximal oxygen deficit must be a function of the muscle mass engaged in the exercise.

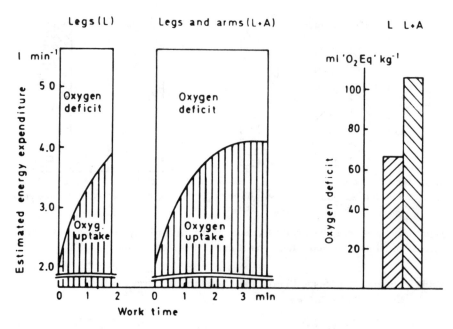

Figure 5. The oxygen uptake and the estimated oxygen deficit are illustrated when exercising with the legs (left) and with the arms and legs (right) in one subject. These data demonstrate that the fraction of the muscle mass involved in the exercise is decisive for the magnitude of the maximal oxygen deficit. Adding arms to leg bicycle exercise increased the oxygen deficit by 60-70% (6).

No measurements are available on top athletes performing whole-body exercise. Thus, the upper range for anaerobic capacity, as in successful rowers or swimmers, is presently unknown. If it is assumed that a top-class 800-m runner has the equivalent of 100 ml "O₂ eq" • kg⁻¹ in anaerobic capacity while running, a top rower should have 150 ml "O₂ eq" • kg⁻¹ or above in an all-out rowing performance.

Critical Contributions by Lars Hermansen

The work of Lars Hermansen has been cited frequently in the above section, and a summary of his scientific contributions is available elsewhere (78). Still, it is appropriate to briefly highlight some of Lars's investigations in the field of anaerobic capacity. What these investigations all have in common is that they were performed at a critical time and on a critical subject. Thus, in addition to the new knowledge they gave us, they initiated new thinking and complementary studies.

In the middle of the 1960s, when muscle biopsies became an acceptable procedure on healthy man, Lars took part in the first direct measurements of muscle glycogen and its utilization in exercise (26). The next significant contribution was the very first measurement of muscle pH at rest and in exhaustive work (28). This was followed by evaluating the role of a reduction in pH for force generation by muscle fibers (17). Equally crucial were the studies of the fate of lactate in the recovery period from intense exercise. He could document that moderate exercise during recovery caused a faster elimination of lactate from the muscle, probably due to enhanced perfusion (29). Further, Lars pointed out the possibility that lactate in skeletal muscle could not only be transferred to pyruvate and oxidized but could also be used as substrate for gluconeogenesis in muscle (30). His last initiative (27), suggesting a more systematic use of the maximal oxygen deficit as a measure of anaerobic capacity, may prove to be most useful in quantifying the maximal anaerobic energy release.

Present

From the previous discussion, it is apparent that the focus has been on whole-body oxygen deficit. This is natural because it is the anaerobic energy release during ordinary exercise that has practical significance. To understand what limits anaerobic energy yield and what mechanisms are involved in its regulation, then other approaches may provide new insights. Thus, we have employed the recently developed knee-extensor exercise model, which allows for a small, well-defined muscle group to perform dynamic contractions (1), and work performed and energy turnover can be expressed per kg muscle weight. Further, precise quantitative measurements can be made of cellular events as well as substrate and gas exchange between the capillary bed and the contracting muscles (2, 77, 81).

Free Energy From ATP Hydrolysis

The exact value for the mechanical efficiency in bicycle work is unknown near or at exhaustive exercise intensities. One reason for this is the difficulty involved in estimating possible energy yield from lactate production. The principal problem is summarized in Figure 6. Oxygen uptake of the exercising muscles increases linearly with elevation in work load, higher work intensities having no tendency for the rate of increase in oxygen uptake to decrease. From the continuous release of lactate and what is accumulated in the muscle, an estimation can be made of the "theoretical" energy yield from glycolysis (Table 3). At approximately 80% of peak knee-extensor oxygen uptake, the estimated energy made available by glycolysis amounts to the equivalent of 8 ml • kg^{-1}, which is only 2% of the observed oxygen uptake. Closer to and at peak exercise, the energy release is equivalent to 56 and 95 ml • kg^{-1}, respectively, which represents 10-15% aerobic metabolism.

Should the results be interpreted to mean that mechanical efficiency is reduced in proportion to the elevation in anaerobic energy release? This is a possibility. However, a more likely explanation is that concomitant with the enhanced lactate production, there is a gradual reduction in free energy from the ATP hydrolysis. The magnitude can be estimated from the equation

$$\Delta G_{ATP} = \Delta G^\circ{}_{ATP} + Rt \cdot T \cdot \ln \left(\frac{ADP \cdot Pi}{ATP} \right),$$

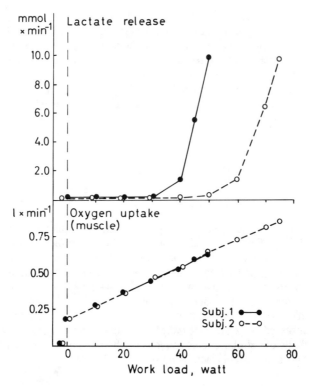

Figure 6. Oxygen uptake of the knee extensor at rest and at various work levels in two subjects with different work capacities (lower panel). The lactate release from the knee extensor is depicted in the upper panel (data are from 2, 81).

where T is the muscle temperature, Rt a constant, and ln the natural logarithm of the ratio for muscle ADP • P_i/ATP (42). Although not considered in this equation, pH influences the situation as well (14).

By introducing appropriate values for the various variables, the reduction in ΔG_{ATP} can be up to 20%. This is the case with reduction in pH to 6.5, increase in muscle temperature to 38.5° C, and an elevation in P_i to 20 mmoles • kg^{-1}, with small changes in ADP (a 2- to 4-fold increase above resting level) and ATP (10-20% reduction from rest). These estimations indicate that the drop in free energy from ATP hydrolysis could be similar in magnitude to the estimated energy obtained from anaerobic glycolysis. It should be emphasized that this in itself does not prove either estimation to be right. Further, the estimations of changes in ΔG for ATP hydrolysis with intense exercise are especially uncertain due to the lack of knowledge of whether the P_i is free or bound. Indeed, it has been suggested that ΔG_{ATP} is unaltered in spite of profound disturbance of the internal milieu (43).

If a lowering of free energy from ATP hydrolysis occurs, we can speculate why lactate is continuously produced at work intensities where the capacity for respiration would be sufficient. A possibility could be that the increased demand of pyruvate for mitochondrial usage at high relative work rates causes an overflow of pyruvate

Table 3 Data on Oxygen Uptake During Knee-Extensor Exercise at High Work Intensities and the Lactate Accumulated in the Thigh Muscles As Well As Released During the Exercise

| Oxygen uptake (approx. % of peak value) | Lactate Production | | Estimated energy yield from lactate production[a] (ml · min^{-1}) | Observed oxygen uptake (ml · min^{-1}) |
	Release (approx. mmol · min^{-1})	Accumulation (mmol · kg^{-1} · min^{-1})		
80	1.5	0	8	400
90-100	5	1.5	56	540
100	9	4	95	620

Note. From refs. 2, 81.

[a]The energy yield from the lactate production is estimated (1 mol of La = 1.5 mol ATP = 5.6 L O$_2$).

to lactate, a view similar to the one proposed by Huckabee (58). The increase in lactate concentration causes pH to become reduced, which in turn affects the CPK reaction and elevates the P_i concentration (69). Concomitantly, heat is accumulating in the muscle, which affects ΔG_{ATP}. In this perspective the initial lactate accumulation can be viewed as the initiation of a circulus vitiosus, where diminished free energy from ATP hydrolysis via the redox stage of the cytosol contributes to enhanced glycolysis in the muscle.

Exercise Protocol

In the experiments to be reported upon, a work intensity was chosen such that exhaustion occurred in the first 8 subjects within 2-4 min. Continuous measurements of whole-body oxygen uptake were performed preexercise, during the exercise, and for the first 60 min of recovery. Blood flow in the femoral vein was measured at rest, as frequently as possible during the exercise period, and repeatedly in the recovery. Concomitantly, blood samples from the femoral artery and vein were drawn and analyzed so that thigh oxygen consumption could be determined as well as a-v_{fem} difference for lactate. In addition, muscle biopsies were taken and analyzed for lactate and pH at rest, at exhaustion, and 3 times in recovery (at 3, 10, and 60 min). Of note is that the calculations of oxygen demand, deficit, and debt are based on a constant energy yield from ATP hydrolysis and without taking into account a possible overestimation of mechanical efficiency during the exercise.

Oxygen Deficit

The resting blood flow of 0.2-0.4 L $\cdot$ min^{-1} increased quickly, reaching 3.0-5.0 L $\cdot$ min^{-1} before exhaustion. Concomitantly, the a-vO$_2$ difference over the leg increased, resulting in up to a 100-fold increase in muscle oxygen uptake. The total amount of oxygen utilized by the muscle during the exercise was 1.9 L. The estimated demand averaged 3.3 L, which resulted in an oxygen deficit of 1.4 L. Lactate production contributed 78% to that oxygen deficit, or the equivalent of 1.1 L of O$_2$.

Lactate Production

The a-v difference for lactate widened markedly during the first minute of the exercise and reached close to 4 mM at exhaustion. Total a-v lactate difference during the exercise amounted to 14.8 mmoles $\cdot$ kg^{-1}. In the same time period, lactate accumulated in the muscle from 1.6 to 29.2 mmoles $\cdot$ kg^{-1} w.w. Thus, of the approximately 45 mmoles $\cdot$ kg^{-1} w.w. of lactate produced, some 1/3 escaped the muscle during the exercise. The efflux of lactate was, in essence, linearly related to the elevation in muscle lactate (Figure 7). Thus, no tendency for a leveling off in lactate release from the muscle, as earlier reported by Jorfeldt et al. (36), was observed. They suggested that the lactate transport mechanisms became saturated and limited

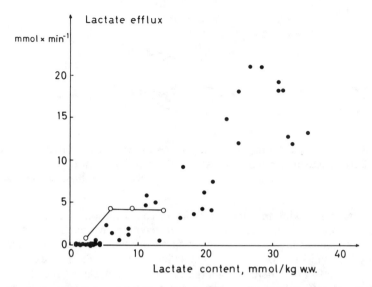

Figure 7. Individual data on 11 subjects for the release of lactate from the muscle in relation to the muscle lactate concentration. The open circles give mean values published by Jorfeldt et al. (36).

the lactate release from muscle. Our peak values for lactate release approached 20 mmoles • min⁻¹, which is 5 times higher than observed by Jorfeldt et al. (36).

The peak lactate release observed during exercise in our study most likely underestimates the release of lactate from the knee-extensor muscle to the blood. A possible explanation may be that the dominant fraction of the blood flow to the thigh muscles perfuses the knee-extensors, but some is directed to the other muscles of the thigh. As the arterial lactate concentration during the exercise becomes markedly elevated, lactate is delivered to and taken up by the hamstrings. No direct measure of lactate concentration in this muscle was performed, but the lactate concentration in the resting contralateral leg demonstrated an elevation to 5-6 mmoles • kg⁻¹ w.w. A schematic illustration of likely values is depicted in Figure 8. These values indicate that the amount of lactate released from the knee extensor to the blood used in our calculations may underestimate the true release by up to 1 mmoles • min⁻¹ at the end of exercise, which makes the difference between the present study and the release values of 4 mmoles • min⁻¹ reported by Jorfeldt et al. (36) even larger. In the latter study, conventional bicycle exercise was performed, and it is likely that skeletal muscle blood flow was markedly lower than in the present study. Perfusion may explain the difference observed in lactate efflux in the two studies and may constitute a limitation to extrusion of lactate from muscle rather than the transport of lactate across the sarcolemma.

Does the reduced pH cause exhaustion? Force and kicking rate were monitored continuously. Either a change in the force tracing, indicating work done by the hamstring (see 1), or a drop in rate were the objective determinants for when the exercise was terminated. At this point muscle pH was reduced, but only to 6.69 (6.50-6.84). The increase in H⁺ concentration that this lowering in pH represents

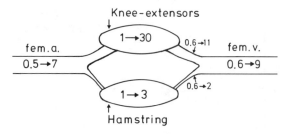

Figure 8. A schematic illustration of likely values for whole blood (artery and vein) and muscle lactate concentration (knee extensors and hamstring) at rest (first value given) and at exhaustion (second value, after the arrow). For further explanation, see the text.

could be associated with impaired ability for force generation (17). In 2 of the subjects, the exercise was repeated after 60 min of recovery. Muscle lactate concentration did not reach as high a level as in the first work bout, and the reduction in pH was only 0.25 units (to 6.79), or 0.10 units less than after the first exercise. This finding and the fact that there was a large variation in muscle pH found among the subjects at exhaustion favor the notion that factors other than muscle pH should be considered as the causes of fatigue and inability to perform at the given exercise intensity. Further, the effect of the lower pH on retarding the rate of glycolysis also appears to be small. Also, ATP resynthesis is probably not a limitation because its concentration in muscle at exhaustion is only slightly below that observed at rest.

Gradients for Lactate

Prior to exercise almost no gradients for lactate in the water phases of muscle cell (interstitial space), plasma, and red blood cells are apparent (Table 4). During exercise the pattern quickly changes. Of note is that there is a gradient not only between muscle and plasma but also in blood between plasma and the red blood cells. This is due to a slow, facilitated diffusion of lactate through the membrane of erythrocytes (only 5% of the lactate enters the red blood cells by simple diffusion; Figure 9). The lactate uptake by red blood cells is so slow that there still is a pronounced difference in lactate concentration in the arterial blood as late as 3 min into the recovery. At the end of exercise, femoral vein plasma concentration of lactate is only half of what is accumulated in the muscle, or 18 mmoles $\cdot$ L^{-1}, but 3 min into recovery, the difference was reduced to 5 mmoles $\cdot$ L^{-1}, and it was nil after 10 min of recovery (Table 4).

Recovery Lactate Efflux

The results in Table 4 demonstrate that the lactate concentration in muscle at the end of the exercise has returned to the normal resting value within 1 hour. The three main routes for the muscle lactate clearance are (a) release into the capillary bed, (b) conversion to pyruvate, and then (c) either oxidation or further conversion to other compounds. Of these three possibilities, we have data for the first because blood flow and a-v difference for lactate over the leg was followed during the 60 min of recovery. The most striking finding is that as much as 82% of the lactate left the muscle as lactate via the blood stream.

Table 4   The Concentration of Lactate in Muscle of the Vastus Lateralis and Femoral Vein Blood at Rest, at End of Exhaustive Exercise, and at Various Times in Recovery

Condition	Gradient For Lactate (mmol · L^{-1})		
	Muscle[a]	Plasma[b]	Erythrocytes[b]
Rest	1.8	1.6	1.6
Exercise	36.2	18.4	12.0
Recovery			
3 min	18.8	13.8	11.0
10 min	9.9	9.0	8.0
60 min	1.8	1.9	1.9

Note. Based on water content of muscle tissue and likely values for its distribution between intra- and extracellular compartments (81) as well as that of plasma and erythrocytes.

[a]Vastus lateralis. [b]Femoral vein.

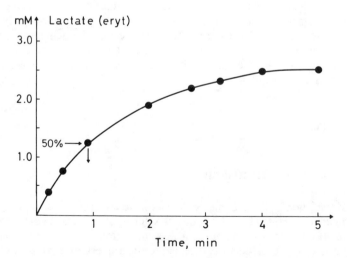

Figure 9.   Lactate concentration of erythrocytes (mmol/L cells) in relation to the time the blood cells have been incubated in a solution containing 4.4 mM lactate. The cells were depleted of ATP by preincubation with iodoacetomide and inosin in order to reduce endogenous lactate production (courtesy of L.O. Simonsen and C. Juel, unpublished data).

Oxygen Deficit and Debt

It can be stated that the oxygen deficit measured in the leg was of the same magnitude as that for the whole body. Further, in recovery the whole-body oxygen debt was markedly larger than the debt found for the leg. This finding is in agreement with the observations that most lactate leaves the muscle in recovery and that the extra energy for the metabolism of lactate is located outside the muscle performing the exercise. The magnitude of the oxygen debt observed for the leg is most likely due to the resynthesis of ATP and CP and the saturation of myoglobin/hemoglobin, which is estimated at 0.5-0.6 L.

Magnitude of the Anaerobic Capacity

The present subjects achieved a maximal oxygen deficit equivalent to from 0.34 to 0.68 L O_2 • kg^{-1} muscle. The human body consists of 40% muscle; some 10-12 L O_2 Eq • kg^{-1} b.w. would then be a reasonable estimate for the maximal oxygen deficit of a sedentary person. A rower with both a larger body weight and a larger muscle mass fraction would be anticipated to achieve perhaps 15 or 20 L O_2 Eq • kg^{-1} b.w. In this context the values for maximal oxygen deficit summarized in Table 2 are noteworthy. They are at most only 1/2-2/3 of the estimated values above. Some recent determinations in rowers indicated that they also are far from reaching the anticipated values. One reason for this is that not all muscles or portions of muscle are engaged in the exercise—not even in rowing—to the limit of the athlete's anaerobic capacity. In addition, the perfusion of the muscle plays a major role for the maximum amount of lactate that is cleared from the muscle during the exercise. In the present experiment when the perfusion was high, it amounted to 30-40% of the lactate produced. Thus, the muscle lactate clearance is a function of the amount of muscle involved in the exercise. If a muscle mass larger than the quadriceps is engaged in the exercise, optimal perfusion of the muscle cannot be achieved because the peripheral blood flow is limited centrally (2, 72). Thus, the larger the muscle mass involved in the exercise, the smaller the fraction of the lactate produced that can leave the muscle (Figure 10).

Prospective

Free Energy From ATP Hydrolysis

In the description of the present results, we have not accounted for a possible alteration in energy release by ATP hydrolysis during short-term exercise to exhaustion. It has been suggested that up to a 20% reduction in free energy may occur. Whether it does or not is unclear. This is a critical question because it affects the estimate of the ATP turnover and, thus, the maximal oxygen deficit. The answer may also give clues to understanding what initiates lactic acid production during exercise.

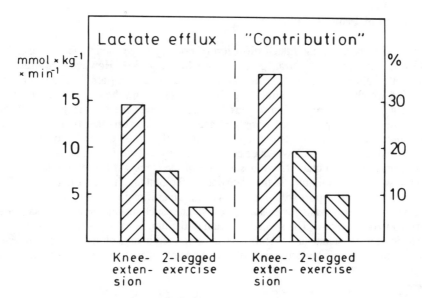

Figure 10. Mean values for the lactate efflux in the present study (knee extension) and two studies in the literature in which ordinary bicycle work has been performed (36, 41). To the right is estimated the relative "contribution" of the efflux of the total lactate production during the exercise.

Can an answer be found? An approach similar to the one used by Edwards may give some insight (19). His subjects performed intense static contraction with the knee extensors. As the circulation through the muscle was arrested, heat accumulated in the muscle. A precise measure of the heat content and the time course for its change during a steady contraction, coupled with detailed measurements of energy utilization, could provide an answer as to whether less energy becomes available from the ATP hydrolysis in the late, as compared to the initial, phase of contraction.

Regulation of Glycolytic Rate

Regarding the question of how fast the anaerobic capacity can be utilized, the factors regulating the rate of glycolysis have provoked special interest. The approach so far has been to measure various compounds and make estimates of free and bound concentrations of key regulators. This approach has its limitations. However, if properly matched with the application of NMR technology, which allows for direct measurements of the free concentrations of some of these compounds, a major breakthrough is possible. A problem that will remain is compartmentalization, where especially cytoplasmic versus mitochondrial concentrations of ADP/ATP and NAD/NADH are critical (23). Mitochondrial volume of muscle fibers can vary from a few to 10-12 volume %, as a function of fiber type and training status (see 75). By careful selection of muscles for study (for example m. soleus and m. gastrocnemius), some insight may be gained on an otherwise difficult problem.

Extrusion of Protons and Lactate

The evidence for a facilitated diffusion of both hydrogen ions and lactate (37), which in part may be a cotransport, is overwhelming (37). However, contrasting views are held (24). A final resolution of this question is a prerequisite to understanding which factors may limit the efflux of lactate from the muscles. It also has a bearing on the pH regulation of muscle cells, although the buffering capacity of the muscle is equally critical. By applying techniques used on other tissues, we may find some answers. For example, by applying inhibitors of facilitated diffusion of lactate and H^+, known to have an effect in erythrocytes (see 15), to isolated muscle fiber preparations, a quantitative description of the transport route(s) in the sarcolemma would be available. If the transport is facilitated, the identification of the mechanisms for transport will give the basis for quantification of flux rates. In turn, this will constitute a basis for evaluation of whether such mechanism(s) may saturate during in vivo exercise. The special problem of the functional significance of muscle perfusion for the lactate and H^+ release can be studied in an isolated, in vitro muscle preparation, where the activation of the muscle, as well as the blood flow, is controlled.

What Is the Cause of Exhaustion?

This question has been raised repeatedly in this century (see 67). As soon as a more universal factor has been proposed to be a likely candidate, it can be shown that the compound or mechanism may be at work only in special circumstances or may co-vary with other candidates which are related to fatigue and exhaustion. As in earlier studies with the knee-extensor model (81), pH is not reduced to a very low level in spite of quite high muscle lactate concentrations. In the investigations of Donaldson et al. (17, 18), a pH of 6.5 at a given Ca^{2+} concentration markedly affected tension development of fast-twitch (FT) fibers, whereas slow-twitch (ST) fibers were affected to a lesser extent. At a pH of 6.7-6.8, as in this study, the pH effect should be minor, especially with an increased activation rate of the motor units resulting in elevated free Ca^{2+} concentration, which could compensate for a reduced pH. However, it may also be argued that the total force developed by the knee-extensor muscle in each contraction represents an unusually large fraction of its force capacity. This may demand a dominant percentage of the available motor unit pool to be recruited at a high rate already at onset of the exercise. As a result, the performance of the muscle is more sensitive to quite small reductions in the peak force development of individual fibers; other fibers cannot compensate because firing rate is already optimal.

What are the critical experiments to be performed? First, we should evaluate whether or not the fatigue is central. This can be investigated by direct electrical stimulation of the muscle at the point of exhaustion. If the fatigue is beyond the motor end plate, sophisticated EMG analyses could be used to evaluate the impairment of propagation of the action potential, including possible alterations of frequency of activation. However, technique problems would probably be encountered, limiting the success of this approach. Electron probe spectra, combined with identifying the location at the ultrastructural level, could reveal ion changes in the T tubuli system, lack of activation, or malfunction of the SR system.

Adaptation

The following brief comments on adaptation are based on speculations on what limits anaerobic work capacity. Various possibilities are outlined in Table 5.

Ad 1. The observed large variation in the time for complete utilization of a person's maximal oxygen deficit may point to the rate of glycolysis as a limitation. A high muscle glycogen content has been shown by some to affect the rate of glycolysis (9, 44), but the results of this study as well as earlier data fail to support this notion (25). Above a certain critical level of muscle glycogen, a further elevation in glycogen has only a little significance on lactate production.

Increase of glycolytic enzymes, including LDH_{4-5}, may be more important. An increase in glycolytic enzymes may reduce the effect of the accumulation of inhibitors such as pH, IMP, and so on, causing better maintenance of the glycolytic rate (22). Can training directly affect the regulators of the glycolytic rate? If Newsholme (64) is correct that the sympathetic nervous system has a significant effect via substrate cycling, then there is a possibility of a training effect.

Ad 2. Several investigations have shown that the buffering capacity of sprint-trained subjects is higher than that of sedentary men (70, 80). Why this is the case is less clear (66). In addition to the role of the CP content and its utilization, none of the protein fractions have definitively been linked with the capacity of muscle to buffer H^+. The role of the bicarbonate system is probably of little significance in muscle (68). Can training cause an improved tolerance to a lowering of muscle pH, as has been suggested (25)? The result of such an adaptation would be that a given drop in pH would cause less impairment of metabolism and force generation. A specifically trained person would then have a lower pH at exhaustion, which has been reported for blood pH but not yet for muscle pH (25).

Ad 3. The present data did not show a decline in efflux rate of lactate at the highest muscle lactate concentration, suggesting that lactate transport mechanisms are sufficient and do not constitute a limitation.

Ad 4. It has been suggested that some fibers within an intensely contracting muscle not only take up lactate from adjacent, more active muscle fibers but are capable of metabolizing the lactate during the exercise (10). The practical role of this pathway is probably negligible. The basis for this statement is that at very intense exercise, most fibers of a muscle would be recruited. This is especially true for the slow-twitch fibers, which have the largest potential for metabolizing lactate. However, these fibers are also quite capable of producing lactate themselves. Thus, the possibility of transfer of lactate within an intensely contracting muscle from a producing fiber to a clearance fiber is mainly of theoretical interest.

Ad 5. Of much greater importance is the clearance of the lactate through the interstitial space into the capillary bed and blood. Of note is that an improvement of this transfer route is the result of pure aerobic-type training.

From the above discussion, it should be clear that there may be two modes of training to improve anaerobic capacity. One is to obtain the highest possible rate of glycolysis, and the other is to maintain the work rate in the face of increasing lactate production. The optimal training pattern may be different for these two variables. Speed and intensity are essential elements for training the rate of glycolysis. The duration of the effort is probably more important for handling the lactate. In this context, it is worthwhile noticing that patients with intermittent claudication do not have a high glycolytic potential in their calf muscles (71), probably because their

Table 5   Schematic Summary of Factors Related to the Lactate Production and the Fate of Produced Lactate in Skeletal Muscle During Exhaustive Exercise

Event	Limiting Factor	Adaptation
Rate of glycolysis and lactate production	Glycogen, key activators, LDH_{4-5}	Elevation of glycogen storage, enhanced glycolytic enzyme content including LDH_{4-5}, enhanced activation/less inhibition
Accumulation in the muscle fiber	Buffer capacity, pH tolerance	Increased breakdown of CP, elevation of specific amino acids
Transport (if facilitated)	Number of lactate transporters	Increased number of lactate transporters
Uptake by adjacent muscle fibers (FT → ST fibers)	"Own" pyruvate and lactate formation, LDH_{1-2}, mitochondrial capacity, NAD:NADH ratio	Enhanced oxygenation of less active adjacent fibers, enhanced oxidative potential and LDH_{1-2}.
Disappearance via interstitial space and blood	Capillary density, muscle perfusion, uptake by other tissues	Capillary proliferation, improved central circulatory capacity, enhanced oxidative potential of nonexercising tissues

walking speed is not a sufficient challenge to glycolytic metabolism. Further, their anaerobic work capacity is low due to a very minor lactate efflux from the muscles because the perfusion of the leg muscles is also low. This is in contrast to athletic training at altitude or hypoxic training. Both procedures appear to result in a pronounced improvement in anaerobic work capacity (62, 63, 82). Maybe "hypoxic" training is more effective than training at sea level.

Conclusion

This presentation is dedicated to the memory of Lars Hermansen. For those of us who were fortunate enough to have known him and to have been close to him, we know what an able and very friendly person he was. Lars could also stimulate and inspire—not only the colleagues in his own laboratory but also the audiences at meetings as well as other investigators in his field of research. Thus, the study we have performed in our laboratory has been initiated solely due to Lars's convincing suggestion that the old problem of oxygen deficit and debt is worth reexamining. I think that the ongoing investigations in Oslo on the anaerobic energy release in exhaustive muscular exercise by Medbø and colleagues demonstrate that he was correct. Hopefully, our efforts on the same subjects will also prove useful.

Acknowledgments

The experiments reported in this article are performed in collaboration with J. Bangsbo, P.D. Gollnick, T. Graham, C. Juel, B. Kiens, and M. Mizuno. The studies have been supported by grants from "TEAM DANMARK."

References

1. Andersen, P.; Adams, R.P.; Sjøgaard, G.; Thorboe, A.; Saltin, B. Dynamic knee extension as a model for the study of an isolated exercising muscle in man. J. Appl. Physiol. 59:1647-1653; 1985.

2. Andersen, P.; Saltin, B. Maximal perfusion of skeletal muscle in man. J. Physiol. (Lond.) 366:233-249; 1985.

3. Araki, T. Ueber die Bildung von Milchäure und Glycose im Organismus bei Sauerstoffmangel. Z. Phys. Chem. 15:335-370; 1891.

4. Araki, T. Ueber die Bildung von Milchäure und Glycose im Organismus bei Sauerstoffmangel. Z. Phys. Chem., Zweite Mitteilung 15:546-561; 1891.

5. Åstrand, P.-O.; Saltin, B. Oxygen uptake during the first minutes of heavy muscular exercise. J. Appl. Physiol. 16(6):971-976; 1961.

6. Åstrand, P.-O. Saltin, B. Maximal oxygen uptake and heart rate in various types of muscular activity. J. Appl. Physiol. 16(6):977-981; 1961.

7. Bang, O. The lactate content of the blood during and after muscular exercise in man. Skand. Arch. Physiol. 74(10):51-82; 1936.

8. Bois-Reymond, E. du. Ueber angeblich saure Reaction des Muskelfleisches. In: Gesammelte Abhandlung zur Allgemeine Muskel- und Nervenphysik. 1877:2-36.

9. Boobis, L.H. Metabolic aspects of fatigue during sprinting. In: Macleod, D.; Maughan, R.; Nimmo, M.; Reilly, T.; Williams, C., eds. Exercise. Benefits, limits and adaptations. London: E. & F.N. Spon; 1987:116-143.

10. Brooks, G.A. The lactate shuttle during exercise and recovery. Med. Sci. Sports Exerc. 18:355-364; 1986.

11. Cheetham, M.E.; Boobis, L.H.; Brooks, S.; Williams, C. Human muscle metabolism during sprint running. J. Appl. Physiol. 61:54-60; 1986.

12. Christensen, E.H.; Hedman, R.; Saltin, B. Intermittent and continuous running. Acta Physiol. Scand. 50:269-286; 1960.

13. Christensen, E.H.; Högberg, P. Steady state, O_2 deficit and O_2 debt at severe work. Arbeitsphysiologie 14:251-254; 1950.

14. Cooke, R.; Franks, K.; Luciani, G.B.; Pate, E. The inhibition of rabbit skeletal muscle contraction by hydrogen ions and phosphate. J. Physiol. 395:77-97; 1988.

15. Deuticke, B.; Beyer, E.; Forst, B. Discrimination of three parallel pathways of lactate in human erythrocyte membranes by inhibitors and kinetic properties. Biochim. Biophys. Acta 6894:96-110; 1982.

16. Dill, D.B.; Edwards, H.T.; Newman, E.V.; Margaria, R. Analysis of recovery from anaerobic work. Arbeitsphysiologie 9:299-307; 1936.

17. Donaldson, S.; Bolitho, K.; Hermansen, L. Differential, direct effects of H^+ on Ca^{2+}-activated force of skinned fibers from the soleus, cardiac and adductor magnus muscles of rabbits. Pflügers Arch. 376:55-65; 1978.

18. Donaldson, S.K.B. Effect of acidosis on maximum force generation of peeled mammalian skeletal muscle fibers. In: Knuttgen, H.G.; Vogel, J.A.; Poortmans, J.R., eds. Biochemistry of exercise. Champaign, IL: Human Kinetics; 1983:126-133. (International series of sport sciences; vol. 13).

19. Edwards, R.H.T. Metabolic changes during isometric contraction of the quadriceps muscle. Thermodynamics of muscular contraction in man. In: Jokl, E., ed. Medicine in sport. Basel, Switzerland: Karger; 1976:114-131. (Vol. 9).

20. Eriksson, B.O.; Gollnick, P.D.; Saltin, B. Muscle metabolism and enzyme activities after training in boys 11-13 years old. Acta Physiol. Scand. 87:485-497; 1973.

21. Gollnick, P.D. Hermansen, L. Biochemical adaptations to exercise: anaerobic metabolism. In: Wilmore, J.H., ed. Exercise and sport sciences reviews. New York: Academic Press; 1973:1-43. (Vol. 1).

22. Gollnick, P.D.; Saltin, B. Hypothesis: significance of skeletal muscle oxidative enzyme enhancement with endurance training. Clin. Physiol. 2:1-12; 1982.

23. Graham, T.E.; Saltin, B. Estimation of the mitochondrial redox state in human skeletal muscle during exercise. J. Appl. Physiol. (in press).

24. Heisler, N. Lactic acid elimination from muscle cells. In: Grote, J. Aktuelle Probleme der Atmungsphysiologie. Mainz, FRG: Akademie der Wissenschaften und der Literatur; (in press).

25. Hermansen, L. Anaerobic energy release. Med. Sci. Sports 1(1):32-38; 1969.

26. Hermansen, L.; Hultman, E.; Saltin, B. Muscle glycogen during prolonged severe exercise. Acta Physiol. Scand. 71:129-139; 1967.

27. Hermansen, L.; Medbø, J.I. The relative significance of aerobic and anaerobic processes during maximal exercise of short duration. In: Marconnet, P.; Poortmans, J.; Hermansen, L. eds. Physiological chemistry of training and detraining. Basel, Switzerland: Karger; 1984:56-57. (Med. sports sci., vol. 17).

28. Hermansen, L.; Osnes, J.-B. Blood and muscle pH after maximal exercise in man. J. Appl. Physiol. 32:304-308; 1972.

29. Hermansen, L.; Stensvold, I. Production and removal of lactate during exercise in man. Acta Physiol. Scand. 86:191-201; 1972.

30. Hermansen, L.; Vaage, O. Lactate disappearance and glycogen synthesis in human muscle after maximal exercise. Am. J. Physiol. 233:E422-E429; 1977.

31. Hill, A.V.; Long, C.N.H.; Lupton, H. Muscular exercise, lactic acid and the supply and utilization of oxygen. Proc. R. Soc. Lond. [Biol.] 96:438-475; 1924.

32. Hill, A.V.; Lupton, H. Muscular exercise, lactic acid and the supply and utilization of oxygen. Q. J. Med. 16:135-171; 1923.

33. Huckabee, W.E. Relationship of pyruvate and lactate during anaerobic metabolism: II. Exercise and formation of oxygen debt. J. Clin. Invest. 37:255-263; 1958.

34. Jacobs, I. Blood lactate implications for training and sports performance. Sports Med. 3:10-25; 1986.

35. Jacobs, I.; Tesch, P.A.; Bar-Or, O.; Karlsson, J.; Dotan, R. Lactate in human skeletal muscle after 10 s and 30 s of supramaximal exercise. J. Appl. Physiol. 55:365-367; 1983.

36. Jorfeldt, L.; Juhlin-Dannfelt, A.; Karlsson, J. Lactate release in relation to tissue lactate in human skeletal muscle during exercise. J. Appl. Physiol. 44(3):350-352; 1978.

37. Juel, C. Intracellular pH recovery and lactate efflux in mouse soleus muscles stimulated in vitro: the involvement of sodium/proton exchange and a lactate carrier. Acta Physiol. Scand. 132:363-371; 1988.

38. Karlsson, J. Lactate and phosphagen concentrations in working muscle of man. Acta Physiol. Scand. Suppl. 358:1-72; 1971.

39. Karlsson, J.; Hermansen, L.; Agnevik, G.; Saltin, B. Energikraven vid löpning. Idrottsfysiologi, rapport nr. 4. Stockholm, Sweden: Trygg-Hansa; 1967.

40. Karlsson, J.; Saltin, B. Lactate, ATP and CrP in working muscles during exhausting exercise in man. J. Appl. Physiol. 29:598-602; 1970.

41. Katz, A.; Broberg, S.; Sahlin, K.; Wahren, J. Leg glucose uptake during maximal dynamic exercise in humans. Am. J. Physiol. 251(14):E65-E70; 1986.

42. Kawai, M.; Guth, K.; Winnikes, K.; Haist, C.; Ruegg, J.C. The effect of inorganic phosphate on ATP hydrolysis rate and the tension transients in chemically skinned rabbit psoas fibers. Pflügers Arch. 408:1-9; 1987.

43. Kentish, J.C.; Nayler, W.G. The influence of pH and Ca^{2+}-regulated ATPase of cardiac and white skeletal myofibrils. J. Mol. Cell. Cardiol. 11:611-617; 1979.

44. Klausen, K.; Sjøgaard, G. Glycogen stores and lactate accumulation in skeletal muscle of man during intense bicycle exercise. Scand. J. Sports Sci. 2(1):7-12; 1980.

45. Knuttgen, H.G. Oxygen debt, lactate, pyruvate, and excess lactate after muscular work. Am. J. Physiol. 17:639-644; 1962.

46. Knuttgen, H.G. Lactate and oxygen debt: an introduction. In: Pernow, B.; Saltin, B., eds. Muscle metabolism during exercise. Advances in Experimental Medicine and Biology 11:361-369; 1971.

47. Knuttgen, H.G.; Saltin, B. Muscle metabolites and oxygen uptake in short-term submaximal exercise in man. J. Appl. Physiol. 32(5):690-694; 1972.

48. Krogh, A.; Lindhard, J. The changes in respiration at the transition from work to rest. J. Physiol. (Lond.) 53:431-437; 1919/1920.

49. Liebig, J. von. Chemische Untersuchungen über das Fleisch und seine Zubereitung zum Nahrungsmittel. Heidelberg, FRG; 1847.

50. Linnarsson, D. Dynamics of pulmonary gas exchange and heart rate changes at start and end of exercise. Acta Physiol. Scand. (Suppl. 415); 1974.

51. Linnarson, D.; Karlsson, J.; Fagraeus, L.; Saltin, B. Muscle metabolites and oxygen deficit with exercise in hypoxia and hyperoxia. J. Appl. Physiol. 36:399-402; 1974.

52. Lohmann, K. Über die enzymatische Aufspaltung der Kreatinphosphorsäure; zugleich ein Beitrag zum Chemismus des Muskelkontraktion. Biochemische Zeitschrift 271:264-277; 1934.

53. Lohmann, K. Konstitution der Adenylpyrophosphorsäure und Adenosindiphosphorsäure. Biochemische Zeitschrift 282:120-123; 1935.

54. Lundsgaard, E. Untersuchungen über Muskelkontraktionen ohne Milchsäurebildung. Biochemische Zeitschrift 217:162-177; 1930.

55. Lundsgaard, E. Weitere Untersuchungen über Muskelkontraktionen ohne Milchsäurebildung. Biochemische Zeitschrift 227:51-83; 1930.

56. Lundsgaard, E. Betydningen af fænomenet mælkesyrefrie muskelkontraktioner for opfattelsen af muskelkontraktionens kemi. Danske Hospitalstidende 75:84-95; 1932.

57. Margaria, R.; Cerretelli, P.; Di Prampero, P.E.; Massari, C.; Torelli, G. Kinetics and mechanism of oxygen debt contraction in man. J. Appl. Physiol. 18:371-377; 1963.

58. Margaria, R.; Edwards, H.T.; Dill, D.B. The possible mechanisms of contracting and paying the oxygen debt and the role of lactic acid in muscular contraction. Am. J. Physiol. 106:689-715; 1933.

59. Medbø, J.I.; Mohn, A.; Tabata, I.; Bahr, R.; Sejersted, O. Anaerobic capacity determined by the maximal accumulated oxygen deficit. J. Appl. Physiol. 64:50-60; (in press).

60. Medbø, J.I.; Tabata, I. Aerobic and anaerobic energy release during shortlasting exhausting bicycle exercise. Acta Physiol. Scand. 129(3):6A; 1987.

61. Meyerhof, O. Die Energieumwandlungen im Muskel. II. Das Schicksal der Milchsäure in der Erholungsperiode des Muskels. Arch. Ges. Physiol. 182:284-317; 1920.

62. Mizuno, M.; Juel, C. Increased skeletal muscle buffer capacity after prolonged sojourn at extreme atltitude (abstract). Can. J. of Sport Sci. p. 25. 1988.

63. Mizuno, M.; Mygind, E.; Lortie, G.; Bro-Rasmussen, T. Is hypoxia the stimulus for skeletal muscle adaptive changes to endurance training? Clin. Physiol. 5(4):22; 1985.

64. Newsholme, E.A.; Leech, A.R. The runner: energy and endurance. Oxford, England: Fitness Books; 1983.

65. Örskov, S.L. Undersøgelser over de aetheropløselige syrer i blod og væv. Copenhagen: Munksgaard; 1931.

66. Parkhouse, W.S.; McKenzie, D.C. Possible contribution of skeletal muscle buffers to enhanced anaerobic performance: a brief review. Med. Sci. Sports Exerc. 16:328-338; 1984.

67. Porter, R.; Whelan, J. Human muscle fatigue: physiological mechanisms. London: Pitman Medical; 1981.

68. Sahlin, K.; Alvestrand, A.; Brandt, R.; Hultman, E. Intracellular pH and bicarbonate concentration in human muscle during recovery from exercise. J. Appl. Physiol. 45:474-480; 1978.

69. Sahlin, K.; Harris, R.C.; Hultman, E. Creatine kinase equilibrium and lactate content compared with muscle pH in tissue samples obtained after isometric exercise. Biochem. J. 152:173-180; 1975.

70. Sahlin, K.; Henriksson, J. Buffer capacity and lactate accumulation in skeletal muscle of trained and untrained men. Acta Physiol. Scand. 122:331-339; 1984.

71. Saltin, B. Physical training in patients with intermittent claudication. In: Cohen, L.S.; Mock, M.B.; Ringqvist, I. eds. Physical conditioning and cardiovascular rehabilitation. New York: J. Wiley & Sons; 1981; 181-196.

72. Saltin, B. Hemodynamic adaptations to exercise. Am. J. Cardiol. 55:42D-47D; 1985.

73. Saltin, B. The physiological and biochemical basis of aerobic and anaerobic capacities in man; effect of training and range of adaptation. In: Mæhlum, S.; Nilsson, S.; Renström, P., eds. An update on sports medicine: proceedings from the second Scandinavian conference in sports medicine. 1987:16-59.

74. Saltin, B.; Gagge, A.P.; Bergh, U.; Stolwijk, J.A.J. Body temperatures and sweating during exhaustive exercise. J. Appl. Physiol. 32:635-643; 1972.

75. Saltin, B.; Gollnick, P.D. Skeletal muscle adaptability significance for metabolism and performance. In: Peachey, L.D.; Adrian, P.H.; Geiger, S.R., eds. Handbook of physiology: skeletal muscle. Bethesda, MD: American Physiology Society; 1983:555-631.

76. Saltin, B.; Gollnick, P.D.; Eriksson, B.O.; Piehl, K. Metabolic and circulatory adjustments at onset of work. In: Gilbert, A.; Guille, P., eds. Proceedings from meeting on physiological changes at onset of work; Toulouse, France. 1971:46-58.

77. Saltin, B.; Gollnick, P.D.; Rowell, L.B.; Sejersted, O.M. Power output of man; the contributions made by Lars Hermansen. In: Jones, N.L.; McCartney, N.; McComas, A.L., eds. Human muscle power. Champaign, IL: Human Kinetics; 1986:183-194.

78. Saltin, B.; Kiens, B.; Savard, G. A quantitative approach to the evaluation of skeletal muscle substrate utilization in prolonged exercise. In: Benzi, G.; Packer, L.; Siliprandi, N., eds. Biochemical aspects of physical exercise. Amsterdam, New York, Oxford. 1986:235-244.

79. Secher, N. The physiology of rowing. J. Sports Sci. 1:23-53.

80. Sharp, R.L.; Costill, D.L.; Fink, W.J.; King, D.S. Effects of eight weeks of bicycle ergometer sprint training on human muscle buffer capacity. Int. J. Sports Med. 7:13-17; 1986.

81. Sjøgaard, G.; Adams, R.P.; Saltin, B. Water and ion shifts in skeletal muscle of humans with intense dynamic knee extension. Am. J. Physiol. 248:R190-R196; 1985.

82. Terrados, N.; Melichna, J.; Sylvén, C.; Jansson, E.; Kaijser, L. Effects of training at simulated altitude on performance and muscle metabolic capacity in competitive road cyclists. Eur. J. Appl. Physiol. 57:203-209; 1988.

List of Invited Speakers

Dr. S.P. Bessman
Department of Pharmacology and
  Nutrition
University of Southern California
2025 Zonal Ave.
Los Angeles, CA
USA

Dr. Arend Bonen
School of Recreation, Physical &
  Health Education
Dalhousie University
Halifax, Canada
B3H 3J5

Dr. Dieter Brdiczka
Faculty of Biology
Universitat Konstanz
D-7750 Konstanz 1
FRG

Dr. R.A.J. Challiss
Department of Biochemistry
University of Oxford
South Parks Road
Oxford, England

Dr. Roger Cooke
Department of Biochemistry &
  Cardiovascular Research Institute
University of California at
  San Francisco
San Francisco, CA
USA

Dr. Sue Donaldson
Department of Physiology
School of Medicine
University of Minnesota
Minneapolis, MN
USA

Dr. David A. Essig
Department of Physical Education
University of Illinois
Chicago, IL
USA

Dr. Henrik Galbo
Institute of Medical Physiology
University of Copenhagen
Blegdamsuej 3 C
Copenhagen 2100 N
Denmark

Dr. Philip D. Gollnick
Department of Veterinary &
  Comparative Anatomy, Pharmacology
  & Physiology
College of Veterinary Medicine
Pullman, WA
USA

Dr. Howard Green
Department of Kinesiology
University of Waterloo
Waterloo, Canada

Dr. Patricia Gregory
Department of Medical Cardiology
University of Chicago
Chicago, IL
USA

Dr. R.G. Haller
Department of Neurology
University of Texas
Health Sciences Center
Dallas, TX
USA

Dr. George Heigenhauser
McMaster University Medical Centre
Box 2000, Station A
Hamilton, Canada

Dr. Peter W. Hochachka
Department of Zoology
University of British Columbia
Vancouver, Canada

Dr. John O. Holloszy
Section of Applied Physiology
Department of Internal Medicine
Washington University School
  of Medicine
St. Louis, MO
USA

Dr. E.W. Holmes
Howard Hughes Medical Institute
  Laboratories
Department of Medicine
Duke University Medical Center
Durham, NC
USA

Dr. Eric Hultman
Department of Clinical Chemistry II
Huddinga University Hospital
Huddinga, Sweden

Dr. C. David Ianuzzo
Departments of Biology and Physical
  Education
York University
Downsview, Canada

Dr. Donald C. Jackson
Laboratoire de Physiologie Respiratoire
Centre National de la Recherche
  Scientifique
67087 Strasbourg
France

Dr. Norman Jones
Ambrose Cardiorespiratory Unit
McMaster University Health Science
  Centre
Hamilton, Canada

Dr. Larry R. Jones
Krannert Institute of Cardiology
Indianapolis, IN
USA

Dr. Martin J. Kushmerick
Department of Radiology
Brigham and Women's Hospital
Boston, MA
USA

Dr. Stephen Lewis
Department of Physiology
University of Texas Health Science
  Center
Dallas, TX
USA

Dr. Michael I. Lindinger
Abteilung Vegetative Physiologie
Zentrum Physiologie
Medizinische Hochschule Hannover
D. 3000 Hannover 61
FRG

Dr. Bernardo Nadal-Ginard
Howard Hughes Medical Institute
Professor of Pediatrics, Physiology
  and Biophysics
Harvard Medical School
The Childrens Hospital, Department
  of Cardiology
Boston, MA
USA

Dr. Jacques Poortmans
Chimie Physiologique
Inst. Super. Educ. Phys. Kines.
Université Libre de Bruxelles
Brussels, Belgium

Dr. Karel J. Rakusan
Department of Physiology
Faculty of Health Sciences
University of Ottawa
Ottawa, Canada

Dr. Heinz Reichmann
Neurologische Universisitas - Klinik
  und Poliklinik im Kopfklinikum
8700 Wurberg
FRG

Dr. Bengt Saltin
August Krogh Institute
University of Copenhagen
Copenhagen, Denmark

Dr. J.-A. Simoneau
Faculty of Biology
Universitat Konstanz
D-7750 Konstanz 1
FRG

Dr. J.T. Stull
Department of Pharmacology
University of Texas Health Science
  Center
Dallas, TX
USA

Dr. John Sutton
Department of Medicine
McMaster University
Hamilton, Canada

Dr. A.W. (Bert) Taylor (Chairman)
Department of Physiology and Faculty
  of Physical Education
The University of Western Ontario
London, Canada

Dr. Glen Tibbits
Department of Kinesiology
Simon Fraser University
Burnaby, Canada

Dr. Milan Vranic
Department of Physiology
University of Toronto
Toronto, Canada

Dr. R. Sanders Williams
Department of Biochemistry
Duke University School of Medicine
Durham, NC
USA

Dr. Radovan Zak
Department of Medicine, Pharmacology
  & Physical Science
University of Chicago
Chicago, IL
USA